THYROID EYE DISEASE

ENDOCRINE UPDATES

Shlomo Melmed, M.D., Series Editor

---

1. E.R. Levin and J.L. Nadler (eds.): Endocrinology of Cardiovascular Function. 1998. ISBN: 0-7923-8217-X
2. J.A. Fagin (ed.): Thyroid Cancer. 1998. ISBN: 0-7923-8326-5
3. J.S. Adams and B.P. Lukert (eds.): Osteoporosis: Genetics, Prevention and Treatment. 1998. ISBN: 0-7923-8366-4.
4. B.-Å. Bengtsson (ed.): Growth Hormone. 1999. ISBN: 0-7923-8478-4
5. C. Wang (ed.): Male Reproductive Function. 1999. ISBN 0-7923-8520-9
6. B. Rapoport and S.M. McLachlan (eds.): Graves' Disease: Pathogenesis and Treatment. 2000. ISBN: 0-7923-7790-7.
7. W. W. de Herder (ed.): Functional and Morphological Imaging of the Endocrine System. 2000. ISBN 0-7923-7923-9
8. H.G. Burger (ed.): Sex Hormone Replacement Therapy. 2001. ISBN 0-7923-7965-9
9. A. Giustina (ed.): Growth Hormone and the Heart. 2001. ISBN 0-7923-7212-3
10. W.L. Lowe, Jr. (ed.): Genetics of Diabetes Mellitus. 2001. ISBN 0-7923-7252-2
11. J.F. Habener and M.A. Hussain (eds.): Molecular Basis of Pancreas Development and Function. 2001. ISBN 0-7923-7271-9
12. N. Horseman (ed.): Prolactin. 2001 ISBN 0-7923-7290-5
13. M. Castro (ed.): Transgenic Models in Endocrinology. 2001 ISBN 0-7923-7344-8
14. R. Bahn (ed.): Thyroid Eye Disease. 2001 ISBN 0-7923-7380-4

THYROID EYE DISEASE

edited by

Rebecca S. Bahn

Mayo Clinic and Foundation

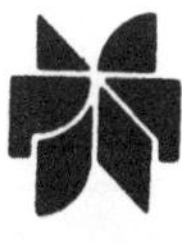

SPRINGER SCIENCE+BUSINESS MEDIA, LLC

Library of Congress Cataloging-in-Publication Data

Thyroid eye disease / edited by Rebecca S. Bahn.
p. ; cm. -- (Endocrine updates ; 14)
Includes bibliographical references and index.
ISBN 978-1-4613-5558-8 ISBN 978-1-4615-1447-3 (eBook)
DOI 10.1007/978-1-4615-1447-3
1. Thyroid eye disease. I. Bahn, Rebecca S. II. Series.
[DNLM: 1. Graves' Disease. WK 265 T5485 2001]
RE715.T48 T48 2001
617.7--dc21

2001029678

Originally published by Kluwer Academic Publishers in 2001
Softcover reprint of the hardcover 1st edition 2001

Printed on acid-free paper.

TABLE OF CONTENTS

Disease Evaluation

Treatment

CONTRIBUTORS

Rebecca S. Bahn
Division of Endocrinology, Department of Internal Medicine, Mayo Clinic, Rochester, Minnesota, USA

Glynn Baker
Department of Ophthalmology, University of Wales College of Medicine, Heath Park, Cardiff, UK

George B. Bartley
Department of Ophthalmology, Mayo Clinic, Rochester, Minnesota, USA

Tomasz Bednarczuk
Department of Medicine, Krume University School of Medicine, Fukuoka, Japan

Elizabeth A. Bradley
Department of Ophthalmology, Mayo Clinic, Rochester, Minnesota, USA

Henry B. Burch
Endocrine Metabolic Service, Walter Reed Army Medical Center, Washington, D.C and Uniformed Services University of the Health Sciences, Bethesda, Maryland, USA

A. J. Dickinson
Department of Ophthalmology, University of Newcastle on Tyne, Newcastle on Tyne, UK

Gregor J. Förster
Department of Nuclear Medicine, Gutenberg-University Hospital, Mainz, Germany

James A. Garrity
Department of Ophthalmology, Mayo Clinic, Rochester, Minnesota, USA

Martin N. Gerding
Department of Endocrinology and Metabolism, Academic Medical Center, University of Amsterdam, The Netherlands

Armin E. Heufelder
Division of Gastroenterology, Endocrinology & Metabolism, Department of Internal Medicine, Philipps-University, Marburg, Germany

Yuji Hiromatsu
Department of Medicine, Krume University School of Medicine, Fukuoka, Japan

Werner Joba
Division of Gastroenterology, Endocrinology & Metabolism, Department of Internal Medicine, Philipps-University, Marburg, Germany

George Kahaly
Department of Endocrinology/Metabolism, Gutenberg-University Hospital, Mainz, Germany

E. Helen Kemp
University of Sheffield Clinical Sciences Centre, Northern General Hospital, Sheffield, UK

Pat Kendall-Taylor
Department of Medicine, University of Newcastle on Tyne, Newcastle on Tyne, UK

Marian Ludgate
Endocrine Section, Department of Medicine, University of Wales College of Medicine, Heath Park, Cardiff, UK

Wolf J. Mann
Department of Otorhinolaryngology, Gutenberg-University Hospital, Mainz, Germany

Maarten Ph. Mourits
Orbital Center, Donders Institute of Ophthalmology, University Hospital, Utrecht, The Netherlands

Wibke Müller-Forell
Department of Neuroradiology, Gutenberg-University Hospital, Mainz, Germany

Natee Munsakul
Division of Endocrinology, Department of Internal Medicine, Mayo Clinic, Rochester, Minnesota, USA

Petros Perros
Department of Medicine, University of Newcastle on Tyne, Newcastle on Tyne, UK

Suzanne Pitz
Department of Ophthalmology, Gutenberg-University Hospital, Mainz, Germany

Mark F. Prummel
Department of Endocrinology & Metabolism and Orbital Center, Academic Medical Center, University of Amsterdam, The Netherlands

Jonathan N. Ridgway
University of Sheffield Clinical Sciences Centre, Northern General Hospital, Sheffield, UK

Hans Peter Rösler
Department of Therapeutic Radiology, Gutenberg-University Hospital, Mainz, Germany

Terry J. Smith
Division of Molecular Medicine, Harbor-UCLA Medical Center, Torrance, California and Department of Medicine and the Jules Stein Eye Institute, University of California Los Angeles School of Medicine, Los Angeles, California, USA

Caroline B. Terwee
Department of Clinical Epidemiology and Biostatistics, Academic Medical Center, Amsterdam, The Netherlands

Philip F. Watson
University of Sheffield Clinical Sciences Centre, Northern General Hospital, Sheffield, UK

Anthony P. Weetman
Department of Medicine, University of Sheffield Clinical Sciences Centre, Northern General Hospital, Sheffield, U.K

Wilmar M. Wiersinga
Department of Endocrinology & Metabolism and Orbital Center, Academic Medical Center, University of Amsterdam, The Netherlands

PREFACE

Patients afflicted with thyroid eye disease or Graves' ophthamopathy (GO) may experience not only pain and visual loss, but also disfigurement. Full understanding of pathogenesis has been elusive, and treatment modalities are imperfect. As with other conditions, more effective intervention will follow only after a better understanding of pathogenesis is reached. The goal of this volume is to give an overview by leaders in the field of the present state of the art both in pathogenesis and clinical aspects of GO.

Much attention has been directed towards determining which cells within the orbit are targets of the autoimmune process, and how these and other cells might participate in the local inflammatory process. It is now generally agreed that orbital fibroblasts, preadipocyte fibroblasts, and adipocytes are the targeted and activated cells in GO and that full-length TSH receptor (TSHr) is expressed in these cells. Further, there is growing consensus that this receptor is up-regulated in the orbit in GO, residing primarily in newly differentiated adipocytes. However, it is also evident, given a sufficiently sensitive assay, that TSHr is detectable in fibroblasts and adipocytes from the normal orbit and other anatomic sites, as well. It will be important to determine whether the observed increase in orbital TSHr expression itself initiates the orbital autoimmune process. Also to be decided is whether orbital lymphocytes from GO patients specifically recognize this receptor, and what factor or factors unique to Graves' disease might stimulate TSHr expression in orbital cells.

Renewed interest has been focused on the concept that patients with Graves' disease may have a generalized autoimmune disease of the connective tissues, with only some patients demonstrating clinically relevant eye and pretibial skin involvement. Severe disease at these sites may reflect mechanical features, including trauma, as well as phenotypic characteristics of regional fibroblasts. It follows that patients with GO may not differ genetically from patients with Graves' hyperthyroidism not having clinically apparent eye disease. This concept highlights the importance of environmental factors in the evolution of this condition. It is likely that the development of animal models of Graves' hyperthyroidism and GO will bring insight into the role of TSHr in disease initiation and into the relative importance of environmental factors in disease expression.

Progress has also been made in diagnosis and treatment. In the past, many studies of potential treatments for GO have suffered from lack of reliable means to assess disease activity and response to treatment. Non-quantitative endpoints and activity scores that obscured, rather than highlighted, important clinical features were frequently used. Exciting new developments include the design of clinically relevant instruments to measure the quality of life in GO patients. Useful means to assess and document disease activity have been validated. In addition, emphasis has been placed on imaging, both for diagnostic precision and for quantitative assessment of therapeutic interventions. It has become apparent that there are clinical subgroups of patients with GO and that treatment must be tailored to the individual patient. Concomitantly, there has been a re-evaluation of the standard treatments for GO, including surgical approaches and orbital radiotherapy, and novel immunotherapies have been proposed.

Many challenges face scientists and clinicians interested in GO and devoted to finding ways to help patients with the condition. This volume was designed to highlight the significant progress being made by many groups of investigators worldwide. The information gained from ongoing laboratory and clinical investigations will lead to new pathophysiology-based treatments and preventive measures that may be equally applicable to other autoimmune diseases. I wish to thank all of my colleagues for their exciting contributions to this volume and for the friendships that have developed through our common interest in this disease.

Rebecca S. Bahn

1

ORBITAL AUTOANTIGENS

Anthony P. Weetman, E. Helen Kemp, Jonathan N. Ridgway, Philip F. Watson.
University of Sheffield Clinical Sciences Centre, Northern General Hospital, Sheffield S5 7AU, United Kingdom.

INTRODUCTION

It is now fully accepted that Graves' ophthalmopathy is an orbital autoimmune disease closely related to Graves' disease and, less commonly, found in autoimmune hypothyroidism (1). These clinical features have led to the hypothesis, discussed at length elsewhere in this volume, that ophthalmopathy is the result of an autoimmune response against one or more orbital autoantigens which are shared by the thyroid. Such antigenic cross-reactivity would explain the known clinical associations and temporal features of the disease but it should still be recognized that any such cross-reactivity could be at the T cell rather than B cell level, and that, so far, this is still not a firmly established fact. Indeed, it remains the case that establishing the nature of autoantigen(s) responsible for ophthalmopathy is the Holy Grail of research in this area, as knowledge of the autoantigen responsible for an autoimmune disease is key to any experiments designed to map pathogenic epitopes or to any autoantigen-based therapeutic endeavors.

In this chapter, the quest for orbital autoantigens is dealt with historically, to allow the reader an understanding of how we have arrived at our present position. To set the scene, most studies have attempted to identify antigens by using patient serum in solid-phase assays designed to identify autoantibodies in crude orbital extracts. This is a simple approach but is likely to be limited in its power; one only has to consider how difficult it would be to detect TSH receptor antibodies by these methods. Furthermore, as subsequent chapters show, there is precious little evidence for a pathogenic role for antibodies in ophthalmopathy. Screening sera against orbital antigens may pick up the orbital equivalent of thyroglobulin, whose importance to the pathogenesis of autoimmune thyroiditis remains obscure. If T cells are responsible for ophthalmopathy, we need assays that detect their orbital antigens, but such methods are still elusive.

EARLY STUDIES

Using bovine, guinea pig and human orbital tissue, including eye muscle and lacrimal gland, no significant binding by antibodies from Graves' ophthalmopathy patients was found by hemagglutination or immunofluorescence (2). A low titer of antibodies was found which bound in around 10% of both controls and patients, the first indication of the background binding of normal serum which has plagued the hunt for antigens subsequently. The same group later reported a new soluble eye muscle antigen, which was recognized by 73% of Graves' ophthalmopathy sera using immunofluorescence, with low reactivity in other patient samples (3). The reasons for this difference from the previous study are not clear.

An alternative, candidate autoantigen-based approach stemmed from the observation that thyroglobulin (TG) or a related protein could be detected in the orbit based on immunoreactivity studies (4). Radioisotope-based lymphography had previously shown a possible connection between the thyroid and orbit as a possible route for the transfer of TG (5). A large panel of monoclonal TG antibodies failed to recognize any component of the orbital contents, arguing against a role for TG as the cross-reactive antigen (6), but later it was found that a quarter of such antibodies did indeed bind to an insoluble membrane fraction of orbital connective tissue (7). Whilst unlikely, therefore, to be TG in the orbit, these results did support the concept of a TG-cross-reactive orbital protein. Further confirmation of this hypothesis arose from experiments in which mice were immunized with eye muscle membranes and then used to derive monoclonal antibodies; one such antibody reacted with mammalian TG but this represented a very low frequency of response (8).

The advent of monoclonal antibodies also prompted their more general use in the investigation of ophthalmopathy. Initial studies showed considerable promise. A monoclonal antibody was obtained from mice immunized with orbital homogenates, which could be used to partially purify a human soluble eye muscle antigen (9). This antigen was then used in an ELISA to demonstrate the binding of antibodies in three-quarters of patients with Graves' ophthalmopathy, but no such reactivity was found in Graves' patients without ophthalmopathy. Subsequent studies were performed with human monoclonal antibodies, which recognized a series of orbital antigens, some of which were not proteins (10). This multiplicity of reactivities, and the possibility of pursuing low-affinity, irrelevant interactions led to this approach being abandoned.

The final set of experiments in the early phase of antigen identification relied on the use of ELISA to identify the presence of antibodies reactive with various orbital homogenates in ELISA. Inevitably, these experiments gave rise to problems in interpretation because different species were used to derive the crude extracts, other components such as blood contaminated the extracts, and background non-specific binding together with low affinity interactions obscured some results. A summary of the results obtained by ELISA up to 1989 is given in Table 1. There is huge variability in these results, ranging from very significant differences between ophthalmopathy patients and those with Graves' disease but no eye involvement at the outset, to no difference at the conclusion. Varying degrees of cross-reactivity were also found, but overall the results indicated that skeletal and orbital muscles shared the same antigens responsible for antibody binding in an ELISA. Such a conclusion seemed counter-intuitive, and this approach gave way to methods, which could identify antigens more precisely, particularly immunoblotting.

Table 1. Summary of Results with ELISA to Detect Antibodies Binding to Orbital Antigens in Graves' Ophthalmopathy

Reference	Orbital tissue	GO +ve	% GD without GO +ve	Comments
11	Porcine EM	64	5	Specific for EM
12	Porcine EM	37	25	Cross-reactive with SM and TM
13	Porcine EM	42	23	Cross-reactive with SM and LM
14	Human and Porcine EM	26	0	Binding present in other thyroid disorders
15	Human EM	11	22	Correlation with SM binding; found in 64% Hashimoto sera
16	Human EM	10	14	Cross-reactive with SM

GD = Graves' ophthalmopathy; GD = Graves' disease; EM = eye muscle (membrane fraction); SM = skeletal muscle; TM = thyroid cell membranes; LM = liver cell membranes

IMMUNOBLOTTING STUDIES USING ORBITAL TISSUE

The simplest method of characterizing antigens in a crude tissue extract is immunoblotting, in which there is size fraction by gel electrophoresis, transfer of antigen to a membrane and probing with antibody. However, only the relative molecular weight can be estimated by this method and the denaturation and modest sensitivity mean that rare antibodies or antigens, or those critically dependent on conformation, will be missed.

A summary of results using orbital antigens is given in Table 2. Essentially, the results can be classified in two groups, one showing no consistent pattern of antigen recognition by antibodies in sera from patients with ophthalmopathy and a smaller group of studies, particularly emanating from Wall and colleagues, showing that ophthalmopathy sera frequently have antibodies which recognize three distinctive components of 55, 64 and 95kD. The 64kD antigen in particular has provoked the most interest as this was recognized by around two-thirds of ophthalmopathy sera, particularly those from patients with active or recent disease, and the antigen appeared to cross-react with a protein in the thyroid but not in skeletal muscle (27). This pattern of reactivity would help explain the distinctive localization of ophthalmopathy, but the discrepancies between the various studies is difficult to reconcile and could only be solved by blinded exchange of sera and antigen samples (which has not happened) or by definitive characterization of the antigen.

Table 2. Summary of the Results with Immunoblotting to Identify Antibodies Binding to Orbital Antigen in Graves' Ophthalmopathy

Reference	Orbital tissue	Reactivity with GO sera	Comments
13	Porcine EM	Multiple bands	64kD reactivity with control sera
16	Human EM	55kD; not disease specific	64kD reactivity with control sera
17-20	Human EM	64kD in >55%; less commonly 50, 58, 85 and 95kD	Controls negative for 64kD reactivity
21	Porcine EM	Multiple bands	64kD reactivity with control sera
22	Human EM	64kD in <40%	64kD reactivity in many tissues and with control sera
23	Porcine EM	55kDa in <48%	No disease-specific 64Da reactivity
24	Rat EM	64kD in 71%	35% of Hashimoto patient without ophthalmopathy also react
25	Porcine and human EM	Multiple bands	No disease-specific 64kD reactivity
26	Porcine EM	64kD in 64% and 95kD in 50%	

IDENTIFICATION OF THE 64kD ANTIGEN

Screening a λgt11 human thyroid cDNA library with a pool of 10 Hashimoto's thyroiditis sera led to the isolation of a clone termed D1, encoding a 97 amino acid peptide (28). The entire sequence of the cDNA was found to have the potential to encode a 63kD protein and the mRNA was expressed in thyroid and extraocular muscle but not skeletal muscle. Although this initial study found that only 24% of sera from patients with autoimmune thyroid disease reacted with the D1 protein, without any clear association with ophthalmopathy, a subsequent study in collaboration with Wall's group provided indirect support for the identity of the 64kD antigen and D1 and indicated that the frequency of antibodies against D1 was 47% in patients with ophthalmopathy and 57% in those with Graves' hyperthyroidism (29).

The potential significance of the D1 antigen was diminished by the discovery of D1 mRNA in a wide variety of tissues including uterus, spleen and parathyroid and by the presence of antibodies to D1 in 53% of controls, 78% of Hashimoto patients and in 63% of Graves' patients, without any correlation between the presence of ophthalmopathy and D1 reactivity (30). Despite this compelling evidence against a role for D1 in ophthalmopathy, further inconclusive attempts were made to examine whether the 64kD antigen and D1 were related (31). Most recently, the D1 cDNA was recloned and expressed in baculovirus-infected insect cells and the denatured material was found to yield a 64kD protein under denaturing conditions by gel electrophoresis, but a 85kD protein under non-denaturing conditions (32). No reactivity was found against the denatured protein but 85% of Graves' ophthalmopathy sera reacted against the non-denatured protein by immunoblotting, contrasting with only 5% of controls. Around a quarter of patients with autoimmune thyroid disease but no ophthalmopathy were also positive, however. It seems remarkable that D1 was originally believed to be the 64kD antigen, only to be proven not to be, and is now being suggested as a novel 85kD orbital autoantigen!

Further attempts to identify the 64kD antigen used gel separation and microsequencing, and initially indicated that this could be calsequestrin, a calcium-binding protein in the sarcoplasmic reticulum of striated muscle, and antibodies against this were detected in 47% of ophthalmopathy sera and 21% of controls (33). However, the most important outcome of this study was a re-estimation of the size of the 64kD protein (now clearly not calsequestrin), which turned out to be around 67kD. Subsequently, this new 67kD protein was partially purified and microsequenced, leading to its identification as the flavoprotein (Fp) subunit of mitochondrial succinate dehydrogenase; 67% of sera from patients with active Graves' ophthalmopathy reacted with Fp by immunoblotting compared to 7% of normal subjects (34). It seems intuitively unlikely that the ubiquitous Fp subunit is the previous 64kD antigen which was cross-reactive with a protein in thyroid yet not skeletal muscle, but further support for this notion was suggested by the close relationship between clinical ophthalmopathy and the detection of these antibodies, as previously reported for 64kD antibodies (35). In contrast, another study failed to find any such relationship (36). Moreover, the sequestered mitochondrial location of the Fp subunit makes it difficult to imagine how it could be a key autoantigen. We have recently established a sensitive and specific immunoprecipitation assay for the Fp protein (37) and have found only a low frequency of antibodies in autoimmune thyroid disease patients and no correlation with the presence of ophthalmopathy (Table 3).

It is difficult to summarize such a complex set of data. Our overall prejudice is that a number of potential antigens around 64kD are present in eye muscle and other tissues, but that these are recognized by healthy as well as patient sera, indicating the frequent occurrence of natural autoantibodies, probably of low affinity and uncertain pathogenic significance. The balance of evidence suggests to us that neither D1 nor Fp is a key autoantigen in ophthalmopathy and that there is no consistent support yet, despite considerable effort, for the crucial importance of an autoantigen around the 64kD size inthis condition. Generation of an animal model of Graves' eye disease by immunization with any of the candidate 64kD antigens would provide a powerful counter argument but has not yet been attempted.

Table 3. Comparison of the Frequency of Antibodies to Succinate Dehydrogenase Flavoprotein Subunit (SDHFp) in Different Patient Groups

Patient Group	Number	% Positive for SDHFp Antibodies
Addison's disease	20	25
Graves' disease	28	21
Autoimmune hypothyroidism	26	19
Systemic lupus erythematosus	20	30
Pretibial myxedema	12	17
Graves' ophthalmopathy	25	12
Controls	20	0

OTHER CANDIDATE AUTOANTIGENS

As well as the efforts directed to identifying the 64kD antigen, other candidate antigens have been explored over the last two decades. Most attention has been paid to the TSH-receptor, as described in the next section, but other candidates have been sought by extrapolation from known potential antigens in muscle, by exploring the orbital fibroblast repertoire of proteins, since this is a key target of the pathogenic process, and by attempts to identify targets for bioactive autoantibodies.

Eye muscle candidate antigens

In one of the first studies to attempt dissection of the orbital antigens responsible for binding antibodies in ELISA, Kadlubowski and colleagues employed myosin, actin and acetylcholine receptor as candidate antigens in a solid phase ^{125}I protein A binding assay (38). Myosin and acetylcholine receptor appeared to be the predominant antigens recognized by antibodies from ophthalmopathy patients in extraocular muscle extract and membrane preparations respectively, with occasional sera reacting against actin. These results certainly explain why so many ELISA studies have shown a close correlation between antibody binding to eye and skeletal muscle homogenates (Table 1), but do not fit with the paradigm of a thyroid cross-reactive (or eye muscle-specific) antigen underlying the pathogenesis of ophthalmopathy. It is also difficult to see why so few patients with Graves' disease have myasthenia gravis if these results are correct. At the least, however, these findings highlight the diversified and non-specific proteins that can be invoked as autoantigens by screening using sera from these patients.

The rationale behind considering TG as a key autoantigen in ophthalmopathy is given in Section 1. A twist to the tale was the discovery that TG shares sequence homology with acetylcholinesterase (AChE), leading the screening of a human thyroid cDNA library with AChE polyclonal antibodies and isolation of two TG segments which had close homology with AChE (39). Ophthalmopathy but not control sera bound to these TG fragments, with only one of 10 Hashimoto sera binding, although the number of samples studied was small.

These elegant studies have only partially been reproduced using whole antigen, which would seem the best substrate for binding antibodies that, when pathogenic, generally recognize conformational epitopes. No correlation was found between human red cell AChE binding and TG binding by sera from patients with autoimmune thyroid disease, one antigen did not absorb out reactivity against the other, and there was no higher frequency of

AChE antibodies in the ophthalmopathy patients than in other thyroid disorders (40). Cross-reactivity between TG and *Electrophorus* AChE was found in another study, raising a question over the species specificity of some of these responses, but the highest frequency of AChE antibodies was found in patients with myasthenia gravis, indicating that AChE autoreactivity alone cannot trigger Graves' ophthalmopathy (41). Moreover, experimentally induced acetylcholinesterase antibodies produce a syndrome of immune-mediated destruction of presynaptic fibres in sympathetic ganglia and the adrenal medulla, which clearly does not accompany ophthalmopathy (42).

The obvious approach to antigen identification is to clone and sequence fragments recognized by antibodies. Human λgt11 eye muscle expression libraries have been screened with no real success (43), which may relate to a low (or absent) frequency of antibody, a low expression of antigen or the need for proper conformational structure before binding can occur. This last point assumes an importance determined by how one interprets the immunoblotting data described in Section 2: our view is that the presence of a frequent antibody detectable by immunoblotting with crude eye muscle extracts should allow molecular cloning, and the failure of this approach (we suspect other negative studies have not been published) argues against the importance of antibodies and antigens detected by immunoblotting.

However, Wall and colleagues have recently cloned a novel protein, termed G2s by screening an eye muscle λgt11 library with an affinity-purified anti-55kD protein antibody from a patient with ophthalmopathy (44). The estimated molecular weight of the entire protein is 220kD and mRNA for this novel protein was strongly expressed in eye muscle, thyroid and skeletal muscle, and less strongly in pancreas, liver, lung and heart muscle. By immunoblotting against the G2s fusion protein, antibodies were found in 70% of ophthalmopathy patients (whose disease was less than 3 years in duration), in 36% of Graves' patients without ophthalmopathy, in 17% of Hashimoto's thyroiditis and in 16% of control subjects. However, by ELISA the frequency of antibodies in ophthalmopathy and Hashimoto patients was the same (54%).

These frequencies do not correspond with the previously reported frequencies for 55kD antibodies in ophthalmopathy (20). This may simply be the result of using a fusion protein which is a fragment of the putative antigen, but the relationship between this fragment, the 55kD protein and the intact 220kD G2s remains to be clarified. Based on the tissue distribution and frequency of antibody binding, we are inclined to the view that this is unlikely to be a major autoantigen in ophthalmopathy.

Fibroblast antigens

As described in detail later in this book, the most likely pathogenesis of Graves' ophthalmopathy involves, at least proximally, stimulation of orbital fibroblasts in extraocular muscle cytokines. The fibroblast is therefore an obvious target cell in which to identify relevant autoantigens and, by culturing fibroblasts, enrichment for this source of antigen is possible. The first study to use this approach utilized immunoblotting and determined the presence of a 23kD fibroblast protein which was recognized by 56% of IgG class antibodies in sera from patients with Graves' disease (but with no distinct bias in favour of the subgroup with ophthalmopathy) compared with 15% of controls (45). Using Graves' patient sera with or without ophthalmopathy, we were unable to detect specific orbital fibroblast antigens by ELISA or immunoblotting although, in the latter, proteins at 80 and 92kD were significantly more frequently with ophthalmopathy sera than with controls (25). Negative whole cell ELISA results have also been reported by others (46).

A somewhat different approach was suggested by the demonstration that IgA class antibodies in ophthalmopathy sera bound to eye muscle antigens in ELISA, although the antigen being recognized was not elucidated (47). Reasoning that the autoimmune response in patients with both ophthalmopathy and thyroid dermopathy is likely to represent the acme of autoreactivity against fibroblast antigens in Graves' disease, we sought IgA antibodies against fibroblast antigens in such patients and detected them in high frequency (Table 4), using both dermal and retrobulbar fibroblasts (48). In immunoblotting studies, these sera reacted with a 54kD dermal fibroblast antigen and a 66kD retrobulbar fibroblast antigen, which are most likely variants of the same protein, based on absorption studies (unpublished).

Table 4. Frequency of IgA Class Antibodies Against Fibroblasts. Adapted from data in (48)

	% Sera positive		
	n	Retrobulbar fibroblasts	Dermal fibroblasts
Controls	17	4	7
Graves' dermopathy and ophthalmopathy	21	47	79
Graves' disease	21	13	19
Autoimmune hypothyroidism	9	16	11
Non-thyroid autoimmunity	19	4	0

Despite these encouraging results, it remains the case that no distinctive fibroblast antigen has emerged which can be invoked as a critical autoantigen in the development of ophthalmopathy. Extracellular matrix proteins are an alternative source of antigens for the inflammation in orbital connective tissue, but although antibodies to collagen, fibronectin and laminin occur in some patients with autoimmune thyroid disease, the pattern of reactivity is not disease-specific (49). Any such responses most likely represent a secondary reactivity of uncertain pathogenic significance.

Receptors as antigens

Autoantibodies can cause disease by fixing complement, by mediating antibody-dependent cell-mediated cytotoxicity and by stimulating or blocking receptors, the latter mechanism having a fundamental role in the pathogenesis of autoimmune thyroid disease. It is, therefore, logical to ask whether ophthalmopathy could be caused by receptor antibodies, in which case the receptor in question would be a key autoantigen. The possible role of the TSH receptor is considered in the next section, but the involvement of other receptors has also been suggested.

Porcine extraocular myoblasts proliferated in response to IgGs from ophthalmopathy patients but this effect showed no correlation with TSH receptor antibody levels, indicating a distinct biological activity (50). Unfortunately, this work has not been followed up, although the same group found that IgG from Graves' patients with or without ophthalmopathy interacted with insulin-like growth factor-1 (IGF-1) binding sites on orbital fibroblasts (51). No biological activity of these IgGs was explored. It, therefore, is unclear whether IGF-1 antibodies are responsible for the myoblast growth effect just described, or for the ability of IgGs from ophthalmopathy sera to stimulate collagen synthesis by human fibroblasts (52). It should be noted, in addition, that neither muscle growth nor collagen synthesis are hallmarks of the initial disease process in ophthalmopathy. The initial event instead appears to be enhanced synthesis of glycosaminoglycans by orbital fibroblasts, and we have been unable to show any effect of IgGs from patients with ophthalmopathy plus dermopathy on this key characteristic, or indeed on total protein or DNA synthesis (53). Whilst the vagaries of bioassays could account for these differences, our view is that, at present, there is no unequivocal and compelling evidence for fibroblast or muscle cell receptors acting as autoantigens that are activated by antibodies from ophthalmopathy patients.

THE TSH RECEPTOR

The close relationship between Graves' disease and ophthalmopathy make the TSH receptor (TSH-R) a logical candidate autoantigen, although this does not necessarily imply that TSH-R antibodies are involved in the pathogenesis of the orbital disease. Several studies have examined the correlation between the presence or level of TSH-R antibodies and the clinical presence of ophthalmopathy with conflicting results (54-57), but this work ignores the likely role of T cell autoreactivity in ophthalmopathy: the absence of TSH-R antibodies in ophthalmopathy would not preclude a role for T cell-mediated responses against the receptor as a cause for the disorder.

The first real attempt to take this idea beyond the correlative level was the demonstration of TSH-R mRNA, by reverse transcription-polymerase chain reaction (RT-PCR) amplification, in the retrobulbar tissue of healthy and Graves' disease subjects (58). This spawned enormous interest and many studies subsequently tended to confirm the presence of TSH-R amplification, reviewed in detail elsewhere (59). However, the power of the RT-PCR to detect minor or even illegitimate transcripts (60), uncertainty over the cell types within retrobulbar tissue expressing TSH-R, and the failure to detect functional, complete TSH-R transcripts in the orbit (61) prevented acceptance of the expression of TSH-R as the key autoantigen in ophthalmopathy.

Demonstration of TSH-R protein in the orbit is a fundamental requirement in postulating a role for this antigen and initial studies used antisera raised against TSH-R peptides to detect TSH-R in ocular fibroblasts (62), although evidence for the absence of staining of non-fibroblast control cells was not provided, limiting the power of this important observation. However, confirmation of TSH-R staining was provided by a study using polyclonal and monoclonal TSH-R antibodies, with the receptor being expressed on fibroblasts within the orbital connective tissue and extraocular muscle; the muscle cells themselves did not express TSH-R and abdominal fibroblasts were also not stained, implying truly specific staining (63).

Despite suggesting that the orbital fibroblast was the cell expressing TSH-R, there remained uncertainty over this being the sole source, particularly as TSH-R mRNA and protein started to appear in a whole host of unexpected sites, such as adrenal, kidney and thymus, when studied by liquid hybridization analysis and immunohistochemistry (64). Such a heterogeneous distribution is difficult to reconcile with the notion of an orbital and thyroidal shared or cross-reactive autoantigen as a cause for Graves' ophthalmopathy. Moreover, fat cells have been known for decades to bind TSH and clear cut evidence for their expression of TSH-R mRNA indicated that orbital adipose tissue, often increased in Graves' disease, could be an additional source of receptor (65,66).

The potential involvement of fat cells and fibroblasts has been tied up with the recognition that a subpopulation of orbital fibroblasts can differentiate into lipid-filled adipocytes, and that these preadipocyte fibroblasts are a major source of the TSH-R in orbital tissue from ophthalmopathy patients (66,67). However, no expression of TSH-R was apparent in normal orbital tissue or in late-passaged preadipocyte fibroblasts in culture (67), suggesting the necessity for a humoral factor in Graves' patients to induce expression. TSH-R stimulating antibodies are one possible factor, as TSH and presumably other ligands enhance preadipocyte TSH-R expression *in vitro* (68). This elegant work shows that TSH-R is expressed by orbital preadipocyte fibroblasts in Graves' ophthalmopathy, but the absence of expression in normal orbital tissue is perplexing, as previous studies have shown TSH-R in normal orbital connective tissue and muscle. Thus, there is either a second source of TSH-R expression or low levels are indeed present in some normal subjects. This issue deserves resolution, as expression of TSH-R only in diseased orbital preadipocytes is compatible with a secondary rather than primary process.

Perhaps the clearest evidence for TSH-R having a role in ophthalmopathy is the development of an animal model based on transfer of TSH-R primed T cells to genetically susceptible mice (69). This is dealt with in detail in a later chapter. Suffice to say here that again this strictly falls short of proof that the TSH-R is the key autoantigen in ophthalmopathy as one could imagine a situation in which the intrathyroidal immune response induced by these T cells led to a diversified response against a second thyroid antigen, cross-reactive with an antigen in the orbit, that in turn caused the pathological changes. Nonetheless, the TSH-R is now the prime suspect in a long list of candidate autoantigens

T CELL AUTOANTIGENS

As already mentioned, a major tenet of the search for the key orbital autoantigens is that patients with ophthalmopathy produce antibodies which, besides having a possible role in pathogenesis, could act as probes in ELISA, immunoblotting or library screening to identify the antigens. However, one only has to reflect on lack of reactivity of TSH-R receptors in such methods, despite their fundamental importance to Graves' disease pathogenesis, to appreciate that all of the foregoing studies will be negated if any antibodies are at too low a level, or depend critically on autoantigen conformation. The lack of any convincing reports of ophthalmopathy in neonates born to mothers with Graves' disease argues against the importance of orbital antibodies in contrast to the well-recorded example of neonatal thyrotoxicosis due to transplacental transfer of TSH-R antibodies, as does the prominent role for T cells in current models of pathogenesis, described in detail later in this book.

It is, therefore, logical to attempt to identify orbital autoantigens by their ability to induce T cell responses, although the lack of sensitive assays for T cell autoactivity is still a fundamental problem with this approach, compounded by the lack of access to the major source of autoreactive T cells, the orbit.

The *in vitro* production of migration inhibition factor by circulating T cells in response to antigen was the first assay to be used, and one set of results indicated that TG or a TG-like molecule was present in a crude extract of retrobulbar fat, muscle and lacrimal gland and reactive with T cells (70). However, other studies, reviewed in detail elsewhere (71), failed to find any consistent T cell response to orbital antigens, using this assay and others. We have identified weak circulating T cell proliferative responses to extraocular muscle extracts in patients with autoimmune thyroid disease, but these responses were not specific for eye muscle, being shared by skeletal muscle, and were not confined to patients with clinically evident ophthalmopathy (15). Candidate antigens, including recombinant D1, were tested in another set of experiments, but no T cell responses were observed, although occasional patients had T cell reactivity to individual eye muscle proteins between 25 - 50kD in size (72). In contrast to these generally disappointing results with eye muscle antigen preparations, orbital fibroblasts induced striking proliferation in circulating T cells from some patients (73).

These results, indicating the existence of fibroblast antigens which could stimulate T cells, were further supported by an important study which examined the functional responses of cloned orbital T cells from patients with ophthalmopathy (74). T cell proliferation in response to autologous fibroblasts was observed, and this appeared to be a property of $CD8^+$ rather than $CD4^+$ T cells. Moreover, fibroblast proteins of 6-10 and 19-26kD caused proliferation of circulating and some $CD4^+$cloned orbital T cells (75). Orbital T cell lines have also been shown to proliferate in response to the TSH-R, as well as thyroid and extraocular muscle membrane preparations (74). Elucidation of the fibroblast antigens responsible for some of these results would be a major step forward in our understanding. The detection of TSH-R-responsive T cells in the orbit is compatible with the local expression of TSH-R by preadipocytes, although this observation does not tell us that such cells are truly pathogenic.

CONCLUSIONS

A huge effort has been made over the last four decades to unravel the complex pathogenesis of Graves' ophthalmopathy. A key step in that process is identification of the orbital autoantigens responsible for triggering the local immune response, and the search has been conducted with the underlying credo that such orbital antigens cross-react with thyroid autoantigens. Many contradictory results have been reported and, whichever turn out to be correct, two unpalatable truths emerge. Firstly, there is unlikely to be any easy answer to the question which can be obtained by simple methodologies such as immunoblotting or library screening, most likely because the autoantibodies which would provide the probes for such techniques are not pathogenic and are present at low levels (or, in some patients, are absent). Secondly, and posing a related methodological problem, the autoimmune response against orbital antigens is heterogeneous, with reactivity to several proteins which, by their distribution in tissues outside the orbit, are difficult to accommodate in any simple model of pathogenesis.

In our view, the proteins D1, AChE, Fp and G2s are too ubiquitous to be key autoantigens. It is possible that local factors could somehow amplify an autoimmune response against one of these proteins that, in other situations, does not lead to a significant change, but this is without precedent in organ-specific autoimmune disease, in which target antigens are distinctively cell-specific proteins such as enzymes and receptors. The TSH-R is currently the best candidate autoantigen but there remain uncertainties concerning the source of TSH-R in the orbit and its biological activity. More work is now urgently needed to address the critical issue that mere detection of the receptor raises: is this the orbital autoantigen that actually triggers the autoimmune response? The animal model that has been developed will undoubtedly address this further.

The orbital fibroblast remains the most likely target cell and the demonstration of TSH-R in the preadipocyte fibroblast population ties together the receptor and this cell type, but the non-preadipocyte fibroblast population could still express important autoantigens, with several studies demonstrating antibody- and T cell-based responses suggesting that this is the case. Orbital fibroblast antigen expression libraries, perhaps utilizing differential display, would be one way to take this idea forward. An additional route is to establish immunoglobulin cDNA libraries to derive rare, locally-produced autoantibodies that could be probes for autoantigen screening (77). Although the work involved will be enormous, the goal of full orbital autoantigen identification makes these approaches worth contemplating, as improvements in prognostic techniques and therapy in ophthalmopathy are likely to depend on it.

Acknowledgements

Work in our laboratory is supported by the Sir Jules Thorn Charitable Trust.

REFERENCES

1. Burch, H.B. and Wartofsky, L. 1993. Graves' ophthamopathy: current concepts regarding pathogenesis and management. Endocrine Rev. 14:747-93.
2. Henderson, J. and Wall, J.R. 1981. Failure of haemagglutination and immunofluorecence methods to detect serum orbital antibodies in patients with Graves' ophthalmopathy. Clin. Endocrinol. 14:153-8.
3. Mengistu, M., Laryea, E., Miller, A. and Wall, J.R. 1986. Clinical significance of a new autoantibody against a human eye muscle soluble antigen, detected by immunofluorescence. Clin. Exp. Immunol. 65:19-27.
4. Konishi, J., Herman, M.N. and Kriss, J.P. 1974. Binding of thyroglobulin and thyroglobulin - antithyroglobulin complex to extraocular muscle membrane. Endocrinology 95:434-66.
5. Kriss, J.P. 1970. Radioisotopic thyroidolyphography in patients with Graves' disease. J. Clin. Endocrinol. Metab. 40:872-5.
6. Kodama, K., Sikorska, H., Bayly, R., Bandy-Dafoe, P. and Wall, J.R. 1984. Use of monoclonal antibodies to investigate a possible role of thyroglobulin in the pathogenesis of Graves' ophthalmopathy. J. Clin. Endocrinol. Metab. 59:67-73.
7. Kuroki, T., Ruf, J., Whelan, L., Miller, A. and Wall, J.R. 1985. Anti-thyroglobulin monoclonal and autoantibodies cross-react with an orbital connective tissue membrane antigen: a possible mechanism for the association of ophthalmopathy with autoimmune thyroid disorders. Clin. Exp. Immunol. 62:361-70.
8. Tao, T.W., Cheng, P.J., Pham, H., Leu, S.L. and Kriss, J.P. 1986. Monoclonal antithyroglobulin antbodies derived from immunizations of mice with human eye muscle and thyroid membranes. J. Clin. Endocrinol. Metab. 63:577-82.
9. Kodama, K., Sikorska, H., Bandy-Dafoe, P., Bayly, R. and Wall, J.R. 1982. Demonstration of a circulating autoantibody against a soluble eye muscle antigen in Graves' ophthalmopathy. Lancet ii:1353-6.
10. Salvi, M., Bingoye, F., Chung, F. and Wall, J.R. 1988. Affinity purification of orbital membrane antigens for the study of the pathogenesis of Graves' ophthalmopathy. J. Clin. Endocrinol. Metab. 66:939-45.
11. Atkinson, S., Holcombe, M. and Kendall-Taylor, P. 1984. Ophthalmopathic immunoglobulin in patients with Graves' ophthalmopathy. Lancet ii:374-6.
12. Kadlubowski, M., Irvine, W.J. and Rowland, C.A. 1986. The lack of specificity of ophthalmic immunoglobulins in Graves' disease. J. Clin. Endocrinol. Metab. 63:990-5.
13. Ahmann, A., Baker, J.R., Weetman, A.P., Wartofsky, L., Nutman, T.B. and Burman, K.D. 1987. Antibodies to porcine eye muscle in patients with Graves' ophthalmopathy: identification of serum immunoglobulin directed against unique determinants by immunoblotting and enzyme-linked immunosorbent assay. J. Clin. Endocrinol. Metab. 64:454-60.
14. Miller, A., Sikorska, H., Salvi, M. and Wall, J.R. 1986. Evaluation of an enzyme-linked immunosorbent assay for the measurement of autoantibodies against eye muscle antigens in Graves' ophthalmopathy. Acta Endocrinol. 113:514-22.

15. Weetman, A.P., Fells, P. and Shine, B. 1989. T and B cell reactivity to extraocular and skeletal muscle in Graves' ophthalmopathy. Brit. J. Ophthal. 73:323-7.
16. Schifferdecker, E., Ketzler-Sasse, U., Boehm, B.O., Ronsheimer, H.B., Shcerbaum, W.A. and Schoffling, K. 1989. Re-evaluation of eye muscle autoantibody determination in Graves' ophthalmopathy: failure to detect a specific antigen by use of enzyme-linked immunoblotting techniques. Acta Endocrinol. 121:643-50.
17. Salvi, M., Hiromatsu, Y., Bernard, N., How, J. and Wall, J.R. 1988. Human orbital tissue and thyroid membrane express a 64kDa protein which is recognized by autoantibodies in serum of patients with thyroid-associated ophthalmopathy. FEBS Lett. 232:125-9.
18. Salvi, M., Bernard, N., Miller, A., Zhang, Z-G, Gardini, E. and Wall, J.R. 1991. Prevalence of antibodies reactive with a 64kDa eye muscle membrane antigen in thyroid-associated ophthalmopathy. Thyroid 1:207-13.
19. Bernard, N.F., Ertung, F., Teboul, N., Zhang, Z-G, Salvi, M. and Wall, J.R. 1991. Isotype and immunoglobulin subclass distribution of eye muscle membrane reactive antibodies in the serum of patients with thyroid-associated ophthalmopathy as detected in Western blotting. Autoimmunity 10:57-63.
20. Miller, A., Arthurs, B., Boucher, A., Liberman, A., Bernard, N., Rodien, P., Salvi, M. and Wall, J.R. 1992. Significance of antibodies reactive with a 64kDa eye muscle membrane antigen in patients with thyroid autoimmunity. Thyroid 2:197-202.
21. Weightman, D. and Kendall-Taylor, P. 1989. Cross-reaction of eye muscle antibodies with thyroid-tissue in thyroid-associated ophthalmopathy. J. Endocrinol. 122:201-6.
22. Kendler, D.L., Rootman, J., Huber, G.K. and Davies, T.F. 1991. A 64kD membrane antigen is a recurrent epitope for natural autoantibodies in patients with Graves' thyroid and ophthalmic diseases. Clin. Endocrinol. 35:539-47.
23. Chang, T.C., Chang, T.J., Huang, Y.S., Su, R.J. and Kao, S.C.S. 1992. Identification of autoantigen recognized by autoimmune ophthalmopathy sera with immunoblotting correlated with orbital computed tomography. Clin. Immunol. Immunopathol. 65:161-6.
24. Hiromatsu, Y., Sato, M., Tanaka, K., Shoji, S., Nonaka, K., Chinami, M. and Fukazawa, H. 1992. Significance of anti-eye muscle antibody in patients with thyroid-associated ophthalmopathy by quantitative Western blot. Autoimmunity 14:9-16.
25. Tandon, N., Yan, S.L., Arnold, K., Metcalfe, R.A. and Weetman, A.P. 1994. Immunoglobulin class and subclass distribution of eye muscle and fibroblast antibodies in patients with thyroid-associated ophthalmopathy. Clin. Endocrinol. 40:629-39.
26. Wu, Y-J, Clarke, S.E.M. and Shepherd, P. 1998. Prevalence and significance of antibodies reactive with eye muscle membrane anrigens in sera from patients with Graves' ophthalmopathy and other thyroid and nonthyroid disorders. Thyroid 8:167-74.
27. Wall, J.R., Hayes, M., Scalise, D., Stolarski, C., Nebes, V., Kiljanski, J., Salvi, M. and Sato, M. 1995. Native gel electrophoresis and isoelectric focusing of a 64-kilodalton eye muscle protein shows that it is an important target for serum autoantibodies in patients with thyroid-associated ophthalmopathy and not expressed in other skeletal muscle. J. Clin. Endocrinol. Metab. 80:1226-32.
28. Dong, Q., Ludgate, M. and Vassart, G. 1991. Cloning and sequencing of a novel 64-kDa autoantigen recognized by patients with autoimmune thyroid disease. J. Clin. Endocrinol. Metab. 72:1375-81.

29. Zhang, Z-G, Dong, Q., Rodien, P., Alcalde, L., Bernard, N., Boucher, A., Salvi, M., Arthurs, B., Vassart, G.M., Ludgate, M. and Wall, J.R. 1992. Antibodies in the serum of patients with autoimmune thyroid disorders react with a recombinant 98 amino acid fragment of a full length 64 kDa eye muscle membrane protein which is also expressed in the thyroid. Autoimmunity 13:151-7.
30. Ross, P.V., Koenig, R.J., Arscott, P., Ludgate, M., Waier, M., Nelson, C.C., Kaplan, M.M. and Baker Jr, J.R. 1993. Tissue specificity and serologic reactivity of an autoantigen associated with autoimmune thyroid disease. J. Clin. Endocrinol. Metab. 77:433-8.
31. Bernard, N.F., Nygen, T.N., Tyutyunikov, A., Stolarski, C., Scalise, D., Genovese, C., Hayes, M.B., Ludgate, M. and Wall, J.R. 1994. Antibodies against $_1$D, a recombinant 64-kDa membrane protein, are associated with ophthalmopathy in patients with thyroid autoimmunity. Clin. Immunol. Immunopathol. 70:225-33.
32. Kromminga, A., Hagel, C., Arndt, R. and Schuppert, F. 1998. Serological reactivity of recombinant 1D autoantigen and its expression in human thyroid and eye muscle tissue: A possible autoantigenic link in Graves' patients. J. Clin. Endocrinol. Metab. 83:2817-23.
33. Kubota, S., Gunji, K., Stolarski, C., Kennerdell, J.S. and Wall, J. 1998. Re-evaluation of the prevalences of serum autoantibodies reactive with "64-kd eye muscle proteins" in patients with thyroid-associated ophthalmopathy. Thyroid 8:175-9.
34. Kubota, S., Gunji, K., Ackrell, B.A.C., Cochran, G., Stolarski, C, Wengrowicz, S., Kennerdell, J.S., Hiromatsu, Y. and Wall, J. 1998. The 64-kilodalton eye muscle protein is the flavoprotein subunit of mitochondrial succinate dehydrogenase: The corresponding serum antibodies are good markers of an immune-mediated damage to the eye muscle in patients with Graves' hyperthyroidism. J. Clin. Endocrinol. Metab. 83:443-7.
35. Gunji, K., De Bellis, A., Kubota, S., Swanson, J., Wengrowicz, S., Cochran, B., Ackrell, B.A.C., Salvi, M., Bellastella, A., Bizzarro, A., Sinisi, A.A. and Wall, J.R. 1999. Serum antibodies against the flavoprotein subunit of succinate dehydrogenase are sensitive markers of eye muscle autoimmunity in patients with Graves' hyperthyroidism. J. Clin. Endocrinol. Metab. 84:1255-62.
36. Joffe, B., Gunji, K., Panz, V., Zouvanis, M., Swanson, J., Ackrell, B.A.C. and Wall, J.R. 1998. Thyroid-associated ophthalmopathy in black South African patients with Graves' disease: Relationship to antiflavoprotein antibodies. Thyroid 8: 1023-7.
37. Kemp, E.H., Ridgway, J.N., Smith, K.A., Watson, P.F. and Weetman, A.P. 2000. Autoantibodies in the flavoprotein subunit of succinate dehydrogenase: Analysis of specificity in autoimmune thyroid disease. Clin. Endocrinol. (in press).
38. Kadluboswki, M., Irvine, W.J. and Rowland, A.C. 1987. Anti-muscle antibodies in Graves' ophthalmopathy. J. Clin. Lab. Immunol. 24:105-11.
39. Ludgate, M., Dong, Q., Dreyfus, P.A., Zakut, H., Taylor, P., Vassart, G. and Soreq, H. 1989. Definition, at the molecular level, of a thyroglobulin-acetylcholinesterase shared epitope: Study of its pathophysiological significance in patients with Graves' ophthalmopathy. Autoimmunity 3:167-76.
40. Weetman, A.P., Tse, C.K., Randall, W.R., Tsim, K.W.K. and Barnard, E.A. 1988. Acetylcholinesterase antibodies and thyroid autoimmunity. Clin. Exp. Immunol. 71:96-9.
41. Mappouras, D.G., Philippou, G., Haralambous, S., Tzartos, S.J., Balafas, A., Souvatzoglou, A. and Lymberi, P. 1995. Antibodies to acetylcholinesterase cross-linking with thyroglobulin in myasthenia gravis and Graves' disease. Clin. Exp. Immunol. 100:336-43.

42. Brimijoin, S. and Lennon, V.A. 1990. Autoimmune preganglionic sympathectomy induced by acetylcholinesterase antibodies. Proc. Natl. Acad. Sci. USA 87:9630-4.
43. Elisei, R., Weightman, D., Kendall-Taylor, P., Vassart, G. and Ludgate, M. 1993. Muscle autoantigens in thyroid associated ophthalmopathy: The limits of molecular genetics. J. Endocrinol. Invest. 16:533-40.
44. Gunji, K., De Bellis, A., Li, A.W., Yamada, M., Kubota, S., Ackrell, G., Wengrowicz, S., Bellastella, A., Bizzarro, A., Sinisi, A. and Wall, J.R. 2000. Cloning and characterization of the novel thyroid and eye muscle shared protein G2s: Autoantibodies against G2s are closely associated with ophthalmopathy in patients with Graves' hyperthyroidism. J. Clin. Endocrinol. Metab. 85:1641-7.
45. Bahn, R.S., Gorman, C.A., Johnson, C.M. and Smith, T.J. 1989. Presence of antibodies in the sera of patients with Graves' disease recognizing a 23 kilodalton fibroblast protein. J. Clin. Endocrinol. Metab. 69:622-8.
46. Stover, C., Otto, E., Beyer, J. and Kahaly, G. 1992. Humoral immunity and retrobulbar fibroblasts in endocrine ophthalmopathy. Acta Endocrinol. 126:394-402.
47. Molnár, I. and Balázs, C.S. 1991. Comparative study on IgG and IgA antibodies against human thyroid and eye-muscle antigens in Graves' ophthalmopathy. Acta Medical Hungarica 48:13-21.
48. Arnold, K., Metcalfe, R. and Weetman, A.P. 1995. Immunoglobulin A class fibroblast antibodies in patients with Graves' disease and prebitial myxedema. J. Clin. Endocrinol. Metab. 80:3430-7.
49. Bednarczuk, T., Stolarski, C., Pawlik, E., Slon, M., Rowinski, M., Kubota, S., Hiromatsu, Y., Bartoszewicz, Z., Wall, J.R. and Nauman, J. 1999. Autoantibodies reactive with extracellular matrix proteins in patients with thyroid-associated ophthalmopathy. Thyroid 9:289-95.
50. Perros, P. and Kendall-Taylor, P. 1992. Biological activity of autoantibodies from patients with thyroid-associated ophthalmopathy: In vitro effects on porcine extraocular myoblasts. Q. J. Med. 84:691-706.
51. Weightman, D.R., Perros, P., Sherif, I.H. and Kendall-Taylor, P. 1993. Autoantibodies to IGF-1 binding sites in thyroid associated ophthalmopathy. Autoimmunity 16:251-7.
52. Rotella, C.M., Zonefrati, R., Toccafondi, R., Valente, W.A. and Kohn, L.D. 1986. Ability of monoclonal antibodies to the thyrotropin receptor to increase collagen synthesis in human fibroblasts: An assay which appears to measure exophthalmogenic immunoglobulins in Graves' sera. J. Clin. Endocrinol. Metab. 62:357-67.
53. Metcalfe, R.A., Davies, R. and Weetman, A.P. 1993. Analysis of fibroblast-stimulating activity in IgG from patients with Graves' dermopathy. Thyroid 3:207-12.
54. Wall, J.R., Strakosch, C.R., Fang, S.L., Ingbar, S.H. and Braverman, L.E. 1979. Thyroid binding antibodies and other immunological abnormalities in patients with Graves' ophthalmopathy: Effect of treatment with cyclophosphamide. Clin. Endocrinol. 10:79-91.
55. McLachlan, S.M., Bahn, R. and Rapoport, B. 1992. Endocrine ophthalmopathy: A re-evaluation of the association with thyroid autoantibodies. Autoimmunity 14:143-8.
56. Nishikawa, M., Yoshimura, M., Toyoda, N., Masuki, H., Yonemoto, T., Gondou, A., Kato, T., Kurokawa, H., Furumura, T. and Inada, M. 1993. Correlation of orbital muscle changes evaluated by magnetic resonance imaging and thyroid-stimulating antibody in patients with Graves' ophthalmopathy. Acta Endocrinol. 129:213-9.

57. Kasagi, K., Hidaka, A., Nakamura, H., Takeuchi, R., Misaki, T., Iida, Y. and Konishi, J. 1993. Thyrotropin receptor antibodies in hypothyroid Graves' disease. J. Clin. Endocrinol. Metab. 76:504-8.
58. Feliciello, A., Procellini, A., Ciullo, I., Vonavolontà, G., Avvedimento, E.V. and Fenzi, G. 1993. Expression of thyrotropin-receptor mRNA in healthy and Graves' disease retro-orbital tissue. Lancet 342:337-338.
59. Heufelder, A.E. 1995. Involvement of the orbital fibroblast and TSH receptor in the pathogenesis of Graves' ophthalmopathy. Thyroid 5:331-40.
60. Aust, G., Crisp, M., Bösenberg, E., Ludgate, M., Weetman, A.P. and Paschke, R. 1998. Transcription of thyroid autoantigens in non-expressing tissues. Exp. Clin. Endocrinol. Diab. 106:319-23.
61. Paschke, R., Metcalfe, A., Alcalde, L., Vassart, G., Weetman, A. and Ludagete, M. 1994. Presence of nonfunctional thyrotropin receptor variant transcripts in retroocular and other tissues. J. Clin. Endocrinol. Metab. 79:1234-8.
62. Burch, H.B., Sellitti, D., Barnes, S.G., Nagy, E.V., Bahn, R.S. and Burman, K.D. 1994. Thyrotropin receptor antisera for the detection of immunoreactive protein species in retroocular fibroblasts obtained from patients with Graves' ophthalmopathy. J. Clin. Endocrinol. Metab. 78:1384-91.
63. Spitzweg, C., Joba, W., Hunt, N. and Heufelder, A.R. 1997. Analysis of human thyrotropin receptor gene expression and immunoreactivity in human orbital tissue. Soc. Eur. J. Endocrinol. 136:599-607.
64. Dutton, C.M., Joba, W., Spitzweg, C., Heufelder, A.E. and Bahn, R.S. 1997. Thyrotropin receptor expression in adrenal, kidney and thymus. Thyroid 7:879-83.
65. Endo, T., Ohta, K., Haraguchi, K. and Onaya, T. 1995. Cloning and functional expression of a thyrotropin receptor cDNA from fat red cells. J. Biol. Chem. 270:10833-7.
66. Crisp, M.S., Lane, C., Halliwell, M., Wynford-Thomas, D. and Ludgate, M. 1997. Thyrotropin receptor transcripts in human adipose tissue. J. Clin. Endocrinol. Metab. 82:2003-5.
67. Bahn, R.S., Dutton, C.M., Natt, N., Joba, W., Spitzweg, C. and Heufelder, A.E. 1998. Thyrotropin receptor expression in Graves' orbital adipose/connective tissues: Potential autoantigen in Graves' ophthalmopathy. J. Clin. Endocrinol. Metab. 83:998-1002.
68. Bahn, R.S., Dutton, C.M., Joba, W. and Heufelder, A.E. 1998. Thyrotropin receptor expression in cultured Graves' orbital preadipocyte fibroblasts is stimulated by thyrotropin. Thyroid 8:193-6.
69. Many, M-C, Costaliola, S., Detrait, M., Denef, J-F, Vassart, G. and Ludgate, M. 1999. Development of an animal model of autoimmune thyroid eye disease. J. Immunol. 162:4966-74.
70. Mullin, B.R., Levinson, R.E., Friedman, A., Henson, D.E., Winand, R.J. and Kohn, L.D. 1977. Delayed hypersensitivity in Graves' disease and exophthalmos: Identification of thyroglobulin in normal human orbital muscle. Endocrinology 100:351-66.
71. Weetman A.P. 1992. The role of T lymphocytes in thyroid-associated ophthalmopathy. Autoimmunity 13:69-73.
72. Arnold, K., Tandon, N., McIntosh, R.S., Elisei, R., Ludgate, M. and Weetman, A.P. 1994. T cell responses to orbital antigens in thyroid-associated ophthalmopathy. Clin. Exp. Immunol. 96:329-34.
73. Stover, C., Otto, E., Beyer, J. and Kahaly, G. 1994. Cellular immunity and retrobulbar fibroblasts in Graves' ophthalmopathy. Thyroid 4:161-5.

74. Grubeck-Loebenstein, B., Trieb, K., Sztankay, A., Holter, W., Anderl, H. and Wick, G. 1994. Retrobulbar T cells from patients with Graves' ophthalmopathy are $CD8^+$ and specifically recognize autologous fibroblasts. J. Clin. Invest. 93:2738-43.
75. Otto, E.A., Ochs, K., Hansen, C., Wall, J.R. and Kahaly, G.J. 1996. Orbital tissue-derived T lymphocytes from patients with Graves' ophthalmopathy recognize autologous orbital antigens. J. Clin. Endocrinol. Metab. 81:3045-50.
76. Pappa, A., Calder, V., Ajjan, R., Fells, P., Ludgate, M., Weetman, A.P. and Lightman, S. 1997. Analysis of extraocular muscle-infiltrating T cells in thyroid-associated ophthalmopathy (TAO). Clin. Exp. Immunol. 109:362-9.
77. Jaume, J.C., Portolano, S., Prummel, M.F., McLachlan, S.M. and Rapoport, B. 1994. Molecular cloning and characterization of genes for antibodies generated by orbital tissue-infiltrating B-cells in Graves' ophthalmopathy. J. Clin. Endocrinol. Metab. 78:348-52.

2

ORBITAL AUTOIMMUNITY IN GRAVES' DISEASE

Armin E. Heufelder and Werner Joba
Department of Internal Medicine, Division of Gastroenterology, Endocrinology & Metabolism, Philipps-University, 35033 Marburg, Germany

INTRODUCTION

Graves' disease (GD) is an autoimmune syndrome characterized by hyperthyroidism and a diffusely enlarged thyroid gland. The most prominent extrathyroidal manifestation of this thyroid disease is thyroid-associated or Graves' ophthalmopathy (GO), a medically incurable and chronic autoimmune process that affects all orbital tissue compartments and leads to various eye complications such as discomfort, lid retraction, proptosis, periorbital swelling, extraocular muscle dysfunction, diplopia, and sight loss. When assessed carefully, GO occurs in about 80-90% of patients with GD. In most instances, the orbital problems appear within 18 months after diagnosis of thyroid disease. The close clinical association of GD with GO and pretibial dermopathy (PTD), a less frequent extrathyroidal manifestation, suggests a common antigen or similar sequence of pathogenic events in these affected tissues (1,2). Enlargement of extraocular muscle bodies together with an increase of orbital connective/fatty tissue within the bony orbits is responsible for most of the orbital complications in patients with severe active GO. Tissue enlargement is effected by marked infiltration of immunocompetent cells, mainly macrophages and T lymphocytes, and some B cells and mast cells, as well as by abundant quantities of collagen and hydrophilic glycosaminoglycans (GAGs). It is entirely possible that the orbital immune process is triggered in a non-specific manner, and that antigen encounter by macrophages and dendritic cells facilitates T cell-dependent propagation and perpetuation of the disease. Once recruitment to the orbital space and transmigration of the endothelial cell barrier have occurred, T cells release numerous cytokines capable of stimulating cell proliferation, GAG synthesis, recruitment of new fat cells from orbital adipose precursor cells, and expression of various immunomodulatory molecules by orbital preadipocyte fibroblasts (3). While these mechanisms may sufficiently explain various aspects of how GO may evolve and be propagated, it is still uncertain whether a primary antigen does indeed exist and what its nature might be.

T-CELL REPERTOIRES IN ORBITAL TISSUES

Histochemical analyses have revealed that, within the orbits of patients with active GO, infiltrating immunocompetent cells are predominantly $CD3^+$ T lymphocytes and macrophages, with only a small proportion of Leu-26^+ B lymphocytes (4,5). Both ($CD4^+$) helper/inducer and ($CD8^+$) suppressor/cytotoxic T lymphocytes are present (6,7). A large proportion of these T lymphocytes, especially those adjacent to blood vessels, are $CD3^+$/$CD45RO^+$ cells reflecting a subset of memory T cells and macrophages. In addition, immunohistochemical analyses have demonstrated that most T cells express T cell receptors (TcRs) carrying the α/β phenotype (8). A central role of T cells in propagating the autoimmune process is emphasized by several studies demonstrating restriction of TcR variable (V) region gene usage both in animal models, in patients with Graves' disease (9,10) and in orbital connective/fatty tissues and eye muscle tissue of patients with active GO, suggesting that relevant antigenic epitopes are shared by these tissue compartments. In contrast, in orbital tissues of patients with longstanding, inactive GO or with unrelated orbital conditions, restriction of TcR V gene usage occurred only to a minor degree or was absent (8). Moreover, in two patients with severe, active GO and PTD, restricted variability of expressed TcR Vα and TcR Vβ genes was detected in thyroid, orbital and pretibial tissues, but not in peripheral blood lymphocytes. Moreover, TcR V gene restriction was not detected in corresponding tissues derived from normal healthy individuals (11). Despite obvious heterogeneity of TcR V gene repertoires between these two patients, striking similarities of restricted Vα and Vβ gene family usage were noted in T cells present at these distinct sites of each patient. Moreover, analysis of the nucleotide sequences coding for the variable regions of dominant TcR Vβ gene families in intra- and extrathyroidal tissues of each patient revealed two major populations (Vβ2 and Vβ6) of clonally expanded TcRs or of TcRs whose junctional regions shared significant homologies at the amino acid level. Several conserved amino acid motives were detected in the CD3 domains of junctional regions in expanded TcR gene families of lymphocytes in the thyroid, orbital and pretibial tissue, but not in peripheral blood lymphocytes (11). Taken together, these observations indicate a limited degree of clonality among certain populations of thyroidal, orbital and pretibial lymphocytes, which are likely to be derived from a small number of clones present at high frequency in these distinct sites. This observation is consistent with, but does not prove, the concept that common antigenic determinants may drive the immune process in Graves' disease. During the earlier stages of the immune response, the antigen-driven T-cell response appears to be highly specific and focused (11,12). By contrast, in later stages of the immune process, recruitment of T-cells with more divergent sets of expressed TcR genes may be elicited by tissue destruction and cytokine-induced antigen expression.

T-CELL AND B-CELL TARGETS AND ANTIGENS

Identification of relevant orbital autoantigens has remained difficult because suitable animal models of GD and ophthalmopathy are not available and because of the limited availability of affected human tissue derived from patients with untreated active GO of recent onset. Much efforts have been concentrated on identifying the cell type against which the autoimmune process is directed. Circulating antibodies against proteins contained in eye muscle (64 kDa) and in orbital fibroblasts (23 kDa) are frequently detected in sera of patients with GO (13,14). Unfortunately, these antibodies lack both tissue and disease specificity (15,16), indicating that they are the products rather than the cause of the inflammatory process within the orbits, and generated secondarily as a result of local inflammation and tissue destruction (17). It is now clear that many of these antibodies are directed against ubiquitous cytoskeletal components that are common to many tissues both within and outside of the orbits (17-19). While new putative autoantigens continue to appear (and disappear) in the literature, many of these studies reveal a striking lack of stringency and reproducibility. As a general note of caution, there is little evidence that a particular primary antigen is indeed necessary to elicit the pathogenic sequence of events that leads to GO.

Several studies have focused on the nature of the effector and target cells in the orbits, as well as on their interaction within other orbital cell types. One study demonstrated that autologous orbital fibroblasts, but not crude eye muscle extract, autologous peripheral blood mononuclear cells, allogeneic cells, or purified protein derivative of mycobacterium tuberculosis are specifically recognized by T cells obtained from the retrobulbar tissue of patients with GO in an MHC class I-restricted manner (20). Further analysis revealed that these T-cells, predominantly those of the $CD8^+$, $CD45RO^+$ phenotype, exhibit little target cell cytotoxic activity, but secrete marked amounts of cytokines upon activation. These observations suggest that stimulation of fibroblasts, rather than their destruction, may be an important pathogenic mechanism. It is likely that both orbital connective/adipose tissue and the stromal cell compartment within extraocular muscles harbor the antigen-bearing cells in GO, and that T cells mainly recognize and stimulate orbital preadipocyte fibroblasts. It was shown that Graves' orbital fibroblasts express, in response to appropriate stimuli, various immunomodulatory molecules such as MHC class I and class II molecules, intercellular adhesion molecule-1 (ICAM-1) and 72 kDa heat shock protein (HSP72) (21-23). In this context, activation of orbital fibroblasts through CD40 appears to be a particularly powerful pathway that stimulates the production of certain pro-inflammatory cytokines (24) as well as hyaluronan synthesis and cyclooxygenase-2 expression (25-27). In addition, similar to their intrathyroidal counterparts, orbital preadipocyte fibroblasts may play a pivotal role in perpetuating the orbital immune process by serving as potent inhibitors of T cell and B cell apoptosis, thereby extending their encounter with immune effector cells (28-31).

TSH RECEPTOR

In recent years, significant efforts have been made to define the nature of the target autoantigen in GO. The hyperthyroidism of Graves' disease results from uncontrolled stimulation of the TSHR by antibodies directed against this autoantigen. Clinically, a close temporal relationship between the onset of GD and development of extrathyroidal manifestations, such as GO, PTD or acropachy, is observed. Although a close correlation between the presence of TSHR-directed antibodies and the presence or severity of GO has not definitively been established, patients with GO and PTD almost uniformly display high titers of TSHR-stimulating antibodies (TSAb). Moreover, severe GO frequently occurs in the presence of high concentrations of TSHR-stimulating immunoglobulins (32), and TSHR autoantibodies have recently been demonstrated to correlate with certain clinical features of GO (33). Therefore, the TSHR has become a favorite candidate autoantigen that is shared between the thyroid gland and the orbital and dermal connective tissue (3,17).

The TSHR is a member of the family of G-protein-coupled receptors with seven transmembrane domains (34,35). Its large extracellular domain serves as a target for thyrotropin, TSHR antibodies (TSAb, TBII) and immune effector cells, and therefore plays a central role in TSHR function and immune recognition (36,37). The TSHR has long been considered a thyroid-specific protein, and expression of TSHR in non-thyroidal tissues has been controversial (38). However, the hypothesis that extrathyroidal adipose cells might express TSHR was already forwarded by Rodbell, who demonstrated

TSH-stimulated lipolysis in rat epididymal fat cells (39). In addition, TSH binding to guinea pig adipose and retro-orbital tissues and the presence of TSHR mRNA in guinea pig brown and white adipose tissues have been reported (40). Using a variety of techniques (Northern blot analysis, ribonuclease protection assay, RT-PCR, in situ hybridization, immunoblotting, immunohistochemical staining, TSH binding assays), several investigators have detected TSHR mRNA and protein expression in various extrathyroidal tissues, cultured cells and membrane preparations (41-48). Nevertheless, TSHR expression in extrathyroidal tissues and its potential role in GO are still being debated (49,50). The capacity of the extrathyroidal TSHR to transmit signals and thereby alter certain metabolic and immunological activities in target cells has been examined by several investigators. These studies suggested that TSH and affinity-purified immunoglobulins with high TSHR stimulating activity indeed alter, in a dose-dependent manner, certain metabolic (e.g. adenylate cyclase activity) and immunological (e.g. expression of human leucocyte antigen HLA-DR and ICAM-1) functions in non-thyroidal cells such as orbital fibroblasts and in transfected, TSHR-expressing CHO cells (49,51). However, whether or not the extrathyroidal TSHR is functional must be clearly distinguished from its potential role to serve as an autoantigen. Although recognition of multiple epitopes of the TSHR extracellular domain by antigen-specific T cells has been demonstrated (52,53) and confirmed in recent studies, it still remains to be assessed whether autoreactive lymphocytes obtained from affected tissues recognize extrathyroidal TSH receptors following processing by local antigen-presenting cells. In addition, doubts have been raised as to whether the low levels of TSHR transcripts detected in extrathyroidal tissues may be biologically relevant and sufficient to trigger an immune response. However, since large amounts of TSHR protein are present within the thyroid gland that can generate large numbers of antigen-specific T cells, even small quantities of TSHR protein in extrathyroidal sites would be sufficient to serve this purpose. Once the autoimmune process is established, circulating sensitized T cells and antibodies could recognize even small quantities of a similar protein at remote sites. Moreover, TSHR expression in orbital tissues may be upregulated locally upon appropriate stimulation and differentiation of adipocyte precursor cells.

TSHR protein expression has been detected in human neonatal adipocytes, where it declines rapidly with advancing age and becomes undetectable in adult adipocytes (54). Additionally, recent reports have shown TSH-induced stimulation of TSHR expression in late-passage cultures of orbital preadipocyte fibroblasts (55). These results suggest that a humoral factor present in certain patients with GD, might stimulate TSHR expression in orbital cells, which then can act as an orbital autoantigen in GO (56-58). Using a monoclonal TSHR antibody generated by genetic immunization (59),

TSHR expression in muscle biopsies and adipose tissue from patients with GO has been compared to that in muscle biopsies obtained from patients undergoing strabismus corrections, in normal orbital fat and in orbital pseudotumour (M. Ludgate, personal communication). In patients with GO, immunostaining was noted on elongated fibroblast-like cells, frequently located adjacent to clusters of adipocytes. No such staining was present in the strabismus or pseudotumour samples, implying that in GO, preadipocytes and mature adipocytes express the TSHR.

Recently, an animal model of GO-like disease has been established by immunization of balb/c mice with recombinant human TSHR. The histopathology of the orbital contents in affected animals appears to parallel that in humans, but some unusual features such as infiltration of mast cells has also been noted. Given the absence of fully developed orbits in these mice, it is likely that the mechanical consequences of GO do not become readily apparent in this species. While the data reported to date are still incomplete and do not prove the TSHR as being the primary antigen in GO, they certainly highlight an important role for TSHR-directed immune mechanisms in the evolution of the orbital pathology in GO.

CYTOKINES IN ORBITAL TISSUES

Elaboration and release of certain cytokines by infiltrating lymphocytes is known to stimulate proliferation of fibroblasts and synthesis of large amounts of GAGs, which results in tissue volume expansion and proptosis. Several studies have demonstrated the presence of various cytokines, especially IFN-γ, TNF-α and IL-1α, mainly located in close proximity to T cell aggregates within the affected connective tissue of patients with active GO. In addition, these cytokines have been detected in extracts of orbital connective tissue and in primary cultures of retroorbital fibroblasts (6,61). Further analysis of cytokine expression by lymphocytes, derived from patients with active GO and propagated in vitro or from patients with longstanding GO, revealed evidence of a T helper cell 1 (Th-1) type cytokine profile of cytotoxic T cells (62) and release of IFN-γ, IL-4 and IL-10 (20,63). In addition, mRNA analysis by RT-PCR demonstrated expression of IL-2, IL-4, IL-5 and IL-10, but not of IFN-γ in orbital tissue from patients with advanced GO (64), suggesting that these cytokines are predominantly produced by activated infiltrating inflammatory cells. Taken together, these observations indicate that Th-1-type cellular immune mechanisms appear to act during the earlier stages, whereas Th-2-type humoral effector mechanisms may propagate the orbital immune process (7). In addition, numerous cytokines and inflammatory mediators, such as IL-1α, IL-6, IL-8, IGF-1,

TGF-β, PDGF, RANTES, MCP-1 and PGE_2 are synthesized by residential connective tissue cells both in an autocrine manner and in response to infiltrating lymphocytes and monocytes/macrophages. These agents have been shown to act as local paracrine and autocrine modulators of cellular immune and metabolic activities within the affected orbital tissues (3,66). Cytokine effects of potential relevance to the orbital autoimmune process involve the induction and stimulation of major histocompatibility complex (MHC) class II molecules (21,22), heat shock proteins (21,23) and adhesion molecules in orbital fibroblasts and in microvascular endothelial cells (66). Chemokines such as RANTES and MCP-1 may play a crucial role in triggering T cells to migrate across activated endothelium along a chemoattractive gradient. In this context, it is of interest that RANTES is abundantly expressed in the perivascular connective tissue in active GO. Furthermore, TNFα and IL-1, two key pro-inflammatory mediators in GO tissue, act to strongly stimulate RANTES expression and release by orbital preadipocyte fibroblasts (Schuessler A et al, unpublished). Of note, RANTES expression, following upregulation by these pro-inflammatory cytokines, was readily suppressed by IL-4 and dexamethasone, respectively, consistent with the concept that Th2-type cytokines and immunosuppressants act to down-regulate or even terminate the pro-inflammatory cascade of events in GO.

Additionally, various cytokines and agents, e.g. IFN-γ, TGF- β, IGF-1, IL-1α, and leukoregulin, in part acting through cyclooxygenase type 2 and hyaluronate synthase (25,26), stimulate GAG synthesis (predominantly hyaluronic acid and chondroitin sulfate) by orbital fibroblasts (67-70). Furthermore, it has been demonstrated that several cytokines and growth factors (IL-1α, IL-4, IGF-1, TGF-β, and PDGF), which are present in situ in the orbital tissue of patients with GO, stimulate cell proliferation in fibroblasts from orbital connective/fatty tissue and from extraocular muscle perimysium (71). Fibroblast proliferation was inhibited by glucocorticoid agonists, suggesting a glucocorticoid receptor-mediated mechanism of action. In addition, it has been demonstrated that certain cytokines stimulate orbital fibroblasts to synthesize various metalloproteinase inhibitors, and, to a lesser degree, metalloproteinases (71-73). These studies suggest that enlargement of ocular tissues in GO not only results from excessive accumulation of extracellular matrix components but also from an impairment of their degradation. A striking role of IL-1 in the pathogenesis of GO is suggested by its pleiotropic pro-inflammatory activities, as orbital fibroblast can be stimulated by IL-1 to express HLA-DR, adhesion molecules, heat shock proteins, metalloproteinase inhibitors and prostaglandins. In addition, there is evidence that impaired synthesis of IL-1 receptor antagonist (IL-1RA) by orbital fibroblasts may in part be responsible for the predominance of IL-1-mediated effects in the orbital tissues in GO (74-77). However, this hypothesis was not reflected by a recent study which measured IL-1RA levels in peripheral blood (78). Taken together, various cytokines act to recruit activated immune and inflammatory cells to the orbital tissues in GO, resulting in an increase and perpetuation in inflammation. These activated cells then produce numerous other mediators of inflammation and fibrogenesis, both by themselves and through their action on adjacent immune effector cells and residential orbital cells such as fibroblasts.

ORBITAL ADIPOGENESIS

Adipose precursor cells such as the preadipocyte fibroblast have long been neglected by many investigators as another potential target cell. An overabundance of adipose tissue both within the contents of the orbits and protruding externally is a prominent feature in many patients with GO (79,80). Preadipocytes have been isolated from the stromal-vascular fraction of neonatal and adult human adipose/connective tissues derived from various regions of the body (81-83). Recent studies have shown that a subpopulation of orbital fibroblasts, preadipocyte fibroblasts, can differentiate into mature adipocytes once exposed to appropriate paracrine stimuli (84). Thus, it is likely that orbital adipose tissue in GO is more cellular and comprises a higher proportion of preadipocytes capable of differentiating into adipocytes. Moreover, the process of adipocyte differentiation appears to be a restricted phenotypic attribute of orbital fibroblasts, as it was not observed in dermal fibroblasts and perimysial fibroblasts from extraocular muscle. Thus, under appropriate conditions of autocrine and paracrine stimulation, orbital preadipocytes may serve as a pool of precursor cells for orbital tissue volume enlargement, and perhaps provide distinct metabolic and immunologic activities of relevance to the evolution of GO. Recently, studies have investigated the link between adipogenesis and the expression of a functional TSHR in orbital preadipocyte fibroblasts (85). When treated according to a differentiation protocol, confluent late-passage GO and normal preadipocyte fibroblasts generated a significant proportion of mature adipose cells, whereas only fibroblast-like cells were apparent in control cultures. Importantly, a robust increase in cAMP production was detected in differentiated cultures following stimulation with rhTSH, which was absent in undifferentiated cultures. These data suggest that cultured orbital preadipocyte fibroblasts express few if any functional TSH receptors, but these cells have the potential to differentiate towards mature orbital adipocytes expressing a higher number of functional TSHR.

SUMMARY

GO it thought to result from a complex interplay of genetic and environmental factors. Various genes including those coding for HLA may determine a patient's susceptibility to the disease and its severity, but in addition numerous and often unknown environmental factors may determine its course. Once established, the chronic inflammatory process within the orbital tissues appears to take on a momentum of its own. Based upon our current state of knowledge, we propose the following working scheme for the pathogenesis of GO (Figure 1): On the background of a permissive immunogenetic milieu, circulating T cells in patients with GD, directed against certain antigens on thyroid follicular cells, recognize antigenic epitopes that are shared by tissues contained in the orbital space. Here, preadipocytes and fibroblasts most likely act as target and effector cells of the orbital immune process. This includes preadipocyte fibroblasts present in the perimysium of extraocular muscles, which do not appear to be immunologically or metabolically different from those located in the orbital connective tissue. Alternatively, GO may be initiated in a non-specific manner by macrophages and dendritic cells that respond to an environmental (e.g. microbial) insult. These cells can efficiently take up antigen, travel to regional lymphoid tissues and present antigenic peptides to T cells, thereby sensitizing T cells to proliferate, to expand in an antigen-specific manner and to recirculate, ready to release abundant quantities of pro-inflammatory mediators upon re-encounter of antigen. Differentiation of orbital preadipocyte fibroblasts into mature adipocytes expressing increased levels of TSHR may be driven by stimulation with circulating or locally produced cytokines or effectors. To date, it is still unknown how autoreactive T cells escape deletion by the immune system and become directed against a self-antigen that is presented by cells residing in the thyroid gland and in certain extrathyroidal locations. Mimicry of a host antigen by a microorganism or presentation of an altered self-antigen may promote proliferation and expansion of autoreactive T cell clones. T cell recruitment into the orbital tissues is facilitated by certain chemokines and cytokines, which help to attract T cells by stimulating the expression of several adhesion molecules (e.g. ICAM-1, VCAM-1, CD44) in vascular endothelium and connective tissue cells.

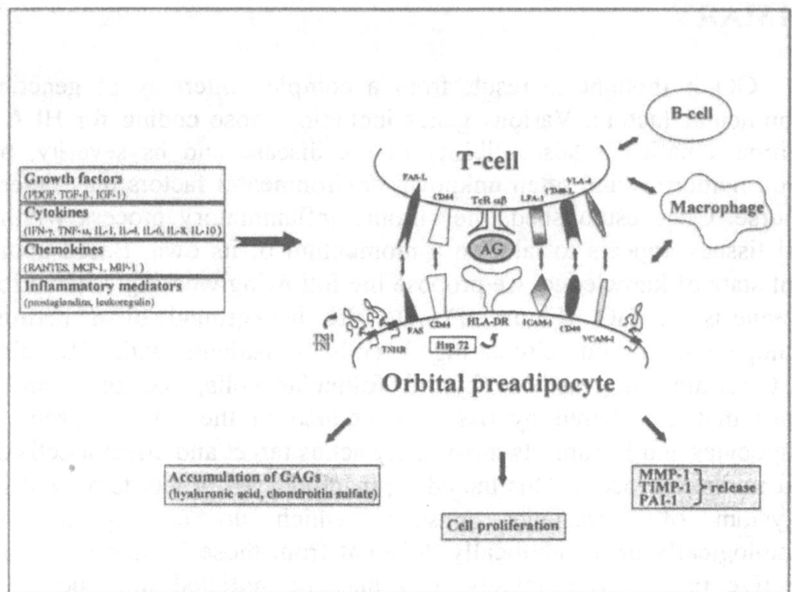

Figure 1: Proposed key steps in the pathogenesis of Graves' ophthalmopathy. TcR: T-cell receptor; LFA-1: leucocyte function associated antigen-1; VLA-4: very late antigen-4; ICAM-1: intercellular adhesion molecule-1; VCAM-1: vascular cell adhesion molecule-1; Hsp 72: Heat shock protein 72; TSI: thyroid-stimulating immunoglobulin; GAGs: glycosaminoglycans; MMP-1: matrix metalloproteinase-1; TIMP-1: tissue inhibitor of metalloproteinase-1; PAI-1: plasminogen activator inhibitor-1; PDGF: Platelet-derived growth factor; TGF-β: Transforming growth factor-β; IGF-1: Insulin-like growth factor-1; IFN-γ: Interferon-γ; TNF-α: Tumor necrosis factor-α; RANTES: ; MCP-1: Monocyte chemotactic protein-1; MIP-1: Macrophage inflammatory protein-1.

Adhesion molecules are known to be important for a variety of interactions between immunocompetent cells, connective tissue cells and extracellular matrix components. In addition, these molecules play a central role in lymphocyte activation and localization, facilitating antigen recognition, T cell costimulation, and various effector-target cell functions at the inflammatory sites, many of which result in amplification of the cellular immune process in active GO. Demonstration of limited variability of T cell receptor V gene usage in patients with early active GO suggests that an antigen-driven selection and/or expansion of specific T cells may occur during the early stages of GO. Macrophage-dependent T cell recruitment to the orbital space may trigger the release of a number of cytokines (most likely a Th-1-type spectrum) into the surrounding tissues. Cytokines, oxygen free radicals and fibrogenic growth factors, released both from infiltrating inflammatory and residential cells, act upon orbital preadipocytes in a paracrine and autocrine manner to stimulate adipogenesis, fibroblast proliferation, glycosaminoglycan synthesis, and the expression of immunomodulatory molecules. Smoking, a well-known aggravating factor in GO with an uncertain mode of action, may aggravate tissue hypoxia and exert important immunomodulatory effects. Local release of certain cytokines, TSHR-directed autoantibodies, or other factors might further enhance adipogenesis, glycosaminoglycan synthesis and expression of immunomodulatory proteins within the orbits. Once the net effect of these changes is to increase the volume of the fatty connective tissues within the orbit, then proptosis, extraocular muscle dysfunction, and periorbital congestion will ensue. Future studies will be aimed at identifying factors that might modulate adipogenesis in orbital cells and clarifying the link between adipogenesis and TSHR expression in the orbit. Taken together, a number of important details in the complex pathogenesis of GO have been deciphered. However, the puzzle is far from being complete, and many challenges are still ahead. Given the recent elucidation of at least some of the key pro-inflammatory mediators in GO, controlled clinical studies will soon be under way to assess whether targeted modulation of the orbital immune process indeed bears the potential to benefit our patients.

Acknowledgments

This work has been supported by grants from Deutsche Forschungsgemeinschaft, Bonn, Germany (He 1485/3-1 and He 1485/5-2 and 5-3, Gerhard-Hess-Program).

REFERENCES

1. Bahn RS, Heufelder AE. Mechanisms of disease Pathogenesis of Graves' ophthalmopathy. N Engl J Med 1993; 329:1468-75.
2. Gorman CA, Heufelder AE, Bartley GB. Ophthalmopathy. In DeGroot LJ (ed.) Endocrinology, Philadelphia PA: Saunders, 712-715, 1994.
3. Heufelder AE. Retro-orbital autoimmunity. Bailliere's Clin Endocrinol Metab 1997; 11:499-520.
4. Weetman AP, Cohen S, Gatter KC , Fells P, Shine B. Immunohistochemical analysis of the retrobulbar tissues in Graves' ophthalmopathy. Clin Exp Immunol 1989; 75:222-7.
5. Heufelder AE, Bahn RS. Elevated expression in situ of selectin and immunoglobulin superfamily adhesion molecules in retroocular connective tissues from patients with Graves' ophthalmopathy. Clin Exp Immunol 1993; 91:381-9.
6. Heufelder AE, Bahn RS. Detection and localization of cytokine immunoreactivity in retroocular connective tissue in Graves' ophthalmopathy. Eur J Clin Invest 1993; 23:10-7.

7. Aniszewski JP, Valyasevi RW, Bahn RS. Relationship between disease duration and predominant orbital T cell subset in Graves' ophthalmopathy. J Clin Endocrinol Metab 2000; 85:776-80.
8. Heufelder AE, Herterich S, Ernst G, Bahn RS, Scriba PC. Analysis of retroorbital T cell antigen receptor variable region gene usage in patients with Graves' ophthalmopathy. Eur J Endocrinol 1995; 132:266-77.
9. Davies TF, Martin A, Concepcion ES, Graves P, Cohen L, Ben-Nun A. Evidence of limited variability of antigen receptors on intrathyroidal T cells in autoimmune thyroid disease. N Engl J Med 1991; 325:238-44.
10. Davies TF, Martin A, Concepcion ES, Graves P, Lahat N, Cohen WL, Ben-Nun A. Evidence for selective accumulation of intrathyroidal T lymphocytes in human autoimmune thyroid disease based on T cell receptor V gene usage. J Clin Invest 1992; 89:157-62.
11. Heufelder AE, Wenzel BE, Scriba PC. Antigen receptor variable region repertoires expressed by T cells infiltrating thyroid, retroorbital and pretibial tissue in Graves' disease. J Clin Endocrinol Metab 1996; 81:3733-9.
12. Pappa A, Lawson JM, Calder V, Fells P, Lightman S. T cells and fibroblasts in affected extraocular muscles in early and late thyroid associated ophthalmopathy. Br J Ophthalmol 2000; 84:517-22.
13. Salvi M, Miller A, Wall JR. Human orbital tissue and thyroid membranes express a 64 kDa protein which is recognized by autoantibodies in the serum of patients with thyroid-associated ophthalmopathy. FEBS Letters 1988; 232:135-9.
14. Bahn RS, Gorman CA, Johnson CM, Smith TJ. Presence of antibodies in the sera of patients with Graves' disease recognizing a 23 kDa fibroblast protein. J Clin Endocrinol Metab 1989; 69:622-8.
15. Kadlubowski M, Irvine MJ, Rowland AC. The lack of specificity of ophthalmic immunoglobulins in Graves' disease. J Clin Endocrinol Metab 1986; 63:990-5.
16. Kendler DL, Rootman J, Huber GK, Davies TF. A 64 kDa membrane antigen is a recurrent epitope for natural antibodies in patients with Graves' thyroid and ophthalmic abnormalities. Clin Endocrinol 1991; 35:539-47.
17. Burch HB, Wartofsky L. Graves' ophthalmopathy: Current concepts regarding pathogenesis and management. Endocr Rev 1993; 14:747-93.
18. Gunji K, Kubota S, Stolarski C, Wengrowicz S, Kennerdell JS, Wall JR. A 63 kDa skeletal muscle protein associated with eye muscle inflammation in Graves' disease is identified as the calcium binding protein calsequestrin. Autoimmunity 1999; 29:1-9.
19. Gunji K, De Bellis A, Li AW et al. Cloning and characterization of the novel thyroid and eye muscle shared protein G2s: autoantibodies against G2s are closely associated with ophthalmopathy in patients with Graves''hyperthyroidism. J Clin Endocrinol Metab 2000; 85:1641-7.
20. Grubeck-Loebenstein B, Trieb K, Sztankay A, Holter W, Anderl H, Wick G. Retrobulbar T cells from patients with Graves' ophthalmoapthy are $CD8^+$ and specifically recognize autologous fibroblasts. J Clin Invest 1994; 3:2738-43.
21. Heufelder AE, Wenzel BE, Gorman CA, Bahn RS. Detection, cellular localization and modulation of heat shock proteins in cultured fibroblasts from patients with extrathyroidal manifestations of Graves' disease. J Clin Endocrinol Metab 1991; 73:739-45.
22. Heufelder AE, Smith TJ, Gorman CA, Bahn RS. Increased induction of HLA-DR by interferon-gamma in cultured retroocular fibroblasts derived from patients with Graves' ophthalmopathy and pretibial dermopathy. J Clin Endocrinol Metab 1991; 73:307-13.

23. Heufelder AE, Wenzel BE, Bahn RS. Cell surface localization of a 72 kilodalton heat shock protein in retroocular fibroblasts from patients with Graves' ophthalmopathy. J Clin Endocrinol Metab 1992; 74:732-736.
24. Sempowski GD, Rozenblit J, Smith TJ, Phipps RP. Human orbital fibroblasts are activated through CD40 to induce proinflammatory cytokine production. Am J Physiol 1998; 274:C707-14.
25. Smith TJ. The putative role of prostaglandin endoperoxidase H synthase-2 in the pathogenesis of thyroid-associated orbitopathy. Exp Clin Endocrinol Metab 1999; 107 (Suppl 5):S160-S163.
26. Kaback LA, Smith TJ. Expression of hyaluronan synthase messenger ribonucleic acids and their induction of interleukin-1beta in human orbital fibroblasts: potential insight into the molecular pathogenesis of thyroid-associated ophthalmopathy. J Clin Endocrinol Metab 1999; 84:4079-84.
27. Cao HJ, Wang HS, Zhang Y, Lin HY, Phipps RP, Smith TJ. Activation of human orbital fibroblasts through CD40 engagement results in a dramatic induction of hyaluronan synthesis and prostaglandin endoperoxide H synthase-2 expression. Insights into potential pathogenic mechanisms of thyroid-associated ophthalmopathy. J Biol Chem 1998; 273:29615-25.
28. Bichlmair AM, Wenzel BE, Scriba PC, Heufelder AE. Thyroid-derived fibroblasts support survival, differentiation and immunoglobulin secretion of cultured Graves' thyroid-derived B lymphocytes. Thyroid 1995; 5 (Suppl. 1):390 (abstract).
29. Mohacsi A, Trieb K, Anderl H, Grubeck-Loebenstein B. Retrobulbar fibroblasts from patients with Graves' ophthalmopathy induce downregulation of APO-1 in T lymphocytes and protect T cells from apoptosis during coculture. Int Arch Allergy Immunol 1996; 109:327-33.
30. Koga M, Hiromatsu Y, Jimi A, Inoue Y, Monaka K. Possible involvement of Fas-mediated apoptosis in eye muscle tissue from patients with thyroid-associated ophthalmopathy. Thyroid 1998; 8:311-8.
31. Ohtsuka K, Hashimoto M. Serum levels of soluble Fas in patients with Graves' ophthalmopathy. Br J Ophthalmol 2000; 84:103-6.
32. Morris J, Hay ID, Nelson RE, Jiang Nai S. Clinical utility of thyrotropin receptor antibody assays: Comparison of radioreceptor and bioassay methods. Mayo Clin Proc 1988; 63:707-12.
33. Gerding MN, van der Meer JW, Broenink M, Bakker O, Wiersinga WM, Prummel MF. Assocation of thyrotrophin receptor antibodies with the clinical features of Graves' ophthalmopathy. Clin Endocrinol 2000; 52:267-71.
34. Nagayama Y, Kaufman KD, Seto P, Rapoport B. Molecular cloning, sequence and functional expression of the cDNA for the human thyrotropin receptor. Biochem Biophys Res Commun 1989; 165:1184-90.
35. Parmentier M, Libert F, Maenhaut C, Lefort A, Gerard C, Perret J, Van Sande J, Dumont JE, Vassart G 1989 Molecular cloning of the thyrotropin receptor. Science 246:1620-2.
36. Murakami M, Mori M. 1990 Identification of immunogenic regions in human thyrotropin receptor for immunoglobulin G of patients with Graves' disease. Biochem Biophys Res Commun 171:512-8.
37. Kosugi S, Akamizu T, Takai O, Prabhakar BS, Kohn LD. The extracellular domain of the TSH receptor has an immunogenic epitope reactive with Graves' IgG but unrelated to receptor function as well as determinants having different roles for high affinity TSH binding and the activity of thyroid-stimulating autoantibodies. Thyroid 1991; 1:321-30.

38. Paschke R, Vassart G, Ludgate M. Current evidence for and against the TSH receptor being the common antigen in Graves-disease and thyroid-associated ophthalmopathy. Clin Endocrinol 1995; 42:565-9.
39. Rodbell M. Metabolism of isolated fat cells. I. Effects of hormones on glucose metabolism and lipolysis. J Biol Chem 1964; 239:375-80.
40. Roselli-Rehfuss L, Robbins LS, Cone RD. Thyrotropin receptor messenger ribonucleic acid is expressed in most brown and white adipose tissues in the guinea pig. Endocrinology 1992; 130:1857-61.
41. Feliciello A, Porcellini A, Ciullo, Bonavolonta G, Avvedimento EV, Fenzi G. Expression of thyrotropin-receptor mRNA in healthy and Graves' retro-orbital tissue. Lancet 1993; 342:337-8.
42. Endo T, Ohno M, Kotani S, Gunji K, Onaya T. Thyrotropin receptor in non-thyroid tissues. Biochem Biophys Res Com 1993; 190:774-9.
43. Heufelder AE, Dutton CM, Sarkar G, Donovan KA, Bahn RS. Detection of TSH receptor RNA in cultured fibroblasts from patients with Graves' ophthalmopathy and pretibial dermopathy. Thyroid 1993; 3:297-300.
44. Crisp MS, Lane C, Halliwell M, WynfordThomas D, Ludgate M Thyrotropin receptor transcripts in human adipose tissue. J Clin Endocrinol Metab 1997; 82:2003-5.
45. Hiromatsu Y, Sato M, Inoue Y, Koga M, Miyake I, Kameo J, Tokisawa S, Yang D, Nonaka K. Localization and clinical significance of thyrotropin receptor mRNA expression in orbital fat and eye muscle tissues from patients with thyroid-associated ophthalmopathy. Thyroid 1997; 6:553-62.
46. Spitzweg C, Joba W, Hunt N, Heufelder AE. Analysis of human thyrotropin receptor gene expression and immunoreactivity in human orbital tissue. Eur J Endocrinol 1997; 136:599-607.
47. Stadlmayr W, Spitzweg C, Bichlmair AM, Heufelder AE. Full length TSH receptor transcripts and TSH receptor-like immunoreactivity in orbital and pretibial fibroblasts of patients with Graves' ophthalmopathy and pretibial dermopathy. Thyroid 1997; 7:3-12.
48. Bahn RS, Dutton CM, Natt N, Joba W, Spitzweg C, Heufelder AE. Thyrotropin receptor expression in Graves' orbital adipose/connective tissues: Potential autoantigen in Graves' ophthalmopathy. J Clin Endocrinol Metab 1998; 83:998-1002.
49. Heufelder AE. Involvement of the orbital fibroblast and TSH receptor in the pathogenesis of Graves' ophthalmopathy. Thyroid 1995; 5:331-40.
50. Bahn RS 1996 A possible role for the thyrotropin receptor in thyroid-associated ophthalmopathy. Orbit 15:119-28.
51. Heufelder AE, Bahn RS. Evidence for the presence of a functional TSH receptor in retroocular fibroblasts from patients with Graves' ophthalmopathy. Exp Clin Endocrinol Diabetol 1992; 100:62-7.
52. Arnold K, Tandon N, McIntosh RS, Elisei R, Ludgate M, Weetman AP. T cell responses to orbital antigens in thyroid-associated ophthalmopathy. Clin exp Immunol 1994; 96:329-34.
53. Akamizu T, Ueda Y, Hua L, Okuda J, Mori T. Establishment and characterization of an antihuman thyrotropin (TSH) receptor-specific CD4+ T cell line from a patient with Graves' disease: evidence for multiple T cell epitopes on the TSH receptor including the transmembrane domain. Thyroid 1995; 5:259-64.
54. Marcus C, Ehren H, Bolme P, Arner P. Regulation of lipolysis during the neonatal period: Importance of thyrotropin. J Clin Invest 1988; 82:1793-7
55. Bahn RS, Dutton CM, Joba W, Heufelder AE. Thyrotropin receptor expression in cultured Graves' orbital preadipocyte fibroblasts is stimulated by thyrotropin. Thyroid 1998; 8:193-6.

56. Costagliola S, Many M-C, Stalmans-Falys M, Tonacchera M, Vassart G, Ludgate M. Recombinant TSHR and the induction of autoimmune disease in BALBc mice, a new animal model. Endocrinology 1994; 135:2150-9.
57. Costagliola S, Many M-C, Stalmans-Falys M, Vassart G, Ludgate M. The autoimmune response induced by immunizing female mice with the human TSHR varies with the genetic background. Mol Cell Endocrinol 1995; 115:119-206.
58. Costagliola S, Many M-C, StalmansFalys M, Vassart G, Ludgate M. Transfer of thyroiditis, with syngeneic spleen-cells sensitized with the human thyrotropin receptor, to naive balb/c and nod mice. Endocrinology 1996; 137:4637-43.
59. Costagliola S, Rodien P, Many M-C, Ludgate M, Vassart G. Genetic immunization against the human thyrotropin receptor causes thyroiditis and allows production of monoclonal antibodies recognizing the native receptor. J Immunol 1998; 160:1458-65.
60. Costagliola S, Many MC, Denef JF, Pohlenz J, Refetoff S, Vassart G. Genetic immunization of outbred mice with thyrotropin receptor cDNA provides a model of Graves' disease. J Clin Invest 2000; 105:803-11.
61. Heufelder AE, Bahn RS, Boergen KP, Scriba PC. Detection, localization and modulation of hyaluronic acid/CD44 receptor expression in patients with endocrine orbitopathy. Med Klin 1993; 88:181-4.
62. de Carli M, D'Elios M, Mariotti S, Marcocci C, Pinchera A, Ricci M, Romagnani S, del Prete G. Cytolytic T cells with Th-1like cytokine profile predominate in retroorbital lymphocytic infiltrates of Graves' ophthalmopathy. J Clin Endocrinol Metab 1993; 77:1120-4.
63. Hiromatsu Y, Yang D, Bednarczuk T, Miyake I, Nonaka K, Inoue Y. Cytokine profiles in eye muscle tissue and orbital fat tissue from patients with thyroid-associated ophthalmopathy. J Clin Endocrinol Metab 2000; 85:1194-9.
64. McLachlan SM, Prummel MF, Rapoport B. Cell-mediated or humoral immunity in Graves' ophthalmopathy? Profiles of T-cell cytokines amplified by polymerase chain reaction from orbital tissue. J Clin Endocrinol Metab 1994; 78:1070-4.
65. Heufelder AE, Eggert K, Ernst G, Bahn RS, Scriba PC. Expression of cytokine and growth factor genes in cultured retroorbital fibroblasts from patients with Graves' ophthalmopathy. Proc. Endocrin Soc 76th Annu Meet 1994; 228 (abstract).
66. Heufelder AE, Bahn RS. Modulation of intercellular adhesion molecule-1 (ICAM-1) by cytokines and Graves' IgGs in cultured Graves' retroocular fibroblasts. Eur J Clin Invest 1992; 22:529-37.
67. Smith TJ, Wang HS, Evans CH. Leukoregulin is a potent inducer of hyaluronan synthesis in cultured human orbital fibroblasts. Am J Physiol. 1995; 268(2 Pt 1):C382-8.
68. Korducki JM, Loftus SJ, Bahn RS. Stimulation of glycosaminoglycan production in cultured human retroocular fibroblasts. Invest Ophthalmol Vis Sci 1992; 33:2037-42.
69. Imai Y, Ibaraki K, Odajima R, Shishiba Y. Effects of dibutyryl cyclic AMP on hyaluronan and proteoglycan synthesis by retroocular tissue fibroblasts in culture. Endocr 1994; J 41:645-54.
70. Cao HJ, Smith TJ. Leukoregulin upregulation of prostaglandin endoperoxidase H synthase-2 expression in human orbital fibroblasts. Am J Physiol 1999; 277:C1075-C1085.
71. Heufelder AE, Bahn RS. Modulation of Graves' orbital fibroblast proliferation by cytokines and glucocorticoid receptor agonists. Invest Ophthalmol Vis Sci 1994; 35:120-7.
72. Cao HJ, Hogg MG, Martino LJ, Smith TJ. Transforming growth factor-beta induces plasminogen activator inhibitor type-1 in cultured human orbital fibroblasts. Invest Ophthalmol Vis Sci 1995; 36:1411-9.

73. Seibold M, Ernst G, Schworm H-D, Heufelder AE. Expression and regulation of matrix metalloproteinase-2 in thyroid and retroorbital tissues of patients with Graves' ophthalmopathy. J Endocrinol Invest 1996; 19 (supplement 6):82 (abstract).
74. Seibold M, Spitzweg C, Joba W, Heufelder AE. Detection and regulation of tissue inhibitor of metalloproteinase-1 (TIMP-1) and matrix metalloproteinase-1 (MMP-1) in Graves' and normal orbital fibroblasts. Exp Clin Endocrinol Diabet 1997; 105 (supplement 1):38-39 (abstract).
75. Hofbauer LC, Mühlberg T, Konig A, Heufelder G, Schworm HD, Heufelder AE. Soluble interleukin-1 receptor antagonist serum levels in smokers and nonsmokers with Graves' ophthalmopathy undergoing orbital radiotherapy. J Clin Endocrinol Metab 1997; 82:2244-7.
76. Mühlberg T, Heberling HJ, Joba W, Schworm HD, Heufelder AE. Detection and modulation of interleukin-1 receptor antagonist messenger ribonucleic acid and immunoreactivity in Graves' orbital fibroblasts. Invest Ophthalmol Vis Sci 1997; 38:1018-28.
77. Muehlberg T, Joba W, Spitzweg C, Schworm HD, Heberling HJ, Heufelder AE. Interleukin-1 receptor antagonist ribonucleic acid and protein expression by cultured Graves' and normal orbital fibroblasts is differentially modulated by dexamethasone and irradition. J Clin Endocrinol Metab 2000; 85:734-42.
78. Bartalena L, Manetti L, Tanda ML et al. Soluble interleukin-1 receptor antagonist concentration in patients with Graves' ophthalmopathy is neither related to cigarette smoking nor predictive of subsequent response to glucocorticoids. Clin Endocrinol 2000; 52:647-51.
79. Peyster RG, Ginsberg F, Silber JH, Adler LP. Exophthalmos caused by excessive fat: CT volumetric analysis and differential diagnosis. Am J Neuroradiol 1986; 7:35-40.
80. Hufnagel TJ, Hickey WJ, Cobbs WH, Jacobiec FA, Iwamoto T, Eagle RC. Immunohistochemical and ultrastructural studies on the exenterated orbital tissues of a patient with GD. Ophthalmology 1987; 91:1411-9.
81. Wiederer O, Löffler G. Hormonal regulation of the differentiation of rat adipocyte precursor cells in primary culture. J Lipid Res 1987; 28:649-58.
82. Chen X, Hausman DB, Dean RG, Hausman GJ. Differentiation-dependent expression of obese (ob) gene by preadipocytes and adipocytes in primary cultures of porcine stromal-vascular cells. Biochim Biophys Acta 1997; 1359:136-42.
83. Hausman GJ, Richardson RL. Newly recruited and pre-existing preadipocytes in cultures of porcine stromal-vascular cells: morphology, expression of extracellular matrix components, and lipid accretion. J Anim Sci 1998; 76:48-60.
84. Sorisky A, Pardasani D, Gagnon A, Smith TJ. Evidence of adipocyte differentiation in human orbital fibroblasts in primary culture. J Clin Endocrinol Metab 1996; 81:3428-31.
85. Valyasevi RW, Erickson DZ, Harteneck DA, Dutton CM, Heufelder AE, Jyonouchi SC, Bahn RS. Differentiation of human orbital preadipocyte fibroblasts induces expression of functional thyrotropin receptor. J Clin Endocrinol Metab 1999; 84:2557-62.

3

ADIPOGENESIS AND TSH RECEPTOR EXPRESSION

Natee Munsakul and Rebecca S. Bahn
Division of Endocrinology, Metabolism and Nutrition, Mayo Clinic/Foundation, Rochester, Minnesota, 55905

INTRODUCTION

The symptoms and signs of Graves' ophthalmopathy (GO) can be explained mechanically by an increase in the volume of tissues within the confines of the bony orbit. Volume measurements of the orbital adipose/connective tissue compartment and the extraocular muscles using computed tomography (CT) scans revealed abnormalities in 87% of Graves' patients with clinically detectable GO (1). Enlarged muscles with normal fat volume was noted in 48% of these patients, while enlargement of both the extraocular muscles and the fat compartment was found in 46% of patients. The converse, or increased fat compartment volume with normal muscle volumes, was found in 8% of GO patients. In another study, measurement of extraocular muscle volumes in 50 patients with GO revealed relatively poor correlation between the extent of muscle enlargement and proptosis measurements. In contrast, another group of investigators found the degree of proptosis to correlate well with orbital fat volumes (2). Taken together, these studies suggest that orbital adipose tissue expansion in GO likely influences the degree of proptosis to a greater extent than does the extraocular muscle enlargement.

Histologic examination of orbital tissues in GO reveals an accumulation of glycoaminoglycans (GAG), both within the extraocular muscle bodies and the posterior orbital adipose/connective tissues (3). These hydrophilic macromolecules are produced by orbital fibroblasts and their presence leads to gross edema and swelling of these tissues. As there is little increase in fat tissue within the extraocular muscles in GO, enlargement of the muscle bodies appears to be due primarily to GAG accumulation. The extraocular muscle cells themselves are intact, but are widely separated by these hydrophilic extracellular matrix components and edema (4). Extensive swelling of the extraocular muscles at the apex of the orbit may result in compressive optic neuropathy and visual loss. In contrast, hydrated GAG appears to contribute little to the increased mass of the non-muscle, adipose/connective tissue compartment. Orbital CT scans of patients with GO suggest that the density (a reflection of water content) of these tissues is indistinguishable from that of normal orbital adipose tissue. It appears therefore, that the expansion of the adipose/connective tissue compartment in GO results primarily from the process of adipogenesis, or the development of new adipose cells.

ADIPOSE TISSUE AND ADIPOGENESIS

Adipose tissue allows for triacylglycerol storage in periods of energy excess and the subsequent release of free fatty acids during energy deprivation. This lipogenic/lipolytic balance is under tight hormonal control. In addition, adipose is a biologically active and dynamic tissue with major endocrine and immunological roles. For instance, adipocytes secrete tumor necrosis factor alpha (TNFα), a cytokine that may act in an autocrine or paracrine fashion to impair insulin action (5). Mature adipocytes represent between one-third and two-thirds of the total number of cells in adipose tissue. The remaining cells comprise the stromal vascular fraction and include blood cells, endothelial cells and adipocyte precursor cells. These preadipocytes are thought to have derived from a pleuripotent embryonic stem cell precursor with the capacity to differentiate to mesodermal cell types, including adipocytes, chondrocytes and myocytes.

The initial observation that the stromal vascular fraction of human omental adipose tissue contains fibroblast-like cells (termed "preadipocytes") having the ability to differentiate into mature adipocytes was made by Poznanski approximately 30 years ago (6). The potential of these cells to become mature fat cells continues throughout life and generally occurs in response to relatively high-carbohydrate or high-fat diets (7). Although several of the individual distinguishing features of adipocytes are shared by other cell types, these cells exhibits a unique and distinctive phenotype. Necessary and sufficient criteria for classifications as an adipocyte include the ability to perform lipogenesis *de novo*, to take up and store circulating triglycerides, and to mobilize and release stored lipids as an energy reservoir (8). In addition, lipid vacuoles are a necessary morphologic characteristic of adipocytes, and cells must express adipocyte-specific (PPARγ2, leptin, aP2) and adipocyte-induced (LPL, PEP-CK, adipsin, C/EBPs, ADD1/SREBP1) gene markers to be so classified.

Adipose tissue develops through a combination of increased cell number (hyperplasia) and cell size (hypertrophy). Because remarkable increases in cell number were first observed in severe obesity of childhood onset, it was generally thought that the capacity to form new adipocytes was present only during the neonatal and childhood years. However, it has now become clear that new adipocyte formation is an ongoing process that plays a role in adipose tissue enlargement throughout life (9). Increases in total body triacylglycerol of more than four-times normal are fairly commonly seen in human obesity. Because individual adipocytes do not have the capacity to increase their triacylglycerol stores to this extent, it is thought that adipogenesis is induced once a critical adipocyte volume is reached (5). Observations of this type have led to the hypothesis that paracrine signals from mature adipocytes to preadipocytes might trigger differentiation (10,11).

Primary culture systems for isolated preadipocytes have been developed using immortalized cell lines such as the 3T3-L1 (26), 3T3-F442A (27), and ob1771 (14) lineages. These preadipocytes resemble fibroblasts and are capable of differentiating into mature adipocytes under appropriate hormonal control or experimental manipulation (15). Sorisky and colleagues demonstrated that cultures derived from human orbital connective tissue contain such adipocyte precursor cells (comprising 5-10% of the total), capable of responding to adipogenic stimuli *in vitro* (16).

Adipocyte differentiation protocols generally include insulin (or IGF-1), glucocorticoid, and isobutylmethylxantine under serum-free conditions. Differentiation rates as high as 70% are sometimes observed (17). The developmental program of the preadipocytes can be divided into four distinct stages that include; 1) preconfluent proliferation; 2) confluence/growth arrest; 3) hormonal induction/clonal expansion; and (4 permanent growth arrest / terminal differentiation (15). During this process, the preadipocytes begin to express genes regulating lipoprotein lipolysis, fatty acid cellular uptake, and synthesis of fatty acids and triglycerides. These genes can be classified as markers either of early (commitment), middle, or late (terminal) differentiation (Table 1). A precise assessment of the stage of differentiation can be obtained by studying the expression of relevant mRNA or protein by Northern/Western blot analysis, or by the measurement of enzyme activities. In addition to these particular genes, it has been estimated by 2-D protein electrophoresis that at least another 200 proteins change their levels of expression during differentiation (18).

Table 1. Gene Markers of Adipocyte Differentiation

Early (commitment) phase	Middle phase
LPL	PPARγ
A2COL6	CEBPα
C/EBPβ,δ	
Actin, Tubulin, Fibronectin	
Late (terminal) phase	
GLUT4	Hormone sensitive lipase
Leptin	Fatty acid synthase
Insulin receptor, IRS-1	GPDH

Adipogenesis involves not only the activation, but also the repression of gene expression (19). Sul was the first to describe preadipocyte factor-1 (pref-1), a gene highly expressed in preadipocytes, but completely absent in adipocytes (20). It has been shown that constitutive expression of pref-1 in 3T3-L1 preadipocytes inhibits induction of differentiation, and that its down-regulation is required for adipocyte differentiation to ensue. Experimental reversal of adipocyte differentiation is accompanied by reemergence of pref-1 expression (21).

TSH-RECEPTOR EXPRESSION IN ADIPOCYTES

The finding of TSH-stimulated lipolysis in rat epididymal adipose cells was the first evidence that TSH receptor (TSH-r) might be expressed in tissues other than the thyroid (22). Subsequently, specific TSH binding to guinea pig adipose and retro-orbital tissues (23) or to porcine orbital connective tissue membranes (24), and lipolysis of rat adipose cells incubated with long-acting thyroid stimulator was reported (25). Following the cloning of TSHr, both guinea pig brown and white adipose tissues were shown to express TSHr (26), and the expression and function of this gene in rat adipocytes was found to parallel the process of adipocyte differentiation in these cells (27).

Determining whether TSHr is expressed in human fat tissue has been more problematic. Some investigators reported low-affinity TSH binding to human fat cell membrane preparations (28), while others found no specific TSH-binding to human adult fat cells (23). Later studies demonstrated lipolysis at physiologic TSH does in neonatal, but not in adult, human fat cells (29). These effects declined rapidly with age, suggesting a role for TSH in human neonatal thermogenesis. Further studies in neonatal adipocytes showed that the lipolytic effect of TSH could be reproduced by treating cells with stimulatory TSHr autoantibodies, and inhibited with TSHr blocking autoantibodies (30).

Our studies have explored the link between adipogenesis and the expression of TSHr in human orbital preadipocyte fibroblasts. In these studies, confluent preadipocyte fibroblasts from patients with GO and normal individuals were exposed for 7-10 days to in vitro conditions shown to stimulate adipogenesis in these cells (31). A significant increase in cAMP production (96-183 fold) following rhTSH stimulation was demonstrated in these differentiated cultures. In addition, we found mature adipose cells staining with antibodies directed against leptin in cultures treated in this manner (32). We interpreted these results to suggest that, while cultured orbital preadipocyte fibroblasts do not express measurable functional TSHr, these cells can be stimulated *in vitro* to differentiate into TSHr-bearing adipocytes. It may be that adipocyte TSHr expression in humans is a function of newly-differentiated cells.

IMPLICATIONS FOR PATHOGENESIS OF GO

The autoantigen involved in the hyperthyroidism of Graves' disease is known to be TSHr. However, whether this antigen plays a role in the pathogenesis of GO is unclear. Certainly, TSHr is a prime candidate to be the orbital autoantigen because its involvement would help to explain the close clinical and laboratory associations between GO and hyperthyroidism. Reports by several laboratories have identified TSHr mRNA, or a variant TSHr transcript, in human GO orbital tissues and cell cultures using the reverse-transcriptase polymerase chain reaction (33-35). However, RNA transcripts detected only by PCR-based amplification of cDNA may have little physiologic relevance. In order to clarify this issue, we performed studies using a ribonuclease protection assay for semi-quantitative detection of this low abundance mRNA. The presence of mRNA corresponding to TSHr extracellular domain was clearly demonstrated in uncultured GO orbital adipose/connective tissue specimens (36). In contrast, TSHr mRNA was just faintly detectable in normal orbital fatty connective tissue samples These results suggest that TSHr expression is significantly augmented in the orbit in GO, potentially making the receptor available to act as an autoantigen.

We wished to determine whether particular inflammatory cytokines, known to be present in the orbit in GO, might impact adipogenesis or TSHr expression in orbital fibroblasts. Accordingly, cells were treated with recombinant human TNF-α, interferon-γ (rhIFN-γ) or transforming growth factor-β (hTGF-β; each 1 ng/mL) for 10-days during culture in conditions known to induce adipocyte differentiation (16). This treatment resulted in profound inhibition of TSH-dependent cAMP production (mean 99%, 95%, and 95% inhibition, respectively). Levels of cAMP in these cultures were even lower than those measured in the control cultures that were maintained for the same period of time in medium lacking several of the components necessary for adipocyte differentiation. In addition to decreased cAMP production, we found morphological differentiation of the cells to be partially inhibited when either IFN-γ or TNF-α was present in cultures during the entire differentiation process. In contrast, TGF-β treatment did not significantly impact morphological differentiation. Further studies involving other cytokines that stimulate TSHr expression in these cells are underway.

CONCLUSION

Expression of TSHr is augmented in newly differentiated orbital adipose cells and in orbital tissues from patients with GO. This process may be stimulated *in vivo* by cytokines present within these tissues and would be expected to lead to an increase in their volume. The enhanced expression of TSHr within the orbit in the setting of Graves' disease might allow the receptor to act there as an autoantigen. Circulating activated T cells, directed against TSHr, would then infiltrate these tissues and secrete cytokines, including IFN-γ and TGF-β. These cytokines have been shown to increase glycosaminoglycan production and to stimulate the expression of immunomodulatory proteins in orbital fibroblasts (37) These effects would likely aid in the development and propagation of GO. However, these same cytokines have been shown to inhibit TSHr expression and adipogenesis within the orbit, effects seeming to favor disease remission. It appears therefore that the initiation and subsequent clinical severity of GO is influenced by many competing inhibitory and stimulatory factors acting simultaneously within the orbit, some of which impact the expression TSHr and stimulate the expansion of orbital adipose tissue.

REFERENCES

1. Forbes G, Gorman CA, Brennan MD, Gehring DG, Ilstrup DM, Earnest F. 1986 Ophthalmopathy of Graves' disease: computerized volume measurements of the orbital fat and muscle. Am J Neuroradiol. 7:651-656.
2. Peyster RG, Ginsberg F, Silber JH, Adler LP. 1986 Exophthalmos caused by excessive fat: CT volumetric analysis and differential diagnosis. Am J Neuroradiol. 7:35-40.

3. Campbell RJ. 1984 Pathology of Graves' ophthalmopathy: IN: Gorman CA, Waller RA, Dyer JA (eds): The Eye and Orbit in Thyroid Disease. New York Raven, pp.25-31.
4. Tallstedt L Norberg R. 1988 Immunohistochemical staining of normal and Graves' extraocular muscle. Invest Ophthalmol Vis Sci. 29:175-184.
5. Sorisky A.1999 From preadipocyte to adipocyte: differentiation-directed signals of insulin from the cell surface to the nucleus. Crit Rev Clin Lab Sci. 36(1) :1-34.
6. Poznanski W, Waheed I, Van R. 1973 Human fat cell precursors. Morphologic and metabolic differentiation in culture. J Lab Invest. 29:570-576.
7. Smas CM, Sul HS. 1995 Control of adipocyte differentiation. Biochem. 309:697-710.
8. Gimble JM, Robinson CE, Clarke SL, Hill MR. 1998 Nuclear hormone receptors and adipogenesis. Crit Rev Eukaryot Gene Expr. 8(2) :141-168.
9. Hirsch J, Fried SK, Edens NK,Leibel RL. 1989 The fat cell. Med Clin N Am. 73:83-96.
10. Alihaud G, Grimaldi P, Negrel R. 1994 Hormonal regulation of adipose differentiation. Trends Endocrinol Metab. 5:132-136.
11. Shillabeer G, Forden JM, Lau DCW. 1989 Induction of preadipocyte differentiation by mature fat cells in the rat. J Clin Invest. 84:381-387.
12. Green H, Kehinde O. 1975 An established preadipose cell line and its differentiation in culture. Factors affecting adipose conversion. Cell. 5:19-27.
13. Green H, Kehinde O. 1976 Spontaneous heritable changes leading to increased adipose conversion in 3T3 cells. Cell. 7:105-113.
14. Negral R, Grimaldi P, Alihaud G. 1978 Establishment of a proadipocyte clonal line from epididymal fat pad of ob/ob mouse that responds to insulin and to lipolytic hormones. Proc Natl Acad Sci USA. 75:6054-6058.
15. Cowherd RM, Lyle RE, McGehee Jr RE.1999 Molecular regulation of adipocyte differentiation. Semin Cell Dev Biol. 10:3-10.
16. Sorisky A, Pardasani D, Gagnon A, Smith TJ. 1996 Evidence of adipocyte differentiation in human orbital fibroblasts in primary culture. J Clin Endocrinol Metab. 81:3428-3431.
17. Hauner H, Entenmann G, Wabitsch M, Gaillard D, Alihaud G, Negerl R, Pfeiffer EF. 1989 Promoting effect of glucocorticoids on the differentiation of human adipocyte precursor cells cultured in a chemically defined medium. J Clin Invest. 84:1663-1670.
18. Cornelius P, MacDougald OA, Lane MD. 1994 Regulation of adipocyte development. Annu Rev Nutr. 14:99-129.
19. Gregoire FM, Smas CM, Sul HS. 1998 Understanding adipocyte differentiation. Physiol Rev. 78:738-809.
20. Smas CM, Sul HS. 1993 Pref-1, a protein containing EGF-like repeats, inhibits adipocyte differentiation.Cell 73: 725-734.
21. Zhou YT, Wang ZW, Higa M, Newgard CB, Unger RH. 1999 Reversing adipocyte differentiation: implications for treatment of obesity. Proc Natl Acad Sci USA. 96:2391-2395.
22. Rodbell M. 1964 Metabolism of isolated fat cells. I. Effects of hormones on glucose metabolism and lipolysis. J Biol Chem 239: 375-380.
23. Davies TF, Teng CS, McLachlan SM, Smith BR, Hall R. 1978 Thyrotropin receptors in adipose tissue, retro-orbital tissue and lymphocytes. Molecular and Cellular Endocrinology 9: 303-310.
24. Perros P, Kendall-Taylor P. 1994 Demonstration of thyrotropin binding sites in orbital connective tissue: Possible role in the pathogenesis of thyroid-associated ophthalmopathy. J Endocrinol Invest 17: 163-170.
25. Kendall-Taylor P, Munro DS. 1971 The lipolytic activity of long-acting thyroid stimulator. Biochem Biophys Acta 231: 314-319.

26. Roselli-Rehfuss L, Robbins LS, Cone RD. 1992 Thyrotropin receptor messenger ribonucleic acid is expressed in most brown and white adipose tissues in the guinea pig. Endocrinol 130: 1857-1861.
27. Haraguchi K, Shimura H, Ling L , Saito T, Endo T, Onaya T. 1996 Differentiation of rat preadipocytes is accompanied by expression of thyrotropin receptor. Endocringology 137 : 3200-3205.
28. Mullin BR, Lee G, Ledley FD, Winand RJ, Kohn LD. 1976 Thyrotropin interactions with human fat cell membrane preparations and the finding of a soluble thyrotropin binding component. Biochemical and Biophysical Research Communications 69:55-62.
29. Marcus C, Ehren H, Bolme P, Arner P. 1988 Regulation of lipolysis during the neonatal period : Importance of thyrotropin. J Clin Invest 82 : 1793-1797.
30. Janssen A, Karlsson FA, Micha- Johansson G, Bolme P, Bronnegard M, Marcus C. 1995 Effects of stimulatory and inhibitory thyrotropin receptor antibodies on lipolysis in infant adipocytes. J Clin Endocrinol Metab 80 : 1712-1716.
31. Valyasevi RW, Erickson DZ, Harteneck DA, et al. 1999 Differentiation of human orbital preadipocyte fibroblasts induces expression of functional thyrotropin receptor. J Clin Endocrinol Metab 84 : 2557-2562.
32. Erickson DZ, Harteneck DA, Erickson BJ, Dutton CM, Bahn RS. Induction of leptin expression in orbital preadipocyte fibroblasts. Thyroid, in press.
33. Heufelder AE, Dutton CM, Sarkar G, Donovan KA, Bahn RS. 1993 Detection of TSH receptor RNA in cultured fibroblasts from patients with Graves' ophthalmopathy and pretibial dermopathy. Thyroid. 3:297-300.
34. Feliciello A, Porcellini A, Ciullo, Bonavolonta G, Avvedimento EV, Fenzi G. 1993 Expression of thyrotropin-receptor mRNA in healthy and Graves' retro-orbital tissue. Lancet 342:337-338.
35. Mengistu M, Lukes YG, Nagy EV, Burch HB, Carr FE, Lahiri S, Burman KD. 1994 TSH receptor gene expression in retroocular fibroblasts. J Endocrinol Invest. 17:437-441.
36. Bahn RS, Dutton CM, Natt N, Joba W, Spitzweg C, Heufelder AE. Thyrotropin receptor expression in Graves' orbital adipose/connective tissues: potential autoantigen in Graves' ophthalmopathy. J Clin Endocrinol Metab 83:998-1002, 1998.
37. Bahn RS, Heufelder AE. 1993 Pathogenesis of Graves' ophthalmopathy. N Engl J Med. 329:1468-1475.

4

ROLE OF CYTOKINES IN THE PATHOGENESIS OF GRAVES' OPHTHALMOPATHY

Yuji Hiromatsu* and Tomasz Bednarczuk†

**Department of Endocrinology and Metabolism, Kurume University School of Medicine, 67 Asahimachi, Kurume, Fukuoka 830-0011 Japan and †Department of Endocrinology, Medical Research Center, Polish Academy of Science. Banacha 1A, 02-097 Warsaw, Poland*

INTRODUCTION

Graves' ophthalmopathy (GO) is generally accepted to be an autoimmune inflammatory disorder of the extraocular muscles (EM) and the orbital fatty/connective tissue (OCT) that is closely associated with Graves' disease (1-3).

Histological examination of retrobulbar tissues obtained from patients with active GO demonstrates an infiltration of mononuclear cells, proliferation of retrobulbar fibroblasts and deposition of glycosaminoglycans (GAG) in the endomysial and perimysial space (4-8). The mononuclear cells consist predominantly of T lymphocytes and less abundant macrophages, B lymphocytes, mast cells or plasma cells. Retrobulbar T cells are mainly activated memory cells ($CD45RO^+$), belonging to both helper/inducer ($CD4^+$) and suppressor/cytotoxic ($CD8^+$) subsets. In the late, inactive stage of GO, the leukocyte infiltration is less evident. In addition to the inflammatory infiltration, the major histopathological findings include the proliferation of connective tissue cells (fibroblasts) and GAG deposition. The GAG have hyaluronic acid as their main substance. This results in increased osmotic pressure which accounts for the profound water binding capacity and interstitial edema of EM and OCT seen in GO. Although there have been reports suggesting damage of EM fibers in end-stage disease when dense orbital scarring is characteristic, the myofibrillar structure is generally normal (8,9).

The clinical symptoms of GO are the consequence of inflammation in the EM and OCT. Based on the clinical findings and computed tomography (CT) or magnetic resonance imaging, GO can be divided into two subtypes: a) GO with prominent eye muscle enlargement, diplopia or visual disturbance; b) GO with prominent soft connective tissue inflammation without evidence of eye muscle enlargement. This latter form is usually associated with proptosis caused by expansion of orbital fat volume (10-12). The immune mechanisms responsible for the development of inflammation in the EM or OCT, and subsequently different subtypes of GO, remain unclear. Molecular analysis of the T cell receptor has suggested that lymphocytes infiltrating EM and OCT are directed against common antigens present in both tissues (13,14). However, studies of autoantibodies have suggested a different humoral response in both subtypes of GO. Patients suffering mainly from "myopathy" had serum antibodies against eye muscle proteins (G2s, SDH), while the other had antibodies against connective tissue proteins (11,15,16).

Cytokines released predominantly by leukocytes infiltrating retrobulbar tissues are likely to play a key role in the initiation and propagation of the autoimmune process in the orbit. In the first part of this chapter, we will discuss the source of cytokines in retrobulbar tissues. We will also consider whether cytokine profiles are differently involved in the two types of GO or in the two major sites of the lesion. This may, in part, explain the immunopathogenesis of the two subtypes of GO. In the second part of the chapter, we will discuss the action of cytokines on the resident-effector cells in GO, namely the orbital fibroblasts, endothelial cells and eye muscle cells.

SOURCE OF CYTOKINES IN GO

Cytokines are protein hormones that serve to regulate immune and inflammatory responses. Although leukocytes participating in the inflammation are the major source of cytokines, resident cells in the affected tissues also participate in the cytokine network (Table 1). It should be also noted that particular cytokines are produced by multiple diverse cells. Therefore, it is often impossible to define the cellular source of cytokines detected in inflamed tissues.

Table 1. Cell Types Contributing the Cytokine Pattern in Graves' Ophthalmopathy

Producer Cell type	Main secreted cytokines
Th1 & Tc1	IL-2, IFN-γ, TNF-β, TNF-α,
Th2 & Tc2	leukoregulin, GM-CSF, Chemokines,
B cells	IL-4, IL-5, IL-6, IL-10, IL-13, TNF-α,
	GM-CSF, Chemokines, IL-4
Macrophages	IL-1, IL-6, IL-10, TNF-α, TGF-β, FGF, Chemokines
Mast cells	IL-3, TNF-α, IL-4, IL-10, IL-13, IL-16, GM-CSF, PAF, Chemokines
Orbital fibroblasts	IL-1, IL-6, IL-8, IL-16, IFN-β, CSF, Chemokines
Endothelial cells	Il-1, IL-6, PDGF, CSF
Eye muscle cells	Not tested

The table includes only cytokines that are so far known to play an important role in the pathogenesis of GO. Abbreviations: IL, interleukin; IFN, interferon; TNF, tumor necrosis factor; GM-CSF, granulocyte-macrophage colony-stimulating factor; TGF, transforming growth factor; FGF, fibroblast growth factor; PAF, platelet activating factor; PDGF, platelet-derived growth factor

T cells

The cytokine profile secreted by involved T cells determines whether the immune response is predominantly humoral or cell-mediated. At least three $CD4^+$ T helper cell (Th) subsets are known to exist: Th1, Th2 and Th0 (17-19). Although Th1 cells secrete IFN-γ, IL-2 and tumor necrosis factor β (TNF-β) upon activation, IFN-γ has several properties that are related to the cell-mediated immune response. IFN-γ is the most potent activator of macrophages. This cytokine also increases the expression of major histocompatibility complex (MHC) class I and II molecules on a variety of cells and it acts, in the hiuman, on B cells to promote immunoglobulin (Ig) class switching to IgG2a and IgG4. The primary cytokine produced by Th2 cells is IL-4, which is responsible for strong antibody responses (including Ig class switching to IgG1 and IgE) and for suppressing the cell-mediated immunity. T cells expressing cytokines of both patterns have been designated Th0. Similarly, $CD8^+$ lymphocytes can be divided into subsets: $CD8^+$ cytotoxic cells (Tc1) that produce significant amounts of IFN-γ and $CD8^+$ suppressor T cells (Tc2) that produce substantial amounts of IL-4. Since the effects of IL-4 and IFN-γ are mutually antagonistic, it is generally believed that the balance between these 2 cytokines determines the type of immune response generated. The Th1/Th2 paradigm may, therefore, play a critical role in the development of immunopathological conditions (18, 19). Overproduction of Th1 cytokines has been implicated in delayed hypersensitivity reactions and in some autoimmune diseases. Th2 cytokines recruit eosinophils and activate mast cells. Thus, dysregulation of Th2 cytokines can lead to allergic and inflammatory conditions. There have been several studies concerning cytokine profiles of retrobulbar T lymphocytes in GO with fairly inconsistent results (12, 20-26).

In situ studies

Because of the difficulties in obtaining tissue specimens from patients with GO, the technical problems related to small specimen size, and the patchy distribution of the lesions, *in situ* studies of cytokine profile in GO have been limited (Table 2). Several groups of investigators have attempted to characterize the cytokine profile of T cells expressed in retrobulbar tissue specimens obtained from patients with GO using the reverse transcriptase-polymerase chain reaction (RT-PCR). RT-PCR is a highly sensitive and specific method to detect RNA, even in small tissue samples, and is expected to directly reflect the *in vivo* cytokine profile. However, this technique has its limitations; it is not quantitative and may not reflect protein expression.

Table 2. Expression of IFN-γ and IL-4 in Retrobulbar Tissues

Authors	Methods	Specimens	Positive IFN-γ	Positive IL-4
Heufelder & Bahn, 1993	Immunohistochemistry Immunoblotting	OCT (n=6)	83%	NA
McLachlan et al., 1994	RT-PCR	OCT (n=5) EM (n=1)	0% 0%	40% 100%
Pappa et al., 1997	RT-PCR	EM (n=12)	0%	67%
Hiromatsu et al., 2000	RT-PCR	OCT (n=29) EM (n=14)	27% 92%	24% 7%

EM, extraocular muscles; OCT, orbital connective tissue; NA, not assessed; RT-PCR, reverse transcriptase-polymerase chain reaction

There have been three reports published to date concerning cytokine profiles in eye muscle tissue from GO. McLachlan et al. (20) studied one eye muscle specimen from a patient with GO and reported the predominance of Th2-like cytokines. Pappa et al. (8) studied 12 eye muscle specimens from 5 patients with GO and found both Th1- and Th2-like cytokine mRNA expression. We studied 14 patients and showed the predominance of a Th1-like profile (12). IFN-γ mRNA was detected in eye muscle tissue from almost all patients with GO, supporting the notion that Th1-like cytokines play an important role in initiating and maintaining the autoimmune response in GO (27). We further showed that pro-inflammatory cytokine gene expression and TNF-α expression in eye muscle tissue was significantly correlated with the degree of enlargement of eye muscle, as assessed by CT scanning (Figure 1). These discrepancies in findings between the previous reports and our study may reflect different patient characteristics such as disease stage and disease activity, patchy distribution of the inflammatory lesion, and differences in the RT-PCR methods employed.

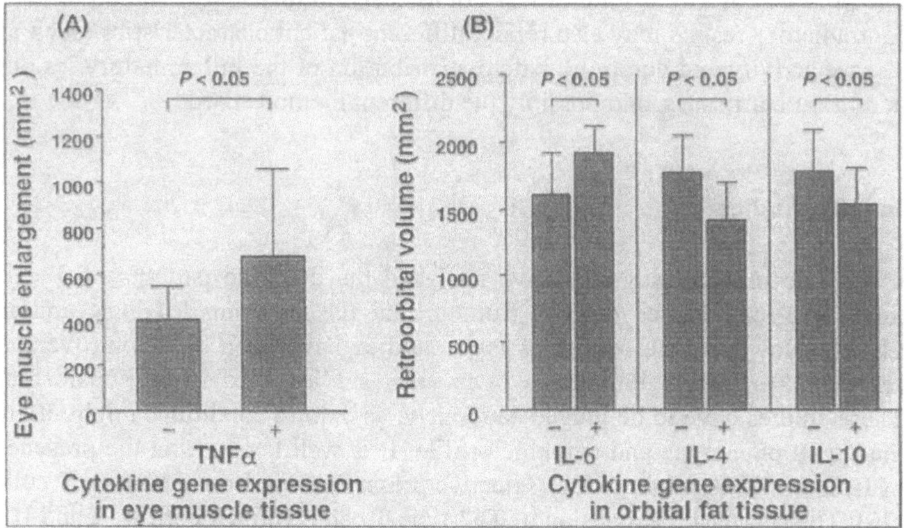

Figure 1. Eye muscle enlargement and orbital volume, assessed by CT, in patients with GO with or without positive detection of TNF-α, IL-4, IL-6 and IL-10 mRNA in eye muscle or orbital fat tissue by RT-PCR (Modified from Reference #12).

With respect to the cytokine profiles in orbital fat tissue, McLachlan et al. (20) studied 5 specimens from 5 patients with GO and showed a predominance of Th2-like cytokine profiles. We have confirmed these findings (12). However, 3 out of 29 (10%) patients showed both Th1 and Th2 profiles, and 5 out of 29 (17%) patients showed Th1 predominance. In those patients, the duration of ophthalmopathy tended to be shorter than in patients with Th2 predominance. We further showed a negative relationship between IL-4 and IL-10 expression and orbital volume, assessed by CT (Figure 1). These results support the hypothesis that Th1-like cytokines may play a role in the acute stage, and Th2-like cytokines may play a role in the chronic stage of GO, mediating the late fibrosis (27). Further studies using a more quantitative method are needed to clarify these issues.

In studies using immunohistochemistry and immunoblotting, particular cytokines involved in cell-mediated immunity, like IFN-γ, TNF-α and IL-1α, have been detected in frozen tissue specimens of OCT from patients with severe GO (5,28). Immunoreactivity was noted both in the cytoplasm of infiltrating mononuclear cells and in adjacent connective tissue. The presence of Th2 cytokines was not assessed in this study. These partially contradictory results may also reflect different patient characteristics (such as disease activity and duration), patchy distribution of the inflammatory lesions in retrobulbar tissues, and possibly the different methods used.

In vitro studies

Several investigators have analyzed the cytokine patterns of T cell lines or T cell clones derived from orbital tissues using RT-PCR and/or ELISA. However, the results of these studies have been also controversial (12, 21-25). Several limitations of *in vitro* studies need to be considered. These studies have to be judged cautiously, as culture conditions might affect the T cell phenotype and cytokine profile. It is well known that the presence of IL-2 and PHA might induce selective pressure away from Th2-type T cells (29). The successful expansion of Th2-type T cells requires both IL-2 and IL-4 in culture (30). In contrast to T cell clones, the phenotype and cytokine profile of T cell lines may change in the course of culture (unpublished data). Finally, cultured lymphocytes might represent bystanders T-cells and thus might not be necessarily tissue antigen specific and responsible for the initiation of the inflammation.

To our knowledge, there has been only one study concerning T cell lines derived from eye muscles. Pappa et al. (21) reported the predominance of $CD4^+$ T cell lines derived from eye muscle tissue from patients with GO. In their study, both Th1 and Th2-like cytokine profiles were present in T cell lines.

Most investigators have used T cell lines or T cell clones derived from orbital connective/fatty tissues to analyze *in vitro* their phenotypes and function. Grubeck-Loebenstein et al. (22) reported a predominance of $CD8^+$ T cells in T cell lines derived from orbital fat tissue, and showed the production of both Th1- and Th2-like cytokines in their T cell lines. De Carli et al. (23) reported the predominance of Th1-like cytokine profile in their T cell clones derived from T cell lines from GO orbital fat tissue. Föerster et al. (24) demonstrated that 10 out of 17 retrobulbar T cell lines consisted predominantly of $CD4^+$ cells. Analysis with RT-PCR of cytokine gene expression revealed both Th1 and Th2 products in all T cell lines: IL-2 signal (100% cell lines), IFN-γ (58%), TNF-β (88%), IL-4 (70%), IL-5 (100%), IL-6 (76%), TNF-α (70%) and IL-10 (23%). All these studies analyzed either the established T cell lines or T cell clones derived from the established T cell lines. In contrast, our phenotypic analysis of T cell clones derived directly from freshly isolated single cell suspension of minced retrobulbar fat tissues of patients with severe GO showed approximately 70 to 80 % were $CD3^+$ $CD4^+$ $CD8^-$ (25). Analysis of the cytokine profile of T cell clones, as documented by the ability to express IFN-γ, IL-2, IL-4 and IL-10, demonstrated that the majority of T cell clones expressed Th1-like profile in both the mRNA and protein levels. A few T cell clones showed Th0-like profile, but no T cell clone showed Th2-like profile. These results suggest that Th1-type $CD4^+$ T cells play important roles in the pathogenesis of GO. More recently Aniszewski et al. (26) reported that Th1-like clones were predominant in cultures from patients with recent onset hyperthyroidism and Th2-like clones were predominant in culture form patients with more remote onset hyperthyroidism. They hypothesized that cell-mediated (Th1-like) immune reactions may predominate in the orbit in early GO, whereas humoral immunity (Th2-like) might play the greater role in later stage of the disease.

The differences in cytokine profiles reported among the studies might be due to differences in sites from which samples were obtained, culture methods, or patients' characteristics. Because of the difficulty in assessing the infiltrating retrobulbar lymphocytes from untreated patients with GO, almost all the specimens studied were in a relatively late phase of the disease.

Therefore, disease activity, stages of the disease, previous treatment for GO and a patchy pattern of the lesion, as well as culture conditions, may also influence the results and explain these apparent discrepancies.

Macrophages

Macrophages are known to act as professional antigen presenting cells. These cells are capable of displaying antigens via class I or II histocompatibility complex (MHC) molecules, and delivering essential co-stimulatory signals to T cells (by B7-1 and B7-2 molecules). Activated macrophages are also one of the principal effectors of cell-mediated immunity. Macrophages are present in normal extraocular muscles (7,8,31). In patients with early GO, and less so with long-standing disease, the number of macrophages infiltrating retrobulbar tissues was found to be significantly increased (8,31). Thus retrobulbar macrophages are likely to play an important role in early phase of inflammation, perhaps by presenting antigen, mounting a Th1 immune response through IL-12 production, and secreting pro-inflammatory cytokines and chemokines.

Pro-inflammatory cytokines such as TNF-α and IL-1α are likely to play an important role in the pathogenesis of the autoimmune inflammation in GO because they have been shown to be present *in situ* in eye muscle and orbital connective tissue specimens from patients with severe GO (8,12,28). Moreover, the enlargement of extraocular muscles, as assessed by CT, was significantly correlated with TNF-α mRNA expression (12). A significant association between a polymorphism of TNF-α promoter gene and severity of ophthalmopathy supports the role of TNF-α in the development of GO (32).

Although other cells like activated T cells and mast cells can secrete TNF-α, macrophages are the major source this cytokine in GO tissues. Since the concentration of this protein is not increased in the serum of patients with GD, it is likely that TNF-α acts locally as a paracrine and autocrine activator of leukocytes and endothelial cells (33,34).

The cellular sources of IL-1, apart from macrophages, include mast cells, fibroblasts and endothelial cells. Like TNF-α, IL-1 principally functions as a mediator of local inflammation. This cytokine exists in 2 forms, namely IL-1α and IL-1β, which bind to the same receptor and have similar biological activities. Proinflammatory effects of IL-1 are counterbalanced by the naturally occurring IL-1 receptor antagonist (IL-1Ra), which competitively binds to IL-1 receptor and inhibits the biological response (35). Serum levels of IL-1 are not increased in patients with GO (36). Whether elevated serum concentrations of IL-1Ra are associated with the presence of GO remains controversial (33, 35-38).

Mast cells

There is now growing evidence of an important role for mast cells in the pathogenesis of GO. IgE, the principal mediator of hypersensitivity reactions, has been reported to be elevated in the sera of patients with Graves' disease (39) and GO (40). Furthermore, deposition of IgE on EM has been described (40). Finally, recent *in vitro* studies have shown that interactions between mast cells and fibroblasts may be, in part, responsible for fibroblast activation and secretion of GAG (41). These interactions are mediated by IL-4. However, mast cells are also a rich source of a variety of other cytokines including TNF-α, IL-1, IL-3, IL-4, IL-5, IL-6 IL-13, granulocyte-macrophage colony-stimulating factor and chemokines.

Resident cells

Resident cells within the orbit have the capacity to actively participate in the initiation and propagation of orbital inflammation. Among resident cells, orbital fibroblasts may function as important immunoregulatory cells. The expression of costimulatory molecules, like intercellular adhesion molecule-1 (ICAM-1) and lymphocyte function-associated antigen-3 (LFA-3), has been demonstrated on orbital fibroblasts (42,43). Orbital fibroblast are also capable of producing IL-6 and chemokines (44). IL-6 is a cytokine that is synthesized by a variety of cells, including T cells, macrophages, endothelial cells, and fibroblasts, in response to IL-1 and, to a lesser degree, TNF. The biological actions of this cytokine are diverse and include costimulation of T cells and macrophages, growth factor for B cells, and systemic reactions (acute phase response). The presence of IL-6 has been demonstrated *in situ* in retrobulbar tissues obtained from patients with GO and *in vitro* using cultured orbital fibroblasts. Interestingly, the volume of OCT, as assessed by CT, was positively correlated with IL-6 mRNA expression and negatively correlated with IL-4 mRNA and IL-10 mRNA expression in OCT (Figure 1). Whether the source of IL-6 in OCT is mainly activated leukocytes or other cells like fibroblasts remains speculative. Moreover several studies have shown increased circulating IL-6 and soluble IL-6 receptor (sIL-6R) in patients with active GO (33,36,38,45). Increased serum concentrations of IL-6 in GO may originate from the autoimmune inflammation in the orbit or thyroid.

Chemokines, superfamilies of small structurally related cytokine molecules, have generated tremendous recent interest. These molecules play major roles in guiding *in vivo* leukocyte migration into and within the inflamed tissue sites (46). However, there are only a limited number of reports concerning chemokines in GO. Studies *in vitro* have demonstrated that orbital fibroblasts are capable of secreting chemokines like IL-8 and monocyte chemotactic protein-1 (47). Locally produced chemokines are crucial for the recruitment of leukocytes to the inflammatory site. In one study, mRNA for IL-8 was detected in EM biopsies obtained from patients with GO, suggesting that this chemokine might play a role in the migration of T cells into retrobulbar tissues (21).

Other resident cells, including endothelial cells, eye muscle cells and adipocytes, may also express immunomodulatory proteins like HLA-DR and heat shock protein (HSP)-70 and secrete important cytokines and chemokines. However, their roles in the regulation of inflammation in the orbit have not been studied in detail.

CYTOKINE ACTION

Cytokines secreted during inflammation act not only on infiltrating leukocytes promoting cell-mediated or humoral mediated immunity, but also affect resident cells. Orbital inflammation in GO appears to result in increased secretory activity by the fibroblasts. Interactions between leukocytes and orbital fibroblasts play a central role in the pathogenesis of GO. Activated fibroblasts secrete GAG and collagen, which are characteristic pathological findings in the perimysial and orbital connective/fatty tissue. Human fibroblasts express numerous regulatory molecules that influence immune function. Therefore, fibroblasts posses the ability to function both as structural elements and as a vital immunoregulatory cells. Cytokine effects on orbital fibroblasts of potential relevance to the autoimmune inflammation include induction of adhesion molecule, HLA-DR, and HSP expression, and stimulation of the secretion of other cytokines. Cytokine effects on other resident cells, like endothelial cells, eye muscle cells and adipocytes, also likely participate in the immunopathogenesis of GO. However, problems in obtaining primary cultures of these cells make it very difficult to analyze *in vitro* the action of cytokines.

Glycosaminoglycan production and proliferation of orbital fibroblasts

Experimental studies have shown that IFN-γ, IL-1α, transforming growth factor-beta (TGF-β), and leukoregulin stimulate GAG secretion by orbital fibroblasts. IFN-γ and especially leukoregulin are potent stimulators of GAG production in orbital fibroblasts, but do not affect GAG synthesis in dermal fibroblasts (48,49). Purified Ig from patients with GO, thyrotropin, IL-2, IL-6, TNF-α, fibroblast growth factor (FGF) or epidermal growth factor (EGF) do not appear to affect the GAG synthesis (48-50). IL-1α, IL-4, platelet-derived growth factor, insulin like growth factor and TGF-β stimulate *in vitro* proliferation of orbital fibroblasts. Glucocorticoid treatment inhibits the cytokine-stimulated proliferation and GAG production of orbital fibroblasts (51).

Recent studies have also demonstrated that a direct interaction between fibroblasts and leukocytes (T cells and mast cells), mediated by CD40/CD40 ligand, may also participate in orbital tissue remodeling (52,53). Orbital fibroblasts, as well as fibroblasts from lungs, express high levels of CD40, a member of the tumor TNF-α superfamily originally found on B cells. Co-culture of orbital fibroblasts with cells expressing a CD40 ligand such as mast cells or T cells leads to a significant increase in GAG synthesis. The CD40/CD40L bridge represents a potentially important conduit for the activation of fibroblasts by both mast cells and lymphocytes. The increase in hyalrunan synthesis by CD40 can be attenuated by dexamethasone, but not by prostaglandin endoperoxide H synthase-2 selective inhibitor.

Immunomodulation

Adhesion molecules

Recruitment of T cells to retrobulbar tissues requires attachment to endothelial cells with subsequent trans-endothelial migration. This process involves a finely tuned cascade cytokine-activated adhesion molecule expression on both endothelial cells and lymphocytes (54,55). The initial attachment and rolling of leukocytes along endothelium is mediated mainly by selectins. Locally produced chemoattractants (chemokines) activate integrins causing firm adhesion of lymphocytes to endothelial cells, followed by rapid migration across the endothelium (56). Further guidance to the site of inflammation is likely provided by adhesion molecules expressed on activated interstitial cells and by chemokines. In one study, the expression of mRNA for IL-8 was detected in EM biopsies obtained from patients with GO, suggesting that this chemokine might play a role in the migration of T cells to retrobulbar tissues (21).

Immunohistochemical studies revealed that the expression of adhesion molecules on endothelial cells from normal orbital tissues was minimal or absent. In contrast, vascular endothelium in retro-bulbar tissues derived from patients with active GO revealed a strong immunoreactivity for ICAM-1, vascular cell adhesion molecule-1 (VCAM-1) and endothelial leukocyte adhesion molecule-1 (ELAM-1, E-selectin) (42,43). The expression of adhesion molecules correlated with the disease activity, being significantly reduced in the later inactive stages.

An *in vitro* study showed that, under baseline conditions, endothelial cells from GO retrobulbar tissues expressed ICAM-1 and CD44 (57). Exposure of endothelial cells to TNF-α, IL-1α and, to a lesser extent, IFN-γ resulted in a marked upregulation or induction of immunoreactivity for ICAM-1, ELAM-1 and VCAM-1. These cytokines are likely to play an important role in the upregulation of adhesion molecules on endothelial cells since they have been detected by immunohistochemistry in OCT from patients with severe GO (28). In addition, blocking experiments using monoclonal antibodies suggested that interactions between endothelial cells and activated T lymphocytes were mediated by β1-and β2-integrin dependent pathways: ICAM-1/LFA-1; VCAM-1/very late antigen-4 (VLA-4, CD49d/CD29) and by integrin independent CD44/hyaluronic acid pathways (57).

The adhesion of lymphocytes to orbital fibroblasts derived from patients with severe GO may be mediated by the interaction of LFA-1 and ICAM-1 (58). Graves' IgG, IFN-γ, IL-1α and TNF-α have been shown to induce the surface expression of ICAM-1 on orbital fibroblasts (58). The effect of Graves' IgG appeared to be specific for orbital fibroblasts from GO patients.

Cytokines and chemokines

In response to pro-inflammatory stimuli, orbital fibroblasts are capable of secreting important mediators of inflammation, like IL-6 and chemokines such as IL-8, IL-16 and RANTES (44,47,59). Orbital fibroblasts lack constitutive expression of IL-6 or IL-8. However, stimulation with IL-

1β, TNF-α and IFN-γ can induce IL-6 gene expression. Dexamethasone can inhibit IL-1-induced IL-6 mRNA expression in a dose-dependent fashion.

There is an alternative pathway for interaction between fibroblasts and CD40 ligand-expressing cells such as T cells and mast cells. Orbital fibroblast express functional CD40, which is upregulated 10-fold by IFN-γ. Fibroblast activation through CD40/CD40 ligand results in induction of pro-inflammatory and chemoattractant cytokines (IL-6 and IL-8) (53).

IL-16, a ligand for CD4, is a chemoattractant molecule expressed by lymphocytes, eosinophils, mast cells, and lung epithelium. In addition, orbital fibroblasts have been shown to express IL-16 (59). Therefore, these cells, and probably other cells such as endothelial cells, likely play a critical role in GO through their secretion of chemokines and recruitment of leukocytes to the inflammatory site.

Prostanoids are important lipid mediators of inflammation and appear to be involved in the physiological regulation of several cellular processes. With regard to the immune system, they impose both immunomodulatory and pro-inflammatory actions, depending on the circumstances. PGE_2 exerts a powerful bias towards the maturation of naïve T lymphocytes from the Th1 to the Th2 subtype, thus potentially modulating the cytokine environment. It participates in B cell maturation and in the activation of mast cells. Wang*et al.* (60) reported that GO orbital fibroblasts exhibited a dramatic upregulation of prostaglandin endoperoxide H synthase-2 (PGHS-2) expression following treatment with leukoregulin, a product of activated T lymphocytes, and IL-1β. The magnitude of the PGHS-2 induction was considerably greater in GO fibroblasts than that in normal orbital fibroblasts or cultures derived from normal-appearing skin. This induction was accompanied by a dramatic increase in PGE_2 production.

As previously mentioned, IL-1Ra is thought to be an important modulator of the pro-inflammatory cascades related to the IL-1 family. When normal orbital and dermal fibroblasts are treated with exogenous IL-1 or leukoregulin, the levels of IL-1Ra are induced dramatically in a time-dependent manner (61). In contrast, the levels of IL-1ra achieved in GO fibroblasts following cytokine exposure are considerably less than those observed in normal cultures (61,62). It is this relative deficiency of IL-1Ra expression in GO cultures that may underlie the exaggerated induction of PGHS-2 and PGE_2 synthesis in these cells. In theory, the actions of IL-1α and IL-1β should be poorly opposed in GO fibroblasts. The molecular basis for the differential induction of IL-1Ra in normal and GO fibroblasts is as yet undetermined, but could provide an important insight into the pathogenic mechanism through which the orbital tissues becomes inflamed. These findings suggest that cyclooxygenase inhibitors and receptor antagonists could have some utility in the therapy of GO.

HLA-DR

The expression of HLA-DR antigen, immunomodulatory molecules such as ICAM-1, and inflammatory cytokines (IL-1β, TNF-α, IFN-γ) has been reported in EM and OCT at early stage of GO in conjunction with lymphocytic infiltration (5-7). Co-stimulatory molecules B7-1 and B7-2 were not expressed in EOM or fibroblasts, which needs full antigen presentation (7,8). The surface expression of HLA-DR was induced *in vitro* on orbital fibroblasts following stimulation with IFN-γ. IFN-γ induced HLA-DR expression was enhanced with concomitant treatment with TNF-α. The induction of HLA-DR by IFN-γ could be blocked by glucocoticoids. Interestingly the expression of HLA-DR increased more when IFN-γ was added in combination with cigarette smoke constituents (63). These findings may, in part, explain the strong association between smoking and GO. Treatment *in vitro* with IFN-γ also induced HLA-DR expression in eye muscle cells and endothelial cells (64).

Heat shock proteins

Heat shock proteins are synthesized by cells undergoing stress and function to maintain cellular homeostasis. The expression of HSP-70 was found on eye muscle cells during the active stage of GO (6). In vitro, HSP-70 expression in orbital fibroblasts could be induced by inflammatory cytokines and various cellular stresses and was suppressed by glucocorticoids and anti-thyroid drugs (65). HSP-70 was detected on the surface of cultured orbital fibroblasts from patients with GO, but not on those from normal subjects(65). Due to high immunogenicity and marked similarities with bacterial proteins, HSPs are thought to play a role in the development of autoimmunity. However, this remains controversial and their definitive role in autoimmne inflammation remains to be established (66).

SUMMARY

Cytokines, released by infiltrating leukocytes and resident orbital cells, are likely to play a crucial role in the initiation and propagation of the autoimmune inflammation in GO. Therefore, studies analyzing the cytokine profiles in EM and OCT are essential to a better understanding of the pathogenesis of GO. However, retrobulbar tissue specimens are generally not available from patients with early, active GO without prior immunomodulatory treatment (with glucucorticoids or radiotherapy). Therefore, the question of whether GO is initiated by a cell-mediated or a humoral-mediated immune response cannot yet be answered. Hopefully, studies using an animal model of GO will help to clarify this issue. Whether the inflammation in EM differs from the inflammation in OCT is also not presently known, because eye muscle surgery is not performed during the active stage of the disease. Nevertheless, a few important details concerning cytokine profiles in these tissues have been recently elucidated.

It is likely that both cell-mediated and humoral immune responses are involved in the pathogenesis of GO because both Th1 and Th2 cytokines have been shown to be present in eye muscles and in orbital connective tissue specimens. The cytokine profile and type of autoimmune activity found in a particular retrobulbar tissue sample likely depends on the activity and the duration of GO. Natt and Bahn (27) postulated that Th1-like cytokines may play a role in the acute stage and that Th2-like cytokines may play a role in chronic late-stage disease. Since IL-4 and IL-10 inhibit Th1 cell proliferation and IFN-γ production, these cytokines may ameliorate the inflammatory lesion and mediate late fibrosis. During the course of inflammation in the EM and OCT, the cytokine pattern might switch from a Th1 to a Th2 response, although the mechanism for the change is presently unknown. Several studies have shown that cytokines involved in cell-mediated immune responses are detected in EM and OCT specimens from patients with active GO, whereas predominantly a Th2 cytokine profile is present in tissues from patients with longstanding GO. There was only one study analyzing the cytokine expression on both tissues in a large number of patients. Differences in cytokine patterns between EM and OCT were described, perhaps reflecting different time courses in switching from Th1 to Th2 between these tissue sites. However, the observations that the enlargement of EM was positively correlated to the expression of TNF-α, and that the orbital volume was positively correlated with an IL-6 signal suggests that there may be distinct differences in inflammation between these two tissues. Further studies using a more quantitative method are needed to clarify these issues.

It is now widely accepted that fibroblasts synthesize extracellular matrix and collagen, and play an important role in various inflammatory and immune reactions. Paracrine/autocrine interactions between orbital fibroblasts and infiltrating lymphocytes/macrophages are thought to play a central role in the evolution of GO. Upon activation, T cells and macrophages populating the retroorbital space are known to secrete a variety of cytokines into the surrounding tissue. IFN-γ, TNF-α and IL-1β have been detected in orbital tissue from patients with GO. Cytokine effects of potential relevance to GO include the stimulation of GAG synthesis and the induction of HLA-DR, HSP, and adhesion molecule expression in orbital fibroblasts. The orbital fibroblasts surrounding EM fibers seem to be extremely sensitive to stimulation by cytokines and other soluble proteins released in the course of an immune reaction. This may explain, in part, the anatomical localization of GO pathology within the orbit.

CONCLUSIONS

Cytokines are thought to play a crucial role in initiating and maintaining the autoimmune response in GO. Th1 cytokines may stimulate proliferation, GAG production and induction of HLA-DR, HSP and adhesion molecules in orbital fibroblasts and endothelial cells. IFN-γ enhances GAG production and protein synthesis by orbital fibroblasts to a greater extent than by dermal fibroblasts, which could account for the apparent localization of the disease process in GO. Furthermore, TNF-α mRNA expression in EM and IL-6 mRNA expression in OCT are positively associated with the enlargement of EM tissue and orbital fat volume, respectively. Since a Th2-dominant cytokine profile has been reported at a later stage of GO, Th2 cytokines may play a role in this stage of GO, mediating remodeling and fibrosis. Indeed, a negative association between IL-4 and IL-10 mRNA expression in OCT with orbital fat volume has been reported. Further studies are needed to clarify this issue. The activation by orbital antigen of T cells within the retrobulbar tissues results in the local release of lymphokines, cytokines, chemokines and growth factors. This leads to the stimulation of cell proliferation, GAG synthesis, and the expression of immunomodulatory molecules by orbital fibroblasts. The particularly robust responses of orbital fibroblasts to pro-inflammatory signals are likely critical to the peculiar tissue reactions associated with GO. Information concerning the involvement of cytokines and chemokines in the pathogenesis of GO may provide a rational new approach to the treatment of GO (35,67,68).

REFERENCES

1. Wall JR, Salvi M, Bernard NF, Boucher A, Haegert D 1991 Thyroid-associated ophthalmopathy: a model for the association of organ-specific autoimmune disorders. Immunol Today 12:150-153.
2. Burch HB, Wartofsky L 1993 Graves' ophthalmopathy, current concepts regarding pathogenesis and management. Endocrine Reviews 14: 747-793.
3. Bednarczuk T, Kennerdell JS, Wall JR 1997 Thyroid-Associated Ophthalmopathy-Pathophysiology and Etiology. In: Falk SA (ed) Thyroid Disease - Endocrinology, Surgery, Nuclear Medicine and Radiotherapy. Raven Press, New York, p 341-358.
4. Weetman AP, Cohen K, Gatter P, Fells, Shine B 1989 Immunohistochemical analysis of retrobulbar tissues in Graves' ophthalmopathy. Clin Exp Immunol 75:222-227.
5. Kahaly G, Hansen C, Felke B, Dienes HP 1994 Immunohistochemical staining of retrobulbar adipose tissue in Graves' ophthalmopathy. Clin Immunol Immunopathol 73:53-62.
6. Hiromatsu Y, Tanaka K, Ishisaka N, et al. 1995 Human histocompatibility leukocyte antigen-DR and heat shock protein-70 expression in eye muscle tissue in thyroid-associated ophthalmopathy. J Clin Endocrinol Metab 80:685-691.
7. Hiromatsu Y 1996 In situ studies of orbital tissue from patients with thyroid-associated ophthalmopathy. Orbit 15: 147-158.
8. Pappa A, Lawson JMM, Calder V, Fells P, Lightman S 2000 T cells and fibroblasts in affected extraocular muscles in early and late thyroid associated ophthalmopathy. Br J Ophthalmol 84: 517-522.
9. Kiljanski JI, Nebes V, Wall JR 1995 The ocular muscle cell is a target of the immune system in endocrine ophthalmopathy. Int Arch Allergy Immunol 106:204-212.
10. Hiromatsu Y, Kojima K, Ishisaka N, Tanaka K, Sato M, Nonaka K, Nishimura H, Nishida H. 1993 Role of magnetic resonance imaging in thyroid-associated ophthalmopathy: its predictive value for therapeutic outcome of immunosuppressive therapy. Thyroid 2:299-305.
11. Gunji K, De Bellis A, Li AW, Yamada M, Kubota S, Ackrell B, Wengrowicz S, Bellastella A, Bizzarro A, Sinisi A, Wall JR 2000 Cloning and characterization of the novel thyroid and eye muscle shared protein G2s: autoantibodies against G2s are closely associated with ophthalmopathy in patients with Graves' hyperthyroidism. J Clin Endocrinol Metab 85:1641-1647.
12. Hiromatsu Y, Yang D, Bednarczuk T, Miyake I, Nonaka K, Inoue Y 2000 Cytokine profiles in eye muscle tissue and orbital fat tissue from patients with thyroid-associated ophthalmopathy. J Clin Endocrinol Metab 85:1194-1199.
13. Heufelder AE, Herterich S, Ernst G, Bahn RS, Scriba PC 1995 Analysis of retroorbital T cell antigen receptor variable region gene usage in patients with Graves' ophthalmopathy. Eur J Endocrinol 132: 266-277.
14. Heufelder AE, Wenzel BE, Scriba PC 1996 Antigen Receptor Variable Region Repertoires Expressed by T Cells Infiltrating Thyroid, Retroorbital, and Pretibial Tissue in Graves Disease. J Clin Endocrinol Metab 81: 3733-3739.

15. Kubota S, Gunji K, Ackrell BA, Cochran B, Stolarski C, Wengrowicz S, Kennerdell JS, Hiromatsu Y, Wall J 1998 The 64-kilodalton eye muscle protein is the flavoprotein subunit of mitochondrial succinate dehydrogenase: the corresponding serum antibodies are good markers of an immune-mediated damage to the eye muscle in patients with Graves' hyperthyroidism. J Clin Endocrinol Metab 83:443-447.
16. Bednarczuk T, Stolarski C, Pawlik E, Slon M, Rowinski M, Kubota S, Hiromatsu Y, Bartoszewicz Z, Wall JR, Nauman J 1999 Autoantibodies reactive with extracellular matrix (ECM) proteins in patients with thyroid-associated ophthalmopathy. Thyroid 9: 289-295.
17. Salgame P, Abrams JS, Clayberger C, et al. 1991 Differing lymphokine profiles of functional subsets of human CD4 and CD8 T cell clones. Science 254:279-282.
18. Liblau RS, Singer SM, McDevitt HO 1995 Th1 and Th2 $CD4^+$ T cells in the pathogenesis of organ-specific autoimmune diseases. Immunol Today 16:34-38.
19. Romagnani S 1997 The Th1/Th2 paradigm. Immunol Today 18:263-266.
20. McLachlan SM, Prummel MF, Rapoport B 1994 Cell-mediated or humoral immunity in Graves' ophthalmopathy? Profiles of T-cells cytokines amplified by polymerase chain reaction from orbital tissue. J Clin Endocrinol Metab 78:1070-1074.
21. Pappa A, Calder V, Ajjan R, et al. 1997 Analysis of extraocular muscle infiltrating T cells in thyroid-associated ophthalmopathy (TAO). Clin Exp Immunol 109:362-369.
22. Grubeck-Loebenstein B, Trieb K, Sztankay A, Holter W, Anderi H, Wick G 1994 Retrobulbar T cells from patients with Graves' ophthalmopathy are CD8+ and specifically recognize autologous fibroblasts. J Clin Invest 93:2738-2743.
23. De Carli M, D'Elios MM, Mariotti S, et al. 1993 Cytolytic T cells with Th1-like cytokine profile predominate in retroorbital lymphocytic infiltrates of Graves' ophthalmopathy. J Clin Endocrinol Metab 77:1120-1124.
24. Forster G, Otto E, Hansen C, Ochs K, Kahaly G 1998 Analysis of orbital T cells in thyroid-associated ophthalmopathy. Clin Exp Immunol 112:427-434.
25. Yang D, Hiromatsu Y, Hoshino T, Inoue Y, Itoh K, Nonaka K 1999 Dominant infiltration of T(H) 1-type CD4+ T cells at the retrobulbar space of patients with thyroid-associated ophthalmopathy. Thyroid. 9:305-310.
26. Aniszewski JP, Valyasevi RW, Bahn RS 2000 Relationship between disease duration and predominant orbital T cell subset in Graves' ophthalmopathy. J Clin Endocrinol Metab 85:776-780.
27. Natt N, Bahn RS 1997 Cytokines in the evolution of Graves' ophthalmopathy. Autoimmunity 26:129-136.
28. Heufelder AE, Bahn RS 1993 Detection and localization of cytokine immunoreactivity in retroocular connective tissue in Graves' ophthalmopathy. Eur J Clin Invest 23:10-17.
29. Hoshino T, Itoh K, Gouhara R, et al. 1995 Spontaneous production of various cytokines except IL-4 from $CD4^+$ T cells in the affected organs of sarcoidosis patients. Clin Exp Immunol 102:399-405.
30. Gup J, Rapoport B, McLachlan SM 1997 Cytokine profiles of in vivo activated thyroid-infiltrating T cells cloned in the presence or absence of interleukin 4. Autoimmunity 26:103-110.
31. Van der Gaag R, Schmidt ED, Zonnerveld FW, Koornneef L 1995 Orbital pathology in thyroid-associated ophthalmopathy. Orbit 15: 109-118.

32. Kamizono S, Hiromatsu Y, Seki N, Bednarczuk T, Matsumoto H, Kimura A, Itoh K. 2000 A polymorphism of the 5' flanking region of tumor necrosis factor alpha gene is associated with thyroid-associated ophthalmopathy in Japanese. Clin Endocrinol (Oxf) 52:759-764.
33. Salvi M, Pedrazzoni M, Girasole G, Giuliani N, Minelli R, Wall JR, Roti E 2000 Serum concentrations of proinflammatory cytokines in Graves' disease: effect of treatment, thyroid function, ophthalmopathy and cigarette smoking. Eur J Endocrinol 143: 197-202.
34. Komorowski J, Jankiewicz J, Robak T, Blasinska-Morawiec M, Stepien H 1998 Cytokine levels as the marker of thyroid activation in Graves' disease. Immunol Lett 60:143-148.
35. Tan GH, Dutton CM, Bahn RS 1996 Interleukin-1 (IL-1) receptor antagonist and soluble IL-1 receptor inhibit IL-1-induced glycosaminoglycan production in cultured human orbital fibroblasts from patients with Graves' ophthalmopathy. J Clin Endocrinol Metab. 81: 449-452.
36. Hofbauer LC, Muhlberg T, Konig A, Heufelder G, Schworm HD, Heufelder AE 1997 Soluble interleukin-1 receptor antagonist serum levels in smokers and nonsmokers with Graves' ophthalmopathy undergoing orbital radiotherapy. J Clin Endocrinol Metab 82: 2244-2247.
37. Mysliwiec J, Kretowski A, Szelachowska M, Mikita A, Kinalska I 1999 Serum pro- and anti-inflammatory cytokines in patients with Graves' disease with ophthalmopathy during treatment with glucocorticoids. Rocz Akad Med Bialymst 44: 160-169.
38. Wakelkamp IM, Gerding MN, Van der Meer JW, Prummel MF, Wiersinga WM 2000 Both Th1- and Th2- derived cytokines in serum are elevated in Graves' ophthalmopathy. Clin Exp Immunol 121: 453-457.
39. Yamada T, Sato A, Komiya I, Nishimori T, Ito Y, Terao A, Eto S, Tanaka Y 2000 An elevation of serum immunoglobulin E provides a new aspect of hyperthyroid Graves' disease. J Clin Endocrinol Metab 85:2775-2778.
40. Raikow RB, Dalbow MH, Kennerdell JS, Compher K, Machen L, Hiller W, Blendermann D 1990 Immunohistochemical evidence for IgE involvement in Graves' orbitopathy. Ophthalmology 97:629-35.
41. Smith TJ, Parikh SJ 1999 HMC-1 mast cells activate human orbital fibroblasts in coculture: evidence for upregulation of prostaglandin E2 and hyaluronan synthesis. Endocrinology 140: 3518-3525.
42. Heufelder AE, Bahn RS 1993 Elevated expression in situ of selectin and immunoglobulin superfamily type adhesion molecules in retroocular connective tissues from patients with Graves' ophthalmopathy. Clin Exp Immunol 91: 381-389.
43. Pappa A, Calder V, Fells P, Lightman S 1997 Adhesion molecule expression in vivo on extraocular muscles (EOM) in thyroid-associated ophthalmopathy (GO). Clin Exp Immunol 108: 309-313.
44. Burnstine MA, Elner SG, Strieter RM, Kunkel SL, Elner VM 1999 Orbital fibroblast interleukin –6 gene expression and immunomodulation. Ophthal Plast Reconstr Surg 15: 306-311.
45. Molnar I, Balzacs C 1997 High circulating IL-6 level in Graves' ophthalmopathy. Autoimmunity 25: 91-96.
46. Melchers F, Rolink AG, Schaniel C 1999 The role of chemokines in regulating cell migration during humoral immune responses. Cell. 99: 351-354.

47. Elner VM, Burnstine MA, Kunkel SL, Strieter RM, Elner SG 1998 Interleukin-8 and monocyte chemotactic protein-1 gene expression and protein production by human orbital fibroblasts. Ophthal Plast Reconstr Surg. 14: 119-125.
48. Smith TJ, Bahn RS, Gorman CA, Cheavens M 1991 Stimulation of glycosaminoglycans by interferon gamma in cultured human retroocular fibroblasts. J Clin Endocrinol Metab 72: 1169-1171.
49. Smith TJ, Wang H-S, Evans CH 1995 Leukoregulin is a potent inducer of hyaluronan synthesis in cultured human orbital fibroblasts. Am J Physiol 268: C382-C388
50. Smith TJ, Bahn RS, Gorman CA 1989 Hormonal regulation of hyaluronate synthesis in cultured human fibroblasts: evidence for differences between retroocular and dermal fibroblasts. J Clin Endocrinol Metab 69: 1019-1023.
51. Heufelder AE, Bahn RS 1994 Modulation of Graves' orbital fibroblasts proliferation by cytokines and glucocorticoid receptor agonists. Invest Ophthalmol Vis Sci 35: 120-127.
52. Cao HJ, Wang HS, Zhang Y, Lin HY, Phipps RP, Smith TJ 1998 Activation of human orbital fibroblasts through CD40 engagement results in dramatic induction of hyaluronan synthesis and prostaglandin endoperoxide H synthase-2 expression. Insights into potential pathogenic mechanism of thyroid associated ophthalmopathy. J Biol Chem 273: 29615-29625.
53. Sempowski GD, Rozenblit J, Smith TJ, Phipps RP 1998 Human orbital fibroblasts are activated by through CD40 to induce proinflammatory cytokine production. Am J Physiol 274: C707-C714.
54. Hynes RO 1992 Integrins: Versatility, Modulation and Signaling in Cell Adhesion. Cell 69: 11-25.
55. Springer TA 1994 Traffic Signals for Lymphocyte Recirculation and Leukocyte Emigration: The Multistep Paradigm. Cell 76: 301-314.
56. Baggiolini M 1998 Chemokines and leukocyte traffic. Nature 392: 565-568.
57. Heufelder AE, Scriba PC 1996 Characterization of receptors on cultured microvascular endothelial cells derived from the retroorbital connective tissue of patients with Graves' ophthalmopathy. Eur J Endocrinol 134: 51-60.
58. Heufelder AE, Bahn RS 1992 Graves' immunoglobulins and cytokines stimulate the expression of intercellular adhesion molecule-1 (ICAM-1) in cultured orbital fibroblasts. European Journal of Clinical Investigation 22: 529-537.
59. Sciaky D, Brazer W, Center DM, Cruikshank WW, Smith TJ 2000 Cultured fibroblasts express constitutive IL-16 mRNA: cytokine induction of active IL-16 protein synthesis through a caspase-3-dependent mechanism. J Immunol 164: 3806-3814.
60. Wang H-S, Cao HJ, Winn VD, Rezanka LJ, Frobert Y, Evans CH, Sciaky D, Young DA, Smith TJ 1996 Leukoregulin induction of prostaglandin-endoperoxide H synthase-2 in human orbital fibroblasts. An *in vitro* model for connective tissue inflammation. J Biol Chem 271: 22718-22728.
61. Cao HJ, Smith TJ 1999 Leukoregulin upregulation of prostaglandin endoperoxide H synthase-2 expression in human orbital fibroblasts. Am J Physiol 277: C1075-C1085.
62. Mühlberg T, Heberling H-J, Joba W, Schworm H-D, Heufelder AE 1997 Detection and modulation of interleukin-1 receptor antagonist messenger ribonucleic acid and immunoreactivity in Graves' orbital fibroblasts. Invest Ophthalmol Vis Sci 38: 1018-1028.

63. Mack WP, Stasior GO, Cao HJ, Stasior OG, Smith TJ 1999 The effects of cigarette smoke constituents on the expression of HLA-DR in orbital fibroblasts derived from patients with Graves ophthalmopathy. Ophthal Plast Reconstr Surg 15: 260-271.
64. Hiromatsu Y, Fukazawa H, How J, Wall JR 1987 Antibody-dependent cell-mediated cytotoxicity against human eye muscle cells and orbital fibroblasts in Graves' ophthalmopathy - roles of Class II MHC antigen expression and □-interferon action on effector and target cells. Clin Exp Immunol 70: 593-603.
65. Heufelder AE, Wenzel BE, Bahn RS 1992 Cell surface localization of a 72 kilodalton heat shock protein in retroocular fibroblasts from patients with Graves' Ophthalmopathy. J Clin Endocrinol Metab 74: 732-736.
66. Eden W, van der Zee R, Paul A, Prakken BJ, Wendling U, Anderton SM, Wauben MHM 1998 Do heat shock proteins control the balance of T-cell regulation in inflammatory diseases. Immunol Today 19: 303-307.
67. Balzacs C, Kiss H, Farid NR 1998 Inhibitory effects of pentoxifylline on HLA-DR expression and glycosaminoglycan synthesis by retrobulbar fibroblasts. Horm Metab Res 30: 496-499.
68. Hiromatsu Y, Yang D, Miyake I, Koga M, Kameo J, Sato M, Inoue Y, Nonaka K 1998 Nicotinamide decreases cytokine-induced activation of orbital fibroblasts from patients with thyroid-associated ophthalmopathy. J Clin Endocrinol Metab 83: 121-124.

5

ANIMAL MODELS OF GRAVES' OPHTHALMOPATHY

Marian Ludgate and Glynn Baker
Departments of Medicine (Endocrine Section) & Ophthalmology, University of Wales College of Medicine, Heath Park, Cardiff CF14 4XN, UK.

INTRODUCTION

Recent years have seen an increase in our understanding of the immunopathogenesis of thyroid eye disease, or Graves' ophthalmopathy (GO), much of which will be discussed in other chapters in this book. GO is an autoimmune disease and progress in other disorders of this type has been greatly accelerated by the establishment of an appropriate animal model. This invariably requires a well-characterised autoantigen, which has been wanting in GO, although progress has also been made in this area. The association with Graves' Disease (GD) immediately implicates the target of the thyroid stimulating antibodies (TSAB), which cause hyperthyroidism, i.e. the thyrotropin receptor (TSHR) and evidence for its role in GO is mounting. The models described in this chapter add further support for the TSHR being an autoantigen in GO, although as will be seen, receptor expression may not be restricted only to the thyroid and orbit.

HISTORICAL MODELS

From the first decades of the twentieth century attempts were made to develop animal models which recapitulated the signs and symptoms of GO. The earliest methods sought to induce exophthalmos and this was achieved by administration of substances which would increase circulating thyrotropin

(TSH) levels such as pituitary extracts or methyl cyanide, or by electrical stimulation to induce smooth muscle contraction, in a variety of species including ducks, guinea pigs and rabbits (1-3). The proptosis induced by methyl cyanide and pituitary extracts could be reversed by cervical ganglion sympathectomy and the mechanism of proptosis assumed to be smooth muscle stimulation primarily of Mullers muscle. The first work, in which exophthalmos was convincingly due to an increase in the volume of the orbital contents, rather than to a nervous mechanism, is probably that of Smelser in 1936. He administered 250-2000mg of pituitary extract to 26 guinea pigs of both sexes, daily over a period of 3 to 9 weeks. All animals lost weight and had signs of thyroid hypertrophy, 3 had slight exophthalmos. When he repeated the experiment, but with the addition of thyroidectomy, 23 developed extreme exophthalmos 12 to 20 days after the first injection. Exophthalmos was present to a lesser extent in eyes that had undergone cervical sympathectomy. The exophthalmos was due to orbital volume expansion and a 40% increase in the weight of the orbital contents was observed, when compared with non-injected thyroidectomized controls. The changes occurred predominantly in the orbital fat and lacrimal gland. The orbital tissues were examined histologically and found to be edematous and infiltrated by lymphocytes and an eosin staining mucopolysaccharide (4).

The approach was extended by Paulson (5), who highlighted the changes in the Harderian lacrimal gland and noted some degeneration and interstitial edema in extra-ocular muscles that were not present in skeletal muscle other than some minor changes in the orbicularis oculi. Increased water content in the orbital fat of injected thyroidectomized guinea pigs was reported by Smelser in 1943 (6). Further progress was made by Dobyns (7) who described a 'Camera Lucida' apparatus for accurate determination of proptosis. This approach involved using bright lighting to startle dark adapted guinea pigs and while transfixed the proptosis could be measured removing the need for restraint or anaesthesia. The effect of the startle would likely produce a high sympathetic drive which may have influenced apparent proptosis.

All of these models required the combination of administration of pituitary extract and thyroidectomy. With the benefit of some 70 years further research this might be explained by the release of thyroid antigens, including the TSHR, into the circulation leading to a break in immunological tolerance with the resulting autoimmune response leading to the orbital lymphocytic infiltration and edema. Additionally, high levels of circulating TSH, both from endogenous sources and the pituitary extract, could stimulate adipogenesis with consequent increase in orbital fat mass. It is tempting to speculate that the non-progressive proptosis described in some patients harbouring a germline gain of function mutation of the TSHR, could be attributed to constitutive activation of the receptor in the adipose compartment mimicking chronic TSH stimulation (8). Indeed the apparent central importance of TSH in the pathogenesis of GO, led to hypophysectomy being adopted as a treatment option for a time. However, despite reports of some success, the therapy was not always effective as exemplified by a patient who developed disease in the contra-lateral eye following surgical hypophysectomy (9) and who had high levels of long acting thyroid stimulator (LATS).

It is slightly more difficult to explain more recent models of GO which have relied solely on the administration of pituitary extracts or TSH preparations and which thus lack an identifiable immune stimulus. In a series of experiments in which exophthalmogenic producing substance (EPS) activity was assayed by its ability to induce proptosis in goldfish and thyreotropic activity was measured in the McKenzie bioassay. Winand and Kohn (10-12) demonstrated that EPS from pituitary extracts is TSH; that not all TSH preparations have EPS; that the EPS was distinct from the thyreotropic activity of TSH and resided in a tryptic fragment of TSH comprising the nearly intact β subunit and the amino terminus of the α subunit. They also reported a 2-fold increase in the glycosaminoglycan (GAG) content of Harderian gland in guinea pigs with exophthalmos following treatment with high doses of TSH or its tryptic fragment. Increases in GAG were also noted in perirenal fat and other retro-orbital tissues but not in skin, kidney or muscle (12). Their conclusion, that EPS resides in TSH, was not supported by the work of Valk and colleagues (13) who induced exophthalmos in male guinea pigs by thyroidectomy coupled with radio-iodine or treatment with propylthiouracil (PTU). The former regimen was more effective than the latter in inducing proptosis but in each case, EPS activity in the serum (measured in the goldfish bioassay) correlated with the severity of exophthalmos (estimated from photographs) but did not correlate with circulating levels of TSH. Thyroxine replacement did not alter exophthalmos and animals administered with thyrotrophin releasing hormone developed no exophthalmos. Once again a surfeit of TSH, as in the PTU treated animals, could stimulate adipogenesis leading to mild proptosis but more severe eye signs require release of thyroid/orbital shared antigens, such as the TSHR, into the circulation, as occurs in the animals receiving thyroid ablation.

In fact none of these models has stood the test of time, in contrast to a range of protocols for inducing thyroiditis involving injection of thyroglobulin (Tg) or transfer of Tg sensitized T cells/clones (14-17). The EPS bioassay was reported to have low specificity, with normal serum able to induce exophthalmos in fish (atlantic minow, *fundus heteroclitus*) and the exophthalmos varied between seasons making reproducibility impossible (18). It was argued that TSH levels are suppressed in patients with GD, even those with severe GO. Even if one accepts that LATS (19), i.e.,TSAB can substitute for TSH, not all patients with GO have TSAB and some are euthyroid. With the growing awareness of the autoimmune nature of GO, it was difficult to envisage how protocols that essentially manipulate the thyroid axis could provide a suitable model of GO. However as mentioned earlier, the addition of thyroid ablation could provide a bolus of thyroid/orbit shared antigen, as has been postulated for the exacerbation of GO which can occur in GD patients treated with radio-iodine (20).

An animal model of GO would probably follow the development of a model for GD. The cloning of the TSHR has resulted in a variety of protocols having this goal and which have been described in an accompanying book in this series and will thus be considered only briefly here.

PROGRESS IN THE DEVELOPMENT OF MODELS OF GRAVES' DISEASE

Convincing animal models of GD should be induced with the TSHR or T cells primed to this antigen, given its central role as the target of TSAB which cause hyperthyroidism. The TSHR is a G protein coupled receptor, with the characteristic seven membrane spanning regions. It is a part of the glycoprotein hormone subfamily and, along with the receptors for luteinizing hormone and follicle stimulating hormone, has a large extracellular domain (ECD) which confers ligand binding specificity (reviewed in 21).

Prior to its cloning, the low level of receptor expression in the thyroid precluded the use of tissue membranes or extracts, as had been achieved with Tg to induce models of thyroiditis. However some success was obtained when immunising five different H-2 mouse strains with detergent extracted and TSH affinity purified receptor from a human thyroid cell line, GEJ (22). Low levels of TBII and mild thyroiditis was observed in H-2s, H-2b and H-2q mice.

Since the cloning of the TSHR, several receptor preparations and fragments have been employed with varying levels of success in mimicking GD.

Several papers have claimed the induction of TSAB, TBAB, TBII and increased thyroxine levels in mice, rabbits and birds treated with synthetic receptor peptides (23-26). To our knowledge lymphocytic thyroiditis was not reported in any of these studies.

We, and others, have produced recombinant receptor fusion proteins in bacteria. We employed the ECD (27) coupled to maltose binding protein (MBP), and reported the induction of TBII in ECD treated BALBc mice (H-2d) mice. We also demonstrated that false positive TBII can be demonstrated using unfractionated sera and that reduced T4 levels were present in both groups after the initial immunizations, but the MBP mice recovered, unlike the ECD-MBP whose thyroids also displayed increased vascularity and focal lymphocytic thyroiditis.

Subsequently we confirmed the induction of TBII and TBAB, accompanied by reduced circulating T4, by the receptor antigen but not MBP, in both males and females. Thyroiditis was induced in 50% of male and 100% of surviving female mice (28).

In mice of differing genetic background (29), particularly in the MHC, H-2b ((C57) and H-2k (CBA) animals did not develop thyroiditis although receptor antibodies were induced. In the same series of experiments, NOD mice, which have a unique H-2g haplotype, developed antibodies to the receptor, destructive thyroiditis and reduced T4 levels, when treated with the ECD-MBP antigen. When comparing the phenotype of the lymphocytic infiltrate, in the BALBc mice B cells and immunoreactivity for IL-4 and IL-10 were found but in the NOD mice there were very few B cells and immunoreactivity for INFγ, indicating the Th2 and Th1 nature of the induced disease respectively.

A major draw back using receptor produced in bacteria was the lack of correct folding and glycosylation and it was hoped that eucaryotic expression in insect cells, using baculovirus vectors, might offer a solution to this problem. Certainly the human ECD produced using the system is superior to the antigen from bacteria in terms of absorbing out TBII activity from GD patients sera (30) but there have been no convincing demonstrations of direct TSH binding to a receptor protein expressed using baculovirus. Never the less useful information has been obtained, with both the human and murine ECD, when injected into animals in combination with various adjuvants. Prabhakar and colleagues (31) studied four different strains of mice treated with the human ECD and observed that antibodies to the receptor, having no biological activity, were induced in all of the mice. In contrast, increased thyroxine levels were present only in the BALBc mice and, despite the absence of thyroiditis, there were changes in the gland, such as budding, indicative of hyperactivity. The same antigen, used by the same group but this time injected into rabbits, induced TBII (32). Perhaps reasoning that an induced immune response to a heterologous antigen is not sufficient to claim autoimmunity, Davies' group have expressed the murine ECD in insect cells and obtained monoclonal antibodies, some of which had TBII and TBAB activities, when measured in vitro on CHO cells expressing the human TSHR (33). Furthermore, when BALBc mice were treated with the same murine antigen and an adjuvant comprised of alum and pertussis toxin (34), TBII and TBAB were induced and mice had reduced levels of T3 accompanied by increased TSH but no signs of thyroiditis or thyroid destruction.

A novel approach involving immunization with the cDNA for the full length human TSHR cloned in a eucaryotic expression vector, was tried (35). It is proposed the cDNA is taken up into the myocytes at the site of injection (usually the anterior tibialis) and subsequently expressed at the surface of these cells. Myocytes do not express MHC-class II or the co-stimulatory molecules necessary to activate T cells. Consequently there must be a phase, perhaps triggered by inflammation of the muscle, in which professional antigen presenting cells become involved, maybe by phagocytosing fragmented receptor released from myocytes. The actual mechanism is unknown, but if this is the whole story, inducing thyroiditis and TSAB using synthetic peptides administered with adjuvants capable of stimulating inflammation at the injection site should have the same effect. However this has not been achieved.

Some success was achieved since 14/15 female BALBc mice treated with receptor cDNA developed antibodies to the TSHR measured by FACS and the majority contained TBII and TBAB activities. One serum contained TSAB resulting in 800% increase in cAMP production and which persisted for 18 weeks. Thyroid hormone levels remained normal throughout the experiment. All mice displayed severe thyroiditis with many infiltrating B cells but no thyroid destruction, quite the opposite with signs of epithelial thickening and budding.

The method was then applied to the NMRI outbred strain of mice with very exciting results (36). 30 male and 30 female mice underwent the genetic immunization protocol and virtually all developed receptor antibodies detectable by FACS. 9/30 males displayed signs of hypothyroidism with TBAB and reduced T4. 4/30 females developed stable hyperthyroidism with circulating TSAB accompanied by increased T3 & T4 but undetectable TSH. In addition thyroiditis and orbital changes (please see below for details) were induced.

One very promising approach has involved treating mice with fibroblasts which express an MHC-class II molecule and the full length, functional human TSHR (37). The mouse strain used was the AKR/N which is H-2^k, homologous to the RT4.15HP murine fibroblast cell line. Recipient mice and cells used as immunogen are MHC-class I identical. The majority of female mice receiving cells expressing MHC-class II and receptor developed TBII. About 20% had increased thyroxine levels and this was shown to be accompanied by TSAB activity. In contrast, TBII positive sera in animals with normal thyroid hormone levels displayed TBAB activity. No TBII, TSAB, TBAB or changes in circulating thyroid hormone were induced in mice receiving cells expressing singly either TSHR or MHC-class II and the thyroids of these animals appeared normal. In contrast, the thyroids of the animals receiving TSHR and MHC-class II expressing fibroblasts were macroscopically enlarged and microscopically displayed changes in architecture e.g. hypertrophy and hypercellularity with follicular cells protruding into the lumen, which are similar to those seen in hyperthyroidism. However, there was no lymphocytic infiltration.

Subsequently the non-MHC genetic control of the induced disease was investigated in five different strains of mice, all H-2^k (38) with the majority of animals developing TBII, irrespective of the strain.

The authors then investigated whether certain regions of the TSHR might be necessary or sufficient to induce disease (39). In previous chimera studies, in which portions of the TSHR were substituted with the equivalent part of the LH receptor, the amino terminal of the protein was found to be required for binding and specific recognition by TSAB (40). A range of such chimeras lacking residues 9-165(mc 1+2); 90-165 (mc1) and 261-370 (mc4) were transfected into the RT4.15Hp and parent cell lines.TBII were induced in mice receiving MHC-class II expressing fibroblasts transfected with the WT and mc4 receptors but not the mc 1 or mc 1+2 constructs. Elevated T4 levels, associated with TSAB were present in 2/9 WT and MHC-class II recipients but not in any of the other treated or control groups. Based on the TBII results, it was concluded that the N terminal segment of the receptor is critical, not only as an epitope for human TSAB but also in the induction of TSHR antibodies in a murine model of GD. However, considering the lack of TSAB in animals receiving the mc4 construct, the participation of the carboxyl end of the ECD should not be overlooked.

This model has recently been confirmed and extended (41) using the same AKR/N mouse strain, receiving the RT4.15HP cell line transfected with the human TSHR (in a slightly different expression vector). There were varying outcomes including TBII and elevated T4 levels accompanied by enlarged thyroids with signs of hypertrophy and colloid droplet formation but no lymphocytic infiltration. Epitope mapping by ELISA revealed that 9/13 sera from mice receiving fibroblasts expressing receptor and MHC-class II, recognised a peptide for residues 97-116 of the N terminal of the ECD but peptides for residues 322-371 in the carboxyl part of the ECD also showed high absorption by experimental but not control sera.

The earliest reported transfer of receptor primed T cells used synthetic peptides shown to be T cell epitopes for GD patients in the in vivo priming step of DBA mice(26). Treatment with 3/4 T cell epitope peptides elicited weak TSAB activity and T cell lines were developed from one TSAB positive and one TSAB negative mouse. When these were transferred to naive syngeneic mice, following a period of in vitro priming with receptor peptides, weak TSAB activity were present in 2/4 mice receiving the line from the TSAB positive donor but no TSAB in the four mice receiving the line from the TSAB negative donor.

We have used unfractionated T cells and a CD4+ enriched population to transfer disease to syngeneic BALBc and NOD recipients. The in vivo priming step could be performed using the receptor produced in bacteria (ECD-MBP) or genetic immunization but in both cases was followed by an in vitro priming period using ECD-MBP. In our first study (42), BALBc and NOD recipients were examined 16 days after transfer of syngeneic receptor primed T cells and both strains of mice displayed thyroiditis similar in phenotype to that induced in the donors using ECD-MBP, i.e. Th2 in the BALBc and Th1 with thyroid destruction in the NOD. Neither strain had developed antibodies to the receptor in the recipient animals at this early stage although these were present in the donor mice.

PROGRESS IN THE DEVELOPMENT OF MODELS OF GRAVES' OPHTHALMOPATHY

Whilst our animal studies were in progress, we and others were able to demonstrate TSHR transcripts and protein in the orbit, particularly in the adipose compartment (43-47).

Consequently in more recent experiments (48), to determine the kinetics of disease induced using unfractionated T cells and a CD4+ enriched population, the mouse orbits were also examined. In both BALBc and NOD recipients the Th2 and Th1 nature of induced thyroiditis respectively was confirmed and found to persist for the 12 week duration of the experiment. At 4 weeks, TSHR antibodies, including TBII, had been induced in both strains and these too persisted throughout the experiment. Changes in thyroid hormone levels were more difficult to evaluate, especially in the BALBc. In NOD recipients of TSHR primed T cells, thyroid hormone levels were reduced, as might be expected from the destructive thyroiditis induced in this strain. 4 weeks after transfer, BALBc recipients of TSHR primed and control non-primed T cells had reduced T4 levels which slowly recovered in the latter. At 8 and 12 weeks, some BALBc recipients of receptor primed T cells had increased T4, relative to the control non-primed recipients.

When examining the orbits, all of the NOD recipients of primed and non-primed cells, displayed normal histology with intact well organised muscle fibre architecture. BALBc orbits of primed (but not non-primed) T cells appeared strikingly different. The muscle fibres were disorganised and separated by periodic acid Schiff positive edema. There was accumulation of adipose tissue and infiltration by immune cells, especially mast cells. These changes were observed in 17 out of 25 (68%) BALBc recipients of receptor primed cells and did not correlate with TBII or T4 levels. However, orbital changes were observed only in mice having the most severe thyroiditis with 25-30% of the gland occupied by interstitium which also correlated with the most skewed Th2 response, B:T cell ratio 1.6-1.9 and IL-4:INF g ratio >2.5.

As mentioned above similar ocular changes, including infiltration by mast cells and macrophages, correlating with the most severe thyroiditis, have been induced by genetic immunization in approximately 20% of the NMRI outbred mice (36).

Currently we lack accurate *in vivo* assessment techniques of the modelled disease. Furthermore, with such small animals, whose skull anatomy lacks the rigid confines of the human orbit, measurement of proptosis is not helpful. In human GO, assessment is aided with computerised tomography (CT) or magnetic resonance imaging (MRI) allowing visualisation of muscle swelling, fat volume expansion and optic nerve compression. Fat suppression MRI techniques are able to differentiate inflammatory from chronic pathology of ocular muscles and can demonstrate changes that occur within orbital fat but in the absence of muscle enlargement (49). In view of this we have investigated orbital MRI as a possible tool for *in vivo* assessment. We see from our images (Figures 1 and 2) that it is possible to distinguish clearly the important structures of the ocular muscles and orbital fat pad where the bulk of the pathology can be demonstrated histologically. With the use of inhalational anaesthesia we will be able to follow changes within individual mice when examining attempts to attenuate disease activity.

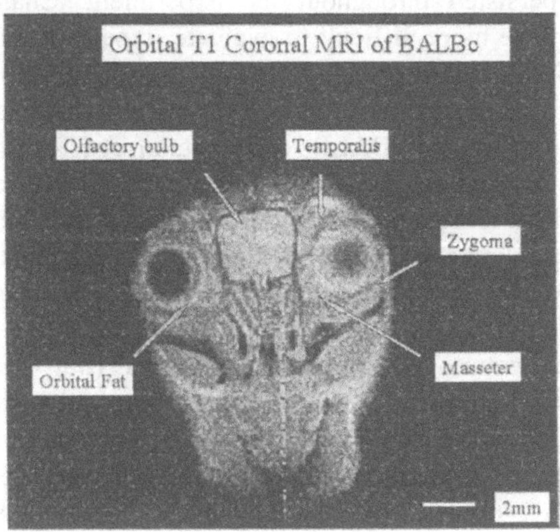

Figure 1.

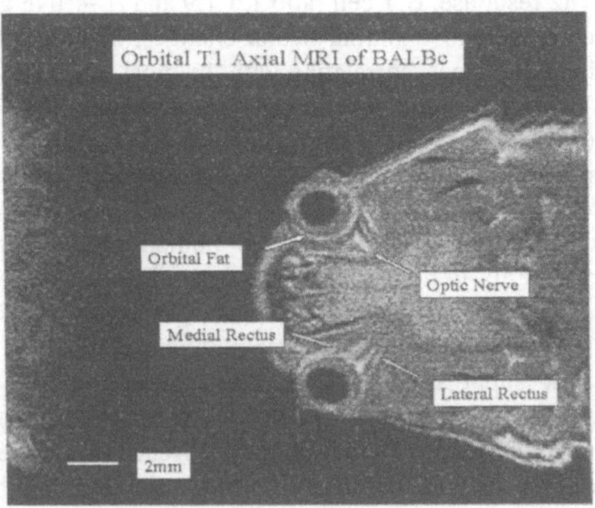

Figure 2.

CONCLUDING COMMENTS

A number of conclusions can be derived from these models. The induction of a GO-like disease using TSHR cDNA or primed T cells is further support for this antigen being an important target in GO as well as in GD. One might reason that release of other thyroid/orbit shared antigens or epitope spreading could occur in the inflammatory process leading to thyroiditis. The non-destructive nature of thyroiditis in BALBc mice argues against this as does the absence of ocular pathology in the NOD mice whose autoimmune response to the TSHR leads to thyroid destruction. Examination of the orbits, for signs of pathology, in mice from thyroiditis models induced with non-TSHR thyroid antigens could resolve this issue.

In the NMRI mice, analysis of their MHC haplotype revealed that they were predominantly H2q, irrespective of whether disease had been induced or not. This highlights the importance of non-MHC genes in the development of GD and also GO and will be a focus for future studies using this model.

In both models information about the involvement of sites outside the thyroid and orbit is limited. We have recently demonstrated that the TSHR is expressed in adipose depots outside the orbit in man (50). The high levels of expression in human GO orbital fat can be explained by an ongoing process of adipogenesis. However we have found that adipocyte differentiation in human non-orbital fat is also associated with increased TSHR expression as has been elegantly demonstrated in rodent fat cells and lines (51-53). Does this imply that edema, GAG and fat accumulation may be occurring in other extra-thyroidal locations? Further studies, of the type reported previously which both support (54) and refute (55) systemic disease, are required and the animal models will prove invaluable in this respect.

Finally the models imply that a Th2 autoimmune response to the receptor can result in GO. This has not been found to be the case in man since most studies have reported a Th1 spectrum of cytokines present in the orbit (56-58). An obvious difference derives from the ability to analyse the mouse disease at an earlier stage than would be possible in man. Of interest, one feature of the Th2 response i.e. the participation of mast cells, has been shown to induce prostaglandin synthesis and GAG production in human orbital fibroblasts, at least in vivo (59). Mast cells have been reported in human GO biopsies (60) but would warrant further investigation. Furthermore increases in circulating IgE, which could activate mast cells (61) and stem cell factor, a mast cell growth factor (62), have been reported in GD. We have not been able to demonstrate IgE antibodies to the TSHR (unpublished observations) but several alternative mechanisms are possible for mast cell activation.

The GO model based on transfer of TSHR primed T cells will be used to evaluate established and novel treatment strategies. We have recently succeeded in performing magnetic resonance imaging of the mouse orbit that will facilitate estimation of GO severity without sacrificing the animal for histological examination.

REFERENCES

1. Code CF & Essex HE. Am J Ophthalmol 1935; 18:1123.
2. Schockaert JA. Hyperplasia of Thyroid and Exophthalmos from treatment with anterior pituitary in young duck. Proc Soc Exp Biol Med 1932; 29:306-308.
3. Marine D, Spence AW, Cipra A. Production of goitre and exophthalmos in rabbits by administration of cyanide. Proc Soc Exp Biol Med 1932; 29:822-823.
4. Smelser GK. Experimental production of exophthalmos resembling that found in Graves' Disease. Proc Soc Exp Biol Med 1936; 35:128-130.
5. Paulson DL. Experimental exophthalmos in the guinea pig. Proc Soc Exp Biol Med 1937; 36:604-605.
6. Smelser GK. Am J Physiol 1943; 140:308.
7. Dobyns BM. The influence of thyroidectomy on the prominence of the eyes in the guinea pig and in man. Surg Gynecol Obstet 1945; 80:526-533.
8. DeRoux N, Polak M, Couet J, Leger J, Czernichow P, Milgrom E, Misrahi M. A neomutation in the thyroid stimulating hormone receptor in severe neonatal hyperthyroidism. J Clin Endocrinol Metab 1996; 81:2023-2026.
9. Furth ED, Becker DV, Ray BS, Kane JW. Appearance of unilateral infiltrative exophthalmos of Graves' Disease after the successful treatment of the same process in the contra-lateral eye by apparently total surgical hypophysectomy. J Clin Endocrinol Metab 1962; 22:518-524.
10. Winand RJ, Kohn LD. Relationship of thyrotropin to exophthalmos producing substance. J Biol Chem 1970; 245:967-975.
11. Kohn LD, Winand RJ. Structure of an exophthalmos producing factor derived from thyrotropin by partial trypsin digestion. J Biol Chem 1975; 250:6503-6508.
12. Winand RJ, Kohn LD. Retrobulbar modifications in experimental exophthalmos: the effect of thyrotropin and an exophthalmos producing substance derived from thyrotropin on the SO_4 incorporation and glycosaminoglycan content of Harderian gland. Endocrinology 1973; 93:670-680.
13. Valk TW, Taylor RE, Barker SB. Production and measurement of exophthalmos producing factor in guinea pigs. Endocrinology 1975; 96:151-159.
14. Vladitui A, Rose N. Autoimmune muirne thyroiditis. Relation to histocompatibility. (H-2) type. Science 1971; 174:1137-1140.
15. Maron R, Zerubavel R, Friedman A, Cohen I. T lymphocyte line specific for thyroglobulin produces or vaccinates against autoimmune thyroiditis. J Immunol 1983; 131:2316-2322.
16. Romball C, Weigle W. Transfer of experimental autoimmune thyroiditis with T cell clones. J Immunol 1987; 138:1092-1098.

17. Hutchings PR, Cooke A, Dawe K, Champion BR, Geysen M, Valerio R, Roitt IM. A thyroxine containing peptide can induce murine experimental autoimmune thyroiditis. J Exp Med 1992; 175:869-872.
18. Dobyns BM, Wright A, Wilson L. Assay of the exophthalmos producing substance in the serum of patients with progressive ophthalmopathy. J Clin Endocrinol Metab 1961; 21:648-662.
19. McKenzie JM. Delayed thyroid response to serum from thyrotoxic patients. Endocrinology 1958; 62:865-870.
20. Bartalena L, Marcocci C, Bogazzi F, Manetti L, Tanda M, DellUnto E, BrunoBossio G, Nardi M, Bartolomei M, Lepri A, Rossi G, Martino E, Pinchera A. Relationship between therapy for hyperthyroidism and the course of Graves' Ophthalmopathy. N Engl J Med. 1998; 338:73-78.
21. Paschke R, Ludgate M. The thyrotropin receptor and thyroid disease. N Engl J Med 1997; 337:1675-1681.
22. Marion S, Braun J, Ropars A, Kohn L, Charreire J. Induction of autoimmunity by immunization of mice with human thyrotropin receptor. Cell Immunol 1994; 158:329-341.
23. Ohmori M, Endo T, Onaya T. Development of chicken antibodies toward the human thyrotropin receptor and their bioactivities. Biochem Biophys Res Comm 1991; 174:399-403.
24. Endo T, Ohmori M, Ikeda M, Onaya T. Thyroid stimulating activity of rabbit antibodies towards the human thyrotropin receptor peptide. Biochem Biophys Res Comm 1991;177:145-150.
25. Sakata S, Ogawa T, Matsui I, Manshouri T, Atassi MZ. Biological activities of rabbit antibodies against synthetic human thyrotropin receptor peptides representing thyrotropin binding regions. Biochem Biophys Res Comm 1992; 182:1369-1375.
26. Hidaka Y, Guimaraes V, Soliman M, Yanagawa T, Okomoto Y, Quintans J, DeGroot L. Production of thyroid stimulating antibodies in mice by immunization with T cell epitopes of human receptor. Endocrinology 1995; 136:1642-1647.
27. Costagliola S, Alcalde L, Tonacchera M, Ruf J, Vassart G, Ludgate M. Induction of thyrotropin receptor (TSH-R) autoantibodies and thyroiditis in mice immunized with the recombinant TSH-R. Biochem Biophys Res Comm 1994; 199:1027-1034.
28. Costagliola S, Many MC, SalmansFalys M, Tonacchera M, Vassart G, Ludgate M. Recombinant thyrotropin receptor and the induction of autoimmune thyroid-disease in BALB/c mice - a new animal-model. Endocrinology 1994; 135:2150-2159.
29. Costagliola S, Many MC, StalmansFalys M, Vassart G, Ludgate M. Autoimmune-response induced by immunizing female mice with recombinant human thyrotropin receptor varies with the genetic background. Mol Cell Endocrinol 1995; 115:199-206.
30. Seetharamaiah GS, Dallas JS, Patibandla SA, Thotakura NR, Prabhakar BS. Requirement of glycosylation of the human thyrotropin receptor ectodomain for its reactivity with autoantibodies in patients' sera. J Immunol 1997; 158:2798-2804.
31. Wagle NM, Dallas JS, Seetharamaiah GS, Fan JL, Desai RK, Memar O, Rajaraman S, Prabhakar BS. Induction of hyperthyroxinemia in BALB/c but not in several other strains of mice. Autoimmunity 1994; 18:103-112.

32. Seetharamaiah GS, Desai RK, Dallas JS, Tahara K, Kohn LD, Prabhakar BS. Induction of TSH binding inhibitory immunoglobulins with the extracellular domain of the human thyrotropin receptor produced using baculovirus expression systems. Autoimmunity 1993; 14:315-320.
33. Davies TF, Bobovnikova Y, Weiss M, Vlase H, Moran T, Graves PN. Development and characterisation of monoclonal antibodies specific for the murine thyrotropin receptor. Thyroid 1998; 8:693-701.
34. Vlase H, Weiss M, Graves PN, Davies TF. Characterization of the murine immune response to the murine TSH receptor ectodomain: induction of hypothyroidism and TSH receptor antibodies. Clin Exp Immunol 1998; 113:111-118.
35. Costagliola S, Rodien P, Many MC, Ludgate M, Vassart G. Genetic immunization against the human thyrotropin receptor causes thyroiditis and allows production of monoclonal antibodies recognizing the native receptor. J Immunol 1998; 160:1458-1465.
36. Costagliola S, Many MC, Denef JF, Pohlenz J, Refetoff S, Vassart G. Genetic immunisation of outbred mice with thyrotropin receptor cDNA provides a model of Graves' disease. J Clin Invest 2000; 105:803-811.
37. Shimojo N, Kohno Y, Yamaguchi KI, Kikuoka S, Hoshioka A, Niimi H, Hirai A, Tamura Y, Saito Y,Kohn LD, Tahara K. Induction of Graves'-like disease in mice by immunization with fibroblasts transfected with the thyrotropin receptor and a class II molecule. Proc Natl Acad Sci USA 1996; 93:11074-11079.
38. Yamaguchi KI, Shimojo N, Kikuoka S, Hoshioka A, Hirai A, Tahara K, Kohn LD, Kohno Y, Niimi H. Genetic control of anti-thyrotropin receptor antibody generation in H-2 (K) mice immunized with thyrotropin receptor transfected fibroblasts. J Clin Endocrinol Metab 1997; 82:4266-4269.
39. Kikuoka S, Shimojo N, Yamaguchi KI, Watanabe Y, Hoshioka A, Hirai A, Saito Y, Tahara K, Kohn LD, Maruyama N, Kohno Y, Niimi H. The formation of thyrotropin receptor (TSHR) antibodies in a Graves' animal model requires the N-terminal segment of the TSHR extracellular domain. Endocrinology 1998; 139:1891-1898.
40. Kohn LD, Shimura H, Shimura Y. The thyrotropin receptor. Vitam Horm 1995; 50:287-384.
41. Kita M, Ahmad L, Marians RC, Vlase H, Unger P, Graves PN, Davies TF. Regulation and transfer of a murine model of thyrotropin receptor antibody mediated Graves' Disease. Endocrinology 1999; 140:1392-1398.
42. Costagliola S, Many MC, StalmansFalys M, Vassart G, Ludgate M. Transfer of thyroiditis, with syngeneic spleen-cells sensitized with the human thyrotropin receptor, to naive BALB/c and nod mice. Endocrinology 1996; 137:4637-4643.
43. Feliciello A, Porcellini A, Ciullo L, Bonavolonta G, Avvedimento E, Fenzi G. Expression of thyrotropin receptor mRNA in healthy and Graves' disease retro-orbital tissue. Lancet 1993; 342:337-338.
44. Paschke R, Vassart G, Ludgate M. Current evidence for and against the TSH receptor being the common antigen in Graves-disease and thyroid-associated ophthalmopathy. Clin Endocrinol 1995; 42:565-569
45. Crisp M, Lane C, Halliwell M, Wynford-Thomas D, Ludgate M. Thyrotropin Receptor Transcripts In Human Adipose Tissue. J Clin Endocrinol Metab 1997; 82:2003-2005.
46 Spitzweg C, Joba W, Hunt N, Heufelder AE. Analysis of Human Thyrotropin Receptor Gene Expression and Immunoreactivity in Human Orbital Tissue. Eur J Endocrinol 1997; 136:599-607.

47. Bahn R, Dutton C, Natt N, Joba W, Spitweg C, Heufelder A. Thyrotropin receptor expression in Graves' orbital adipose/connective tissues; potential autoantigen in Graves' Ophthalmopathy. J Clin Endocrinol Metab 1998; 83:998-1002.
48. Many MC, Costagliola S, Detrait M, Denef JF, Vassart G, Ludgate M. Development of an animal model of autoimmune Thyroid Eye Disease. J Immunol 1999; 162:4966-4974.
49. Laitt RD, Hoh B, Wakeley C, Kabala J, Harrad R, Potts M, Goddard P. The value of the short tau inversion recovery sequence in magnetic resonance imaging of thyroid eye disease. BJR 1994; 67:244-247.
50. Crisp M, Starkey K, Ham J, Lane C, Ludgate M. Adipogenesis in thyroid eye disease. Invest Ophthalmol Vis Sci 2000; *in press.*
51. Haraguchi K, Shimura H, Lin L, Saito T, Endo T, Onaya T. Functional expression of thyrotropin receptor in differentiated 3T3-L1 cells: A possible model cell line of extrathyroidal expression of thyrotropin receptor. Biochem Biophys Res Comm 1996; 223:193-198.
52. Haraguchi K, Shimura H, Lin L, Endo T, Onaya T. Differentiation of rat preadipocytes is accompanied by expression of thyrotropin receptors. Endocrinology 1996; 137:3200-3205.
53. Shimura H, Miyazaki A, Haraguchi K, Endo T, Onaya T. Analysis of differentiation induced expression mechanisms of thyrotropin receptor gene in adipocytes. Mol Endocrinol 1998; 12:1473-1486.
54. Hansen C, Fraiture B, Rouhi R, Otto E, Forster G, Kahaly G. HPLC Glycosaminoglycan analysis in patients with Graves' Disease. Clin Sci 1997; 92:511-515.
55. Peacey SR, Flemming L, Messenger A, Weetman AP. Is Graves' Dermopathy a generalised disorder? Thyroid 1996; 6:41-45.
56. Yang D, Hiromatsu Y, Hoshino T, Inoue Y, Itoh K, Nonaka K. Dominant infiltration of TH1-type CD4+ T cells at the retrobulbar space of patients with thyroid-associated ophthalmopathy. Thyroid 1999; 9:305-309.
57. Hiromatsu Y, Yang D, Bednarczuk T, Miyake I, Nonaka K, Inoue Y. Cytokine profiles in eye muscle tissue and orbital fat tissue from patients with thyroid-associated ophthalmopathy. J Clin Endocrinol Metab 2000; 85:1194-1199.
58. Aniszewski JP,Valyasevi RW, Bahn RS. Relationship between disease duration and predominant orbital T cell subset in Graves' ophthalmopathy. J Clin Endocrinol Metab 2000; 85:776-780.
59. Smith TJ, Parikh SJ. HMC-1 mast cells activate human orbital fibroblasts in coculture: Evidence for up-regulation of prostaglandin E_2 and Hyaluronan synthesis. Endocrinology 1999; 140:3518-3525.
60. Hufnagel TJ, Hickey WF, Cobbs WH, Jakobiec FA, Iwamoto T & Eagle RA. Immunohistochemical and ultrastructural studies on the exenterated orbital tissues of a patient with Graves' disease. Ophthalmology 1984; 91:1411-1419.
61. Sato A, Takemura Y, Yamada T, Ohtsuka N, Sakai K, Miyahara Y, Aizawa T, Terao A, Onuma S, Junun K, Kanamori A, Nakamura Y, Tejima E, Ito Y, Kamijo K. A possible role of immunoglobulin E in patients with hyperthyroid Graves' disease. J Clin Endocrinol Metab 1999; 84:3602-3605.
62. Yamada T, Sato A, Aizawa T, Ootsuka H, Miyahara Y, Sakai H, Terao A, Onuma S, Ito Y, Kanamori A, Nakamura Y & Tejima E. An Elevation of Stem Cell Factor in Patients with Hyperthyroid Graves' Disease. Thyroid 1998; 8:499-504.

6

PARTICIPATION OF ORBITAL FIBROBLASTS IN THE INFLAMMATION OF GRAVES' OPHTHALMOPATHY

Terry J. Smith
Division of Molecular Medicine, Harbor-UCLA Medical Center, Torrance, CA 90502 and Department of Medicine and the Jules Stein Eye Institute, University of California Los Angeles School of Medicine, Los Angeles, CA 90095

INTRODUCTION

Graves' ophthlamopathy (GO) is a disease process where the orbital connective tissue and musculature undergo a complex remodeling. Certain aspects of the tissue changes associated with GO are unusual, such as the disordered accumulation of the glycosaminoglycan, hyaluronan (1). Other changes resemble several other diseases inside and distant from the orbit. In early GO, the muscles and fat/connective tissue are inflamed and this inflammation appears to be driven through the infiltration of bone marrow-derived cells including lymphocytes and mast cells (2). It is this population of recruited cells that is currently believed to be the source of pro-inflammatory cytokines that provoke in orbital fibroblasts the expression of several important lipid mediators and cytokines. Later, scar formation is common and probably leads to the irreversible damage seen in advanced disease. We hypothesize that the unusual phenotype of the orbital fibroblast underlies the particular susceptibility of the orbit to the inflammatory reaction and tissue remodeling that are characteristic of GO. Specifically, it would appear that orbital fibroblast activation is a critical step in the pathogenesis of GO and many of the aspects of the disease can be attributed directly to the phenotype of these cells. In this chapter, I will briefly review those aspects of orbital fibroblast biology which appear to set these cells apart from fibroblasts residing in other anatomic regions of the human body and render them particularly adept at mediating inflammation and fibrosis.

ORBITAL FIBROBLASTS ARE HETEROGENEOUS AND EXHIBIT A DISTINCTIVE MORPHOLOGY

In culture, fibroblasts from most tissues faithfully maintain their phenotype. They proliferate for a finite number of population doublings and then become senescent. The shape of fibroblasts derived from orbital tissue differs from that of dermal fibroblasts (3). Orbital fibroblasts are fusiform (spindle shaped with two or three dendritic processes) or angular, with three or more cytoplasmic processes and exhibit a stellate shape. The perinuclear cytoplasmic areas contain prominent granular features. Dermal fibroblasts, in contrast, are largely angular cells, the cytoplasm of which is generally less granular. When the fine structure of orbital fibroblasts was examined using transmission electron microscopy, it exhibited extensive thin cytoplasmic processes (4). The perinuclear cytoplasm contains multiple assemblies of Golgi membranes, modest amounts of rough endoplasmic reticulum, intermediate filaments and many lysosome-like structures. Glycogen deposits are found in the perinuclear areas and in thin processes. Thus they have similar ultrastructural features to those of other fibroblast types.

When orbital fibroblasts are exposed to PGE_2, they undergo a dramatic change in cell morphology and this effect can be attenuated with serum (5). The action of PGE_2 is stereospecific and appears to be mediated through the binding and activation of EP_2 prostaglandin receptors (6). It involves the generation of cyclic adenosine monophosphate and is transient. The shape-change is far more pronounced in fibroblasts from patients with GO than in those with normal orbital connective tissue. Moreover, dermal fibroblasts harvested from normal appearing skin fail to respond substantially to PGE_2 in this manner.

The varied appearance of orbital fibroblasts in a typical culture suggested that discrete populations of cells might exist. Moreover, some biochemical parameter might be found that would help characterize these populations further. Thy-1 is a glycoprotein that is displayed on the surface of several cell types and is involved in the transduction of extracellular signals. Dermal fibroblasts uniformly express and display Thy-1. Orbital fibroblasts were also found to express Thy-1 but not uniformly (7). When they were analyzed by flow cytometry, approximately 50% were found to recognize an anti-Thy-1 antibody. The two phenotypes could be separated by cell sorting. When each subset was then subjected to culture, the phenotypes were maintained over several population doublings. In murine lung fibroblast cultures, a similar pattern of Thy-1 expression was found and each was associated with a different pattern of IL-1α and IL-1ß expression (8). Whether this will be the case in human orbital cultures has yet to be determined. But the role of Thy-1 in cell signaling suggests that Thy-1^+ cells may have a very different set of roles in normal and pathological function than those not expressing the glycoprotein. A subpopulation of orbital fibroblasts retains the potential to undergo adipogenic differentiation in long-term culture (9). When incubated in culture medium containing, among other factors, insulin, transferrin, PGI_2, isobutylmethylxanthone and dexamethasone, 5-10% of the cells accumulate cytoplasmic droplets containing triacylglycerol as assessed by Oil Red O staining (9). In contrast, dermal fibroblasts fail to undergo differentiation under the same culture conditions.

THE INDUCTION OF KEY PRO-INFLAMMATORY GENES AND THEIR PRODUCTS IS EXAGGERATED IN ORBITAL FIBROBLASTS, ESPECIALLY THOSE FROM PATIENTS WITH GO

Several laboratory groups have been engaged in a systemic examination of various aspects of the phenotype exhibited by orbital fibroblasts. While orbital fibroblasts appear to express most of the same genes and display similar metabolic patterns to those from outside the orbit, there appears to be a common theme emerging from many of the studies thus far completed. Orbital cells express a profile of gangliosides (10) and receptors (11) that potentially facilitate their participation in tissue remodeling and inflammation. Unlike some other fibroblasts, they express endothelin receptors and respond to endothelin (11). This is noteworthy because that polypeptide has been implicated in the initiation of inflammatory responses and as an important signaling mechanism between endothelial cells and components of the interstitium. It would seem that orbital cultures, especially those from patients with GO, are particularly susceptible to the actions of pro-inflammatory cytokines such as interferon-γ, IL-1α, ILα-1ß and leukoregulin. With regard to interferon-γ, the cytokine induces HLA-DR expression dramatically in orbital and pretibial fibroblasts from patients with GO and the magnitude is considerably greater than that observed in normal orbital or skin fibroblasts or fibroblasts from irrelevant regions of patients with Graves' disease (12). IL-1 and CD154 can induce the expression of IL-6 and IL-8 in orbital fibroblasts (13). These inductions are apparently mediated through the activation of the NF-κB transcriptional factor (13). The levels of both chemokines are very high following fibroblast activation and suggest a potentially important pathway through which fibroblasts could signal and activate immunologically competent cells.

An important aspect of the immune response relates to the synthesis and action of PGE_2. This prostanoid is the product of a cascade involved in the conversion of arachidonate to a variety of bioactive lipids. The rate-limiting steps in the synthesis of PGE_2 are catalyzed by prostaglandin endoperoxide H synthase, a membrane-associated enzyme which is expressed as two isoforms, each encoded by a separate gene. IL-1 and leukoregulin induce the inflammatory cyclooxygenase, PGHS-2 or COX-2, in GO orbital fibroblasts (Figure 1) (14,15). The magnitude of the response is many fold greater than that occurring in parallel studies with normal orbital fibroblasts or dermal fibroblasts (14). This induction is isoform-specific in that the level of PGHS-1 (the constitutive enzyme) expression is unaltered. Moreover, the levels of PGE_2 production following treatment with these cytokines is dramatically increased (Figure 1) and the up-regulation in prostanoid synthesis can be completely inhibited with SC58125, a PGHS-2-specific competitive inhibitor.

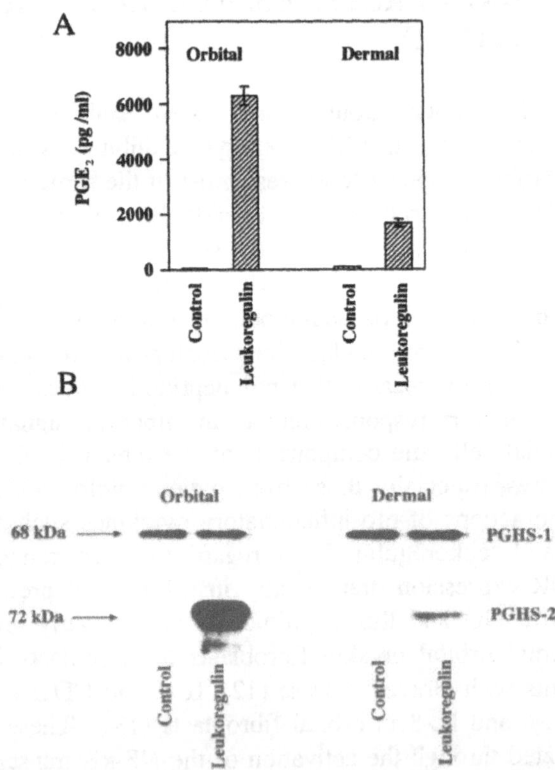

Figure 1. Leukoregulin induces PGE_2 synthesis (A) and prostaglandin endoperoxide H synthase-2 protein (B) in fibroblasts. The magnitude of induction is considerably greater in GO orbital fibroblasts than in dermal cultures. Reprinted from Cao and Smith with permission (16).

The induction of PGHS-2 in orbital fibroblasts involves an up-regulation of the steady-state levels of PGHS-2 mRNA. This transcript migrates as a 5 kb band on northern analysis (Figure 2). Under standard basal culture conditions, orbital fibroblasts from normal tissue and those derived from patients with GO fail to express detectable levels of PGHS-2 mRNA. In contrast, PGHS-1 mRNA which appears in these cells as a 5.2 kb band, is abundant under untreated conditions and is generally invariant with cytokine exposure. When the fibroblasts are treated with IL-1ß or leukoregulin, PGHS-2 mRNA achieves extraordinary levels (14). The magnitude of this induction is probably several-hundred fold and is transient. Levels generally peak at 6-12 hr. and then begin to decline. It would appear, on the basis of nuclear runon studies, that PGHS-2 gene transcription is up-regulated by pro-inflammatory cytokines 2-3 fold above baseline (Figure 3) (14). The human PGHS-2 promoter contains two recognizable NF-κB sites. When GO orbital fibroblasts are treated with leukoregulin, the cytokine induces the translocation of both p50/p50 and p50/p65 dimers to the nucleus (16). Moreover, the induction of PGHS-2 is attenuated with the NF-κB inhibitor, pyrrolidinedithiocarbamate (PDTC) (Figure 2).

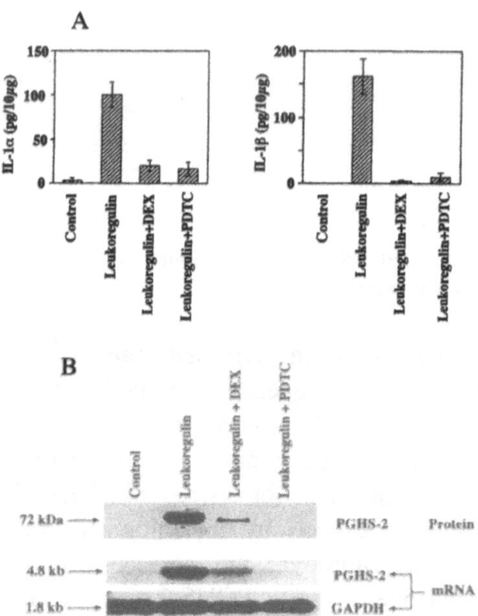

Figure 2. Leukoregulin induces the steady-state levels of PGHS-2 mRNA, IL-1α and IL-1ß protein. These actions can be blocked by inhibition of NF-κB with PDTC. Reprinted from Cao and Smith with permission (16).

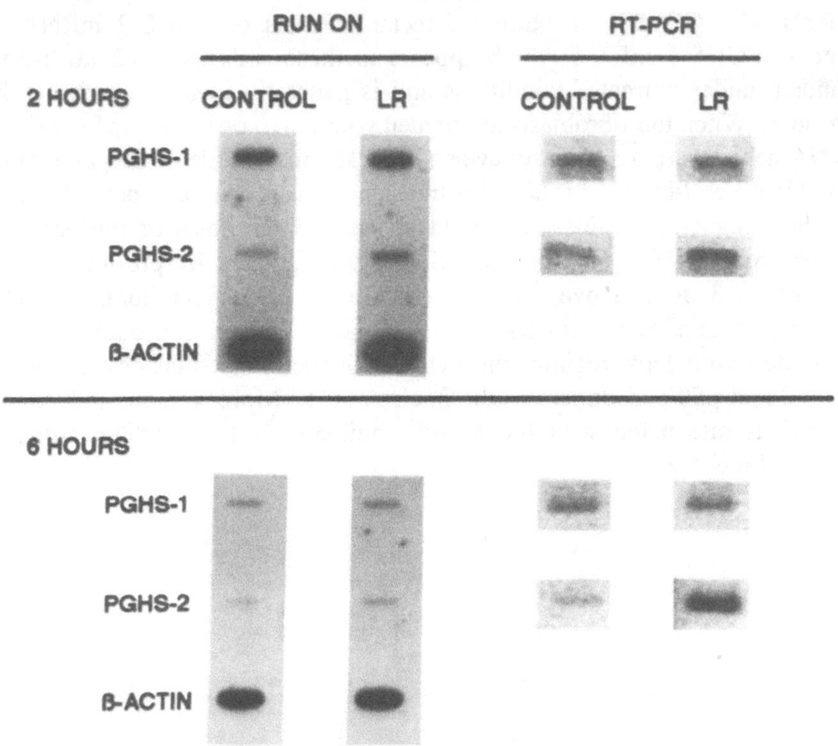

Figure 3. Leukoregulin induces PGHS-2 gene transcription in GO orbital fibroblasts by 2-3 fold. Reprinted from Wang et al with permission (14).

The steady-state levels are increased many fold above the fractional increases in gene transcription, suggesting that PGHS-2 mRNA stability might be enhanced substantially by the cytokines. Indeed, the $T_{1/2}$ is greatly increased (Figure 4) (16) and thus cytokine enhancement of transcript stability represents the major mechanism for increased PGHS-2 expression. The induction is blocked almost entirely by physiologically relevant concentrations of glucocorticoids (14-16). Moreover, the increase in PGE_2 production is also blocked by dexamethasone. While PGHS-2 and its activity are increased following cytokine treatment and inhibited by the actions of glucocorticoids, PGHS-1 mRNA, protein and prostanoid production attributable to the isoform are unaffected by these agents, consistent with the proposed physiological role for PGHS-1 as a "housekeeping" enzyme.

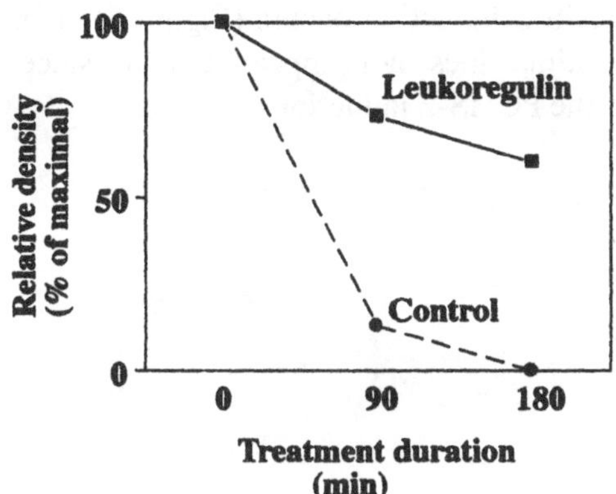

Figure 4. Leukoregulin enhances PGHS-2 mRNA stability in GO orbital fibroblasts. Reprinted from Cao and Smith with permission (16).

The finding that GO fibroblasts exhibit particularly robust PGHS-2 inductions and that these cells, when provoked by cytokines, produce large amounts of PGE_2, is noteworthy. PGE_2 biases the differentiation of naive (Th_0) T lymphocytes toward the Th_2 phenotype at the expense of Th_1 cell development. Moreover, PGE_2 is an important determinant of B cell maturation and influences mast cell activation. It can induce IL-5 synthesis in some lymphocytes while decreasing IL-2 transcript levels in others. Thus in the setting of inflammation in the orbit, the fibroblast by virtue of its capacity to generate PGE_2 can modify the cytokine environment and the make-up of infiltrating cell populations, thus modulating the nature of tissue remodeling occurring in the orbit.

THE BASIS FOR THE EXAGGERATED RESPONSES TO LEUKOREGULIN AND IL-1 IN GO ORBITAL FIBROBLASTS MAY RESIDE, AT LEAST IN PART, IN A DEFECTIVE IL-1 RECEPTOR ANTAGONIST RESPONSE

The induction of PGHS-2 mRNA in orbital fibroblasts by cytokines such as IL-1ß and leukoregulin may be mediated through the intermediate up-regulation of other proteins, as is suggested by a partial susceptibility to cycloheximide blockade (14). A number of proteins are induced by leukoregulin, including IL-1. PGHS-2 induction by leukoregulin appears dependent on endogenous IL-1 expression. When leukoregulin-treated GO fibroblasts are incubated with high concentrations of exogenous IL-1 receptor antagonist (IL-1ra) or specific IL-1α neutralizing antibodies, substantial attenuation of the PGHS-2 induction occurs (Figure 5) (16). IL-1ß, while also induced by leukoregulin, does not appear critical since neutralizing that cytokine fails to alter the PGHS-2 induction.

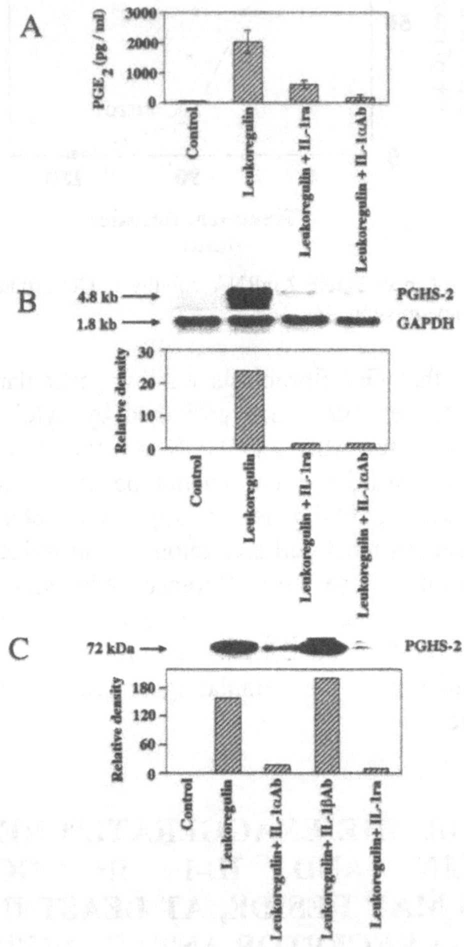

Figure 5. Anti-IL-1Ab and exogenous IL-1ra block inductions by leukoregulin of (A) PGE_2, (B) PGHS-2 mRNA and (C) protein. Reprinted from Cao and Smith with permission (16).

The exaggerated induction of PGHS-2 observed in orbital fibroblasts, particularly in GO orbital fibroblasts, may be related to cytokine actions upstream of the cyclooxygenase. While these fibroblasts, derived from patients with the disease, manifest extraordinary IL-1α and IL-1ß responses, the upregulation of IL-1ra in these cells is considerably less robust than that found in normal cells (16). This diminished level of IL-1ra might underlie the substantial differences in the levels of PGHS-2 achieved following treatment with IL-1 or leukoregulin. While the nature of the defect has not been elucidated, it would help explain the dramatic differences in response to exogenous IL-1 and the cytokines that utilize intermediate IL-1 expression in the intracellular signaling.

CYTOKINE-ACTIVATED ORBITAL FIBROBLASTS SYNTHESIZE HIGH LEVELS OF HYALURONAN AND EXPRESS THREE HYALURONAN SYNTHASE ISOFORMS AND THE UDP GLUCOSE DEHYDROGENASE MRNAS

The most unusual aspect of the tissue remodeling associated with GO is the disordered accumulation of the glycosaminoglycan, hyaluronan. This increase in hyaluronan content has substantial implications for the function of the orbital contents by virtue of its great water binding capacity. Because the orbit is confined by the dimensions of the bony limits, expansion of orbital volume forces the anterior displacement of the contents and increased intraocular pressure. One issue awaiting definition is the mechanism through which the increased hyaluronan content occurs. The question of whether abnormal synthesis or degradation of hyaluronan accounts for the accumulation has yet to be addressed adequately.

Among the early studies utilizing orbital fibroblasts in culture were those assessing their capacity to synthesize glycosaminoglycans such as hyaluronan. Interferon-γ can increase the synthesis of hyaluronan modestly in orbital fibroblasts (17). This effect is not found in dermal fibroblasts. IL-1ß and leukoregulin induce glycosaminoglycan production far more robustly and this action is of a considerably greater magnitude in orbital fibroblasts than in cells from other anatomic areas (18). In a typical study, leukoregulin induced hyaluronan levels by as much as 15-fold above baseline while the cytokine induced hyaluronan less than half as much in dermal cultures (Figure 6). The increase in hyaluronan accumulation is the result of increased synthesis on the basis of pulse-chase studies and can be partially blocked by glucocorticoids (18). Unlike the effects on hyaluronan, incorporation of [^{35}S]sulfuric acid is uninfluenced suggesting that the production of chondroitin sulfate, dermatan sulfate and heparan sulfate production is not altered.

The expression and cytokine-inducibility of all three HAS family members in orbital fibroblasts has recently been examined. While the induction of HAS1 and HAS3 mRNAs appeared to be restricted to certain culture strains,

HAS2 mRNA was invariably expressed at relatively high levels in all fibroblasts tested following treatment with IL-1ß (19). The induction was time-dependent and related to the density of the cultures at the time of cytokine challenge. Moreover, using an antibody directed specifically at HAS2, western analysis confirmed the enzyme protein was also induced by IL-1ß. The overall abundance of HAS2 mRNA was greater than that of the other isoforms on the basis of relative signal strength on northern analysis. The induction of HAS2 mRNA was partially susceptible to treatment with cycloheximide, suggesting that intermediate protein induction(s) may be involved in the upregulation of the HAS2 transcript. They were blocked substantially by dexamethasone.

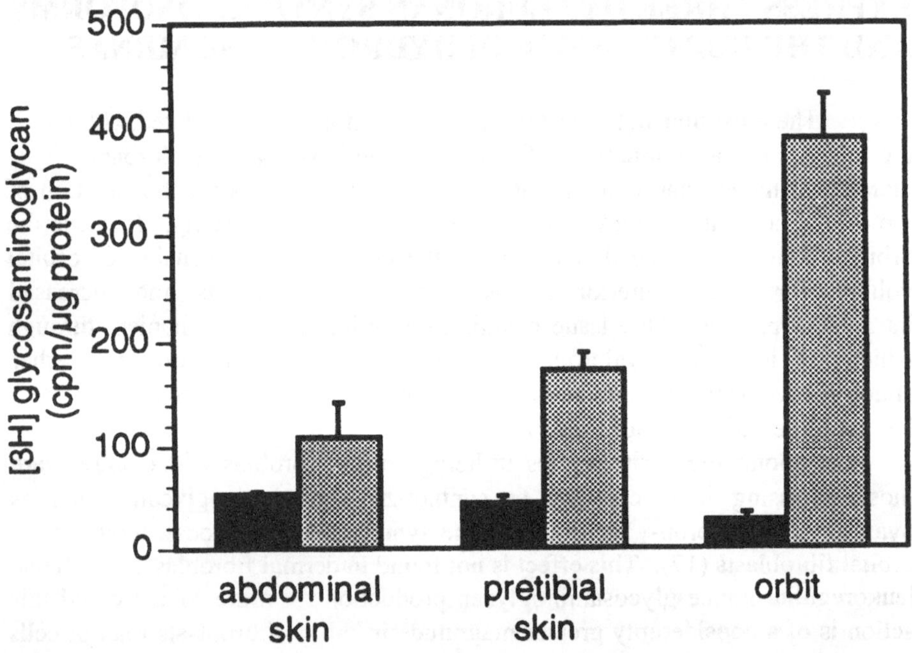

Figure 6. Leukoregulin induces hyaluronan synthesis dramatically in orbital fibroblasts. The magnitude of the upregulation is greater than in dermal cultures. From Smith et al, with permission (18).

UDP-glucose dehydrogenase is inducible in orbital fibroblasts treated with IL-1ß (20). This is important because it suggests that an enzymatic step upstream of the HAS family can also be regulated. UDP-glucose dehydrogenase is involved in the conversion of UDP glucose to UDP glucuronate. This is a critical step in the synthesis of hyaluronan as well as chondroitin sulfate and heparan sulfate. It remains to be determined whether any of the key enzymes in the glycosaminoglycan synthetic pathways are expressed or regulated in a manner that differs in orbital and non-orbital fibroblasts.

ORBITAL FIBROBLASTS DISPLAY CELL-SURFACE CD40 AND WHEN LIGATED WITH CD154, THIS RECEPTOR INITIATES FIBROBLAST ACTIVATION

CD40, a cell surface determinant first recognized on B lymphocytes (21), is expressed on the surface of orbital fibroblasts regardless of whether they were harvested from patients with GO or were obtained from normal orbital connective tissue (13). CD40 is a member of the tumor necrosis factor- (TNF-) receptor superfamily of proteins and in the B cell serves a critical role in immunological activation. It has been found to be displayed on epithelial and endothelial cells. CD40 itself is activated through the binding of CD40 ligand (CD154) which is expressed by T lymphocytes, mast cells, platelets and probably many other types of cells. When cells expressing the CD40 receptor are engaged by CD154, a number of genes are activated. Fibroblasts from several areas of the body frequently involved with autoimmune disease, such as the lung and synovial lining, have been shown to express CD40. Ligation of the receptor can culminate in the upregulation of multiple down-stream targets. With regard to orbital fibroblasts, the synthesis of IL-6 and IL-8 has been shown to be induced (13). This activation of cytokine expression has been associated with NF-κB translocation. The CD40/CD154 bridge also activates the expression of PGHS-2 in orbital and lung fibroblasts and this action involves an intermediate induction of IL-1 (22,23). Interruption of the IL-1 pathway, either by neutralizing the cytokine with an antibody specific for it or by adding high concentrations of exogenous IL-1ra, results in a substantial blockade of the CD40-dependent activation of cyclooxygenase expression (23). Associated with the increase in PGHS-2 levels are elevations of PGE_2 production. Hyaluronan synthesis is also increased through the CD40/CD154 bridge in orbital fibroblasts (23). This upregulation, unlike that of the prostanoid biosynthetic pathway, is apparently not dependent on IL-1 induction. It would appear that multiple NF-κB dimers may be involved in the induction of PGHS-2 by CD40 ligation: both p50/p65 heterodimer and p65/p65 homodimer forms of the transcriptional factor are translocated to the nucleus following CD40 ligation and the induction of PGHS-2 can be attenuated with inhibitors of the NF-κB activation (22,23). Moreover, the mitogen activated protein kinase pathway has been implicated in the intracellular signaling utilized by the CD40/CD154 receptor/ligand pair in the activation of PGHS-2 gene expression.

Finding functional CD40 expressed on orbital fibroblasts, as well as fibroblasts from other anatomic areas frequently involved in autoimmune inflammation, has important implications. It suggests a previously unrecognized mechanism through which non-immune cells can "cross-talk" with lymphocytes and potentially activate both cells. Moreover the strategies currently under development for interrupting the CD40/CD154 bridge could represent important therapeutic opportunities for modifying the natural course of GO and other autoimmune diseases. The restricted expression of CD40 on fibroblasts from particular anatomic regions or on fibroblast subsets in certain tissues could underlie the peculiar distribution of connective tissue disease manifestations.

HUMAN FIBROBLASTS FROM SEVERAL ANATOMIC REGIONS EXPRESS FUNCTIONAL TSH RECEPTORS

The key autoantigen expressed by the thyrocyte that is directly relevant to the pathogenesis of Graves' disease is the thyrotropin receptor (TSHr). It was thus a logical progression to examine the expression of the TSHr in orbital tissues and fibroblasts. The working hypothesis tested was that TSHr expression is anatomically restricted to those tissues manifesting Graves' disease but absent in tissues not usually involved. This receptor distribution might explain the pattern of disease. Indeed, Feliciello *et al* reported the detection of TSHr mRNA in normal orbital tissues as well as those affected by GO (24). Those measurements were made using non-quantitative PCR and thus some concerns were expressed over the validity of that study. Subsequently, several other groups have verified the presence of TSHr transcripts and protein, using several techniques (25-28). Early reports also demonstrated that TSHr mRNA was expressed by cultured orbital fibroblasts (29) and these important observations have been confirmed by later reports (30-32) and included the detection of receptor protein in those cells. A very recent report by Bell *et al* has provided evidence that functional TSHr is expressed by cells of the preadipocyte/fibroblast lineage from anatomic areas not implicated in Graves' disease such as abdominal wall fat and the omentum (33). The authors of that study demonstrated that when preadipocytes are treated with TSH, the $p70^{S6k}$ pathway is activated. This is noteworthy because the Akt/$p70^{S6k}$ pathway, important for signaling a number of down-stream targets involved in protein translation, has been established as a mediator of some TSH-dependent events in thyrocytes (34). Thus, the anatomic distribution of TSHr expression by fibroblasts does not appear to explain the pattern of disease manifestations. The peculiar targeting of the orbit and skin of the leg may rather relate to potential functional differences in the TSHr in various fibroblast subpopulations. This might involve tissue-specific utilization of intracellular signaling pathways. Alternatively, the distribution of the receptor may be unrelated to the pattern of disease manifestations. Assessment of the relative merits of these possibilities will necessarily await further studies examining the relationship between the TSHr and the immune system.

SUMMARY

Orbital fibroblasts exhibit a phenotype that sets them apart from other fibroblasts. In particular orbital fibroblasts from patients with severe GO are particularly responsive to proinflammatory cytokines and ligation of the CD40/CD154 bridge. When activated, these fibroblasts express a set of genes and their products that may play important roles in the inflammatory response found in GO. Moreover, orbital fibroblasts participate in tissue remodeling that can culminate in scar formation and muscle dysfunction. This activity derives from the wide array of molecules they can express, some of them structural. Others can participate in the recruitment of lymphocytes and other immunocompetent cells to the orbit (35). Some of the lipid mediators synthesized by these fibroblasts are known to bias the development of lymphocytes. Recognition of the contribution of the fibroblast in conditioning the orbital response to immune reactivity in the orbit may allow us to formulate effective strategies for interrupting the natural course of GO thereby limiting the morbidity associated with it.

ACKNOWLEDGEMENTS

I am grateful to the dedicated members of my laboratory group and to my many collaborators whose hard work is summarized here. This work was supported in part by grants RO1 EY8976 and RO1 011708 from the National Institutes of Health and by a Merit Review award from the Research Service of the Department of Veterans Affairs.

REFERENCES

1. Smith, T.J., Bahn, R.S., and Gorman, C.A. Connective tissue, glycosaminoglycans, and diseases of the thyroid. Endocrine Rev 1989; 10:366-391.
2. Hufnagel, T.J., Hickey, W.F., Cobbs, W.H., Jakobiec, F.A., Iwamoto, T., and Eagle, R.C. Immunohistochemical and ultrastructural studies on the exenterated orbital tissues of a patient with Graves' disease. Ophthalmol 1984; 91:1411-1419.
3. Smith, T.J., Bahn, R.S., and Gorman, C.A. Hormonal regulation of hyaluronate synthesis in cultured human fibroblasts: evidence for differences between retroocular and dermal fibroblasts. J Clin Endocrinol Metab 1989; 69:1019-1023.
4. Henrikson, R.C., and Smith, T.J. Ultrastructure of cultured orbital fibroblasts. Cell Tissue Res 1994; 278:629-631.
5. Smith, T.J., Wang, H.-S., Hogg, M.G., Henrikson, R.C., Keese, C.R., and Giaever, I. Prostaglandin E_2 elicits a morphological change in cultured orbital fibroblasts from patients with Graves ophthalmopathy. Proc Natl Acad Sci USA 1994; 91:5094-5098.
6. Wang, H.-S., Keese, C.R., Giaever, I., and Smith, T.J. Prostaglandin E_2 alters human orbital fibroblast shape through a mechanism involving the generation of cyclic adenosine monophosphate. J. Clin Endocrinol Metab 1995; 80:3553-3560.
7. Smith, T.J., Sempowski, G.D., Wang, H.-S., Del Vecchio, P.J., Lippe, S.D., and Phipps, R.P. Evidence for cellular heterogeneity in primary cultures of human orbital fibroblasts. J Clin Endocrinol Metab 1995; 80:2620-2625.
8. Phipps, R.P., Baecher, C., Frelinger, J.G., Penney, D.P., Keng, P., and Brown, D. Differential expression interleukin 1 by Thy-1^+ and Thy-1^- lung fibroblast subpopulations: enhancement of interleukin 1 production by tumor necrosis factor-. Eur J Immunol 1990; 20:1723-1727.
9. Sorisky, A., Pardasani, D., Gagnon, A., and Smith, T.J. Evidence for adipocyte differentiation in human orbital fibroblasts in primary culture. J. Clin. Endocrinol. Metab 1996; 81:3428-3431.
10. Berenson, C.S. and Smith, T.J. Human orbital fibroblasts in culture express ganglioside profiles distinct from those in dermal fibroblasts. J Clin Endocrinol 1995; 80:2668-2674.
11. Smith, T.J., Kottke, R.J., Lum, H., and Andersen, T.T. Human orbital fibroblasts in culture bind and respond to endothelin. Am J Physiol 1993; 265:C138-C142.
12. Heufelder, A.E., Smith, T.J., Gorman, C.A., and Bahn, R.S. Increased induction of HLS-DR by interferon-γ in cultured fibroblasts derived from patients with Graves' ophthalmopathy and pretibial dermopathy. J Clin Endocrinol Metab 1991; 73:307-313.
13. Sempowski, G.D., Rozenblit, J., Smith, T.J., and Phipps, R.P. Human orbital fibroblasts are activated through CD40 to induce proinflammatory cytokine production. Am J Physiol 1998; 274:C707-C714.
14. Wang, H.-S., Cao, H.J., Winn, V.D., Rezanka, L.J., Frobert, Y., Evans, C.H., Sciaky, D., Young, D.A., and Smith, T.J. Leukoregulin induction of prostaglandin-endoperoxide H synthase-2 in human orbital fibroblasts. An in vitro model for connective tissue inflammation. J Biol Chem 1986; 271:22718-22728.
15. Young, D.S., Evans, C.H., and Smith, T.J. Leukoregulin induction of protein expression in human orbital fibroblasts: evidence for anatomical site-restricted cytokine-target cell interactions. Proc Natl Acad Sci USA 1998; 95:8904-8909.

16. Cao, H.J., and Smith, T.J. Leukoregulin upregulation of prostaglandin endoperoxide H synthase-2 expression in human orbital fibroblasts. Am J Physiol 1999; 277:C1075-C1085.
17. Smith, T.J., Bahn, R.S., Gorman, C.A., and Cheavens, M. Stimulation of glycosaminoglycan accumulation by interferon gamma in cultured human retrocular fibroblasts. J Clin Endocrinol Metab 1991; 72:1169-1171.
18. Smith, T.J., Wang, H.-S., and Evans, C.H. Leukoregulin is a potent inducer of hyaluronan synthesis in cultured human orbital fibroblasts. Am J Physiol 1995; 268:C382-C388.
19. Kaback, L.A., and Smith, T.J. Expression of hyaluronan synthase messenger ribonucleic acids and their induction by interleukin-1ß in human orbital fibroblasts: potential insight into the molecular pathogenesis of thyroid-associated ophthalmopathy. J Clin Endocrinol Metab 1999; 84:4079-4084.
20. Spicer, A.P., Kaback, L.A., Smith, T.J., and Seldin, M.F. Molecular cloning and characterization of the human and mouse UDP-glucose dehydrogenase genes. J Biol Chem 1998; 273:25117-25124.
21. Banchereau, J., Bazan, F., Blanchard, D., Brière, F., Galizzi, J.P., van Kooten, C., Liu, Y.J., Rousset, F., and Saeland, S. The CD40 antigen and its ligand. Ann Rev Immunol 1994; 12:881-922.
22. Zhang, Y., Cao, H.J., Graf, B., Meekins, H., Smith, T.J., and Phipps, R.P. Cutting edge. CD40 engagement up-regulates cyclooxygenase-2 expression and prostaglandin E_2 production in human lung fibroblasts. J Immunol 1998; 160:1053-1057.
23. Cao, H.J., Wang, H.-S., Zhang, Y., Lin, H.-Y., Phipps, R.P., and Smith, T.J. Activation of human orbital fibroblasts through CD40 engagement results in a dramatic induction of hyaluronan synthesis and prostaglandin endoperoxide H synthase-2 expression. J Biol Chem 1998; 273:29615-29625.
24. Feliciello, A., Porcellini, A, Ciullo, I., Bonavolonta, G., Avvedimento, E.V., and Fenzi, G. Expression of thyrotropin receptor mRNA in healthy and Graves' disease retro-orbital tissue. Lancet 1993; 342:337-338.
25. Wu, S.-L., Yang, C.-S.J., Wang, H.-J., Liao, C.-L., Chang, T.-J., and Chang, T.-C. Demonstration of thyrotropin receptor mRNA in orbital fat and eye muscle tissues from patients with Graves' ophthalmopathy by in situ hybridization. J Endocrinol Invest 1999; 22:289-295.
26. Crisp, M.S., Lane, C., Hallwell, M, Wynford-Thomas, D., and Ludgate, M. Thyrotropin receptor transcripts in human adipose tissue. J Clin Endocrinol Metab 1997; 82:2003-2005.
27. Spitzweg, C., Joba, W., Hunt, N., and Heufelder, A.E. Analysis of human thyrotropin receptor gene expression and immunoreactivity in human orbital tissue. Eur J Endocrinol 1997; 136:599-607.
28. Bahn, R.S., Dutton, C.M., Natt, N., Joba, W., Spitzweg, C., and Heufelder, A.E. Thyrotropin receptor expression in Graves' orbital adipose/connective tissues: potential autoantigen in Graves' ophthalmopathy. J Clin Endocrinol Metab 1998; 83:998-1002.
29. Heufelder, A.E., Dutton, C.M., Sarkar, G., Donovan, K.A., and Bahn, R.S. Detection of TSH receptor RNA in cultured fibroblasts from patients with Graves' ophthalmopathy and pretibial dermopathy. Thyroid 1993; 3:297-300.
30. Mengistu, M., Lukes, Y.G., Nagy, E.V., Burch, H.B., Carr, F.E., Lahiri, S., Burman, K.D. TSH receptor expression in retroocular fibroblasts. J Endocrinol Invest 1994; 17:437-441.

31. Burch, H.B., Sellitti, D., Barnes, S., Nagy, E.V., Bahn, R.S., and Burman, K.D. Thyrotropin receptor antisera for the detection of immunoreactive protein species in retroocular fibroblasts obtained from patients with Graves' ophthalmopathy. J Clin Endocrinol Metab 1994; 78:1384-1391.
32. Valyasevi, R.W., Erickson, D.Z., Harteneck, D.A., Dutton, C.M., Heufelder, A.E., Jyonouchi, S.C., and Bahn, R.S. Differentiation of human orbital preadipocyte fibroblasts induces expression of functional thyrotropin receptor. J Clin Endocrinol Metab 1999; 84:2257-2262.
33. Bell, A., Gagnon, A., Grunder, L., Parikh, S.J., Smith, T.J., and Sorisky, A. Functional TSH receptor in human abdominal preadipocytes and orbital fibroblasts. Am J Physiol 2000; 279:C335-C340.
34. Cass, L.A., and Meinkoth, J.L. Differential effects of cyclic adenosine 3',5'-monophosphate on p70 ribosomal S6 kinase. Endocrinol 1998; 139:1991-1998.
35. Smith, R.S., Smith, T.J., Blieden, T.M., and Phipps, R.P. Fibroblasts as sentinel cells. Synthesis of chemokines and regulation of inflammation. Am J Pathol 1997; 151:317-322.

7

GENETIC AND ENVIRONMENTAL CONTRIBUTIONS TO PATHOGENESIS

Wilmar M. Wiersinga
Dept. of Endocrinology & Metabolism, Academic Medical Center, University of Amsterdam, The Netherlands

INTRODUCTION

The clinical manifestations of Graves' disease comprise Graves' hyperthyroidism, Graves' ophthalmopathy, localized myxedema and thyroid acropachy. Graves' hyperthyroidism is the most prevalent phenotype with a strong female-to-male preponderance of about 8:1 (1). Among patients with Graves' hyperthyroidism, only 34% have clinical manifestations of Graves' ophthalmopathy (2). Orbital imaging demonstrates, however, enlarged extra-ocular muscles in up to 90% of those without clinically apparent ophthalmopathy, indicating involvement of orbital tissues in the vast majority of patients with Graves' hyperthyroidism (3). Graves' ophthalmopathy has a lower prevalence and a lower female-to-male ratio of 5.5:1 (4). Among patients with Graves' ophthalmopathy, 80% have a past or present history of Graves' hyperthyroidism. Evidence of autoimmune thyroid disease is, however, found in the vast majority of patients who are euthyroid upon presentation of eye signs, and about 15% of them will progress to overt Graves' hyperthyroidism within a few years (3-5). Localized (mainly pretibial) myxedema is relatively rare; the female-to-male ratio is 3.5:1 (6). Among patients with localizedmyxedema, over 90% has Graves' hyperthyroidism and most have also Graves' ophthalmopathy; 7% has thyroid acropachy. Localized myxedema occurs in 4% of all patients with Graves' ophthalmopathy, and in 12-15% of those with severe ophthalmopathy. Thyroid acropachy is the rarest of all Graves' disease manifestations, in which the female preponderance has been lost (female to male ratio of 1:1). Thyroid acropachy occurs almost always in association with Graves' ophthalmopathy and localized myxedema (6).

The epidemiological data summarized in Table 1, indicate that Graves' hyperthyroidism is the preferred clinical expression of Graves' disease, followed by Graves' ophthalmopathy, whereas the phenotypes of localized myxedema and thyroid acropachy are rare. The hallmark of Graves' disease is the presence of TSH-receptor stimulating antibodies, which play a causal role in the generation of the thyroid hormone excess. TSH receptor antibodies are also related to the severity and even more so to the activity of Graves' ophthalmopathy (7), and virtually all patients with localized myxedema have high serum concentrations of TSH receptor stimulating antibodies(6). The severity of the autoimmune attack in Graves' disease is apparently greater if Graves' ophthalmopathy develops next to Graves' hyperthyroidism, and is most severe in the patients who besides ophthalmopathy also develop localized myxedema and thyroid acropachy (5,6). A stronger clinical expression of Graves' disease (as evident from the co-existence of two or more of the four phenotypes) seems thus related to a more severe auto-immune attack, interestingly associated with a dampening of the female preponderance (Table 1). This is remarkable in view of the preferential occurrence of autoimmune diseases in women. It looks like male sex protects against autoimmunity, but once the safeguard mechanism has failed the autoimmune response in males might follow a more severe course. Indeed, male sex and older age predipose to more severe eye changes in patients with Graves' ophthalmopathy (8-9).

Table 1. The Phenotypic Appearances of Graves' Disease

Phenotype	**Prevalence**	**Mean interval between occurrence of hyperthyroidism and other phenotypes**	**Female to male ratio**
Graves' hyperthyroidism	most prevalent		8:1
Graves' ophthalmopathy	less prevalent	0-12 months	5.5:1
localized myxedema	rare	12-24 months	3.5:1
thyroid acropachy	very rare	24-36 months	1:1

The question arises which factors determine the severity of the autoimmune attack, and possibly thereby the heterogenesity in the clinical expression of Graves' disease. Graves' disease is generally viewed as a multifactorial disease in which the autoimmune reaction to thyroidal antigens arises against a certain genetic background, probably provoked by environmental factors. In this chapter we will evaluate genetic and environmental factors which render a patient with Graves' disease susceptible to contract Graves' ophthalmopathy. Such factors should be qualitatively or quantitatively different from those observed in Graves' hyperthyroid patients in whom the ophthalmopathy has not become clinically manifest.

GENETIC FACTORS

Autoimmune thyroid disease clusters in families, and the concordance rate for Graves' disease is higher for monozygotic than for dizygotic twins. The genetic basis for Graves' disease is, however, still largely unknown, and a fair number of genes is likely involved. Association studies have demonstrated that *HLA* (human leukocyte antigen), *IgH* (immunoglobulin heavy chain), *CTLA-4* (cytotoxic T-lymphocyte antigen 4) and *TCRβ* (T-cell receptor β-chain) genes confer susceptibility to Graves' disease (10). The relative risk of particular polymorphisms in these genes is, however, rather small, in the order of 2 to 3 (11). For example, the HLA susceptibility haplotype DQA1*501/DQB1*02/DRB1*0304 is present in 47% of Graves' patients and 24% of controls, and carries a RR of 2.72 (95% CI 1.91-3.87) (12). Linkage studies have indeed indicated that stronger genetic susceptibility loci for Graves' disease must be located elsewhere in the genome (10,11). There have been relatively few studies addressing the question of genetic differences between Graves' hyperthyroid patients with or without clinical manifestations of ophthalmopathy. The results of such studies are often conflicting (Table 2). One study indicates clear ethnic differences: the risk of Europeans developing ophthalmopathy relative to Asians is 6.36 (95% CI 1.78-22.7) (13).

MHC Genes

MHC class I

HLA-A antigens have not found to be independently related to Graves' ophthalmopathy (GO) (14-18). In Japanese patients, two HLA-A antigens modify the risk on GO in combination with class II antigens: the HLA-A11 positive and HLA-DPw2 negative pair is associated with GO, negative family history and early onset of Graves' disease, whereas the HLA-A31 negative and HLA-DQw4 positive pair is related to GO, negative family history and late onset of Graves' disease (RR 3.17) (17).

HLA-B antigens in whites are not related to Graves' disease except HLA-B8. HLA-B8 does not distinguish between Graves' hyperthyroid patients with or without GO (12,15), although a higher frequency of HLA-B8 in GO patients has been noted in early studies (39% vs 19%) (19,22) It was also observed that HLA-DR7 enhances the risk for ophthalmopathy in the presence of B8 but has a protective influence in its absence: using the phenotype B8-DR7- as reference (odds ratio 1), the odds ratios were 16.7 for B8+DR7+, 8.7 for B8+DR7- and 0.28 for B8-DR7+ (21,22). In Japanese hyperthyroid patients, the frequencies of HLA-B35 and HLA-B54 were lower in the group with severe GO than in the group without GO (18). Another Japanese study describes that the HLA-B5 positive and HLA-Dw12 positive pair is associated with ophthalmopathy, positive family history and early onset of Graves' disease (RR 6.57) (17). HLA-C antigens have a similar prevalence in patients with or without ophthalmopathy (14, 16-18).

MHC class II

LA-DPB alleles in whites do not differ in frequency between patients with or without GO except HLA-DPB2.1 (or 8) which was less prevalent in GO patients (3%) than in non-GO patients (21%) or controls (30%) (23). This particular allele may thus confer a protective effect with respect to ophthalmopathy. In Japanese patients, the absence of HLA-DPw2 in combination with the presence of HLA-A11 was associated with GO (17), but HLA-DPw2 was more prevalent in euthyroid GO than in Graves' disease (16). HLA-DQB alleles in whites have the same frequency in patients with or without GO (23). The frequency of DQw3.1 in the ophthalmopathy patients was lower than in controls but the difference was lost after correction for the number of Dqw variables tested, questioning the presumed protective effect of this allele (23). In Japanese patients, HLA-DQw4 had a slightly higher frequency in GO than in non-GO patients (17), but the opposite was observed in another study (18).

Table 2. Association studies between genetic markers and susceptibility to Graves' ophthalmopathy in patients with Graves' disease.

	Gene	Group	Association	Reference
MHC class I	HLA-A	Whites	no	14,15
		Japanese	no	16,17,18
	HLA-B	Whites	no	14,15
		Whites	yes (B8)	19-22
		Japanese	yes (B35, B54)	18
	HLA-C	Whites	no	14
		Japanese	no	16-18
MHC class II	HLA-DP	Whites	yes (DPB2.1/8)	23
		Japanese	yes (DPw2)	16,17
	HLA-DQ	Whites	no	23
		Japanese	yes (DQW4)	17,18
	HLA-DR	Whites	no	14,15,25,28
		Whites	yes (DR4)	19,24
		Whites	yes (DR4)	26,27
		Japanese	no	30
		Japanese	yes (DR4, DRw8, DR14)	17,18
MHC class III	complement	Whites	no	15
	TNF	Whites	no	25
		Japanese	yes (TNFα)	30
non-MHC	blood groups	Whites	no	31
		Whites	yes (P1)	15
	IgH	Whites	no	28
		Whites	yes (Gm)	21
	TCR	Whites	no	28
	CTLA-4	Whites	no	32,33
	TSH.R	Whites	no	34,35
		Whites	yes (C253A)	36,37
	IL1RA	Whites	no	38,39,40
	IFN-γ	Whites	no	41

HLA-DR alleles have been studied extensively in view of the association of HLA-DR3 with Graves' disease in whites. DRB3*0101/*0202 heterozygosity revealed a RR of 5.5 in Graves' disease patients with ophthalmopathy (24). HLA-DR3 was indeed more prevalent in Graves' patients with GO than in those without GO (48% vs 22%) (19), but this finding has not been confirmed (25). The genotype A1B8DR3 is present in 24% of all patients with Graves' disease, and in 23% of those who had eye disease (25). Early studies also reported a protective effect of HLA-DR4 against eye disease (26,27), but later studies did not find any differences in HLA-DR alleles between Graves' patients with or without GO (14,15,28). One study reports that the presence of HLA-DR4 is associated with a good response to corticosteroids in severe ophthalmopathy, whereas nonresponders were all HLA-DR4 negative[29]. In Japanese patients, the frequency of HLA-DR4 was lower and of HLA-DR14 higher in patients with GO than in Graves' patients without GO (18); another study reports an association of HLA-DRw8 with no ophthalmopathy, no family history and late onset of Graves' disease (RR 2.71) (17).

MHC class III

Non-HLA genes on chromosome 6, particularly those encoding for completement proteins (such as C3 and properdine factor B) and TNFβ, are not related to occurrence of GO in Graves' patients (15,25). In Japanese, a polymorphism of the 5' flanking region of the TNFα gene is related to the presence or absence of GO (odds ratio 2.30), but not to Graves' hyperthyroidism (30). The strength of the association of the polymorphism-1031C increased with the severity of ophthalmopathy. The results suggest that the polymorphism constitutes a risk through its higher promoter activity of TNFα production. Graves' disease patients with ophthalmopathy had a higher frequency of the combination DRB1*0901(-)/TNFα-1031C (+) than those with no or mild ophthalmopathy (odds ratio 4.59), although the frequency of DRB1*0901 was not different among Graves' disease patients.

NON-MHC Genes

An extensive survey of blood group systems in Graves' patients did not disclose differences between those with or without ophthalmopathy, with the exception of an increased frequency of blood group P_1 in GO (15). A subsequent study was, however, unable to confirm this result (31).

Immunoglobulin polymorphism has been evaluated with respect to the heavy-chain constant region (Gm allotype). One study finds no association with ophthalmopathy, also not in relation to HLA-DR3 (28). Likewise, Gm had no association with eye disease in another study, but seemed to modify the risk for ophthalmopathy associated with HLA-B8: odds ratios were 20.9 for B8+fb- (Gmfb homozygosity), 15.3 for B8+fb- and 1.7 for B8-fb- (B8-fb-=1.0) (21,22).

The T cell receptor β chain gene is associated with Graves' disease, but the distribution of polymorphisms in the T-cell receptor Cα, Vα, Cβ and Jγ genes was not different between Graves' patients with or without eye disease (28).

CTLA-4 alleles have been found associated with Graves' disease in whites and in Japanese. No specific association with ophthalmopathy was observed in two studies (32,33), but one study reported that the biallelic polymorphism CTLA-4 A/G at codon 17 confers susceptibility to GO (87). The strenght of the association of the G allele with GO increased with the severity of the eye disease: odds ratio's are 1.49 for class 1 and 2, 1.67 for class 3 and 4, and 3.06 for class 5 and 6 of eye changes, compared with Graves' disease patients without orbital signs (86).

A TSH receptor polymorphism in the extracellular domain has been described, associated with Graves' disease (at least in females) according to some studies but denied in other papers. An association with GO is reported (36,37), but has not been confirmed (34,35).

Polymorphisms in the interleukin-1 receptor antagonist (IL-1RA) gene have been linked to Graves' disease (38), but this finding has not been corfirmed (39,40). IL-1RA A2 allele frequencies and carriage rates did not differ between Graves' patients with or without eye disease (38-40), although one study noted a tendency towards a higher prevalence of the IL-1RA allele in Graves' patients with extrathyroidal manifestations of the disease (39).

Polymorphisms in the interferon-γ (IFN-γ) gene may play a minor role in the susceptibility to Graves' disease, but the frequency of IFN-γ2 and IFN-γ5 alleles were very similar in patients with or without GO (41).

SUMMARY OF GENETIC CONTRIBUTIONS

The search for genetic susceptibility loci in Graves' ophthalmopathy has been disappointing so far. The results summarized in Table 2, are mostly negative: the proportion of polymorphisms in candidate genes is similar in Graves' patients with or without clinically apparent eye disease. The few positive results could not be confirmed in most cases in subsequent studies. Reasons for the conflicting results may have been incomplete penetrance (not all affected subjects express the phenotype of Graves' ophthalmopathy), a too small sample size (causing insufficient power for confidence in the results), and improvements in the accuracy of genotyping (nowadays determined on PCR-amplified DNA products using allele-specific oligonucleotide probes, whereas HLA molecules were defined in the past serologically using antibodies and by the mixed lymphocyte reaction) (42). The superior methods derived from molecular biology possibly explain why the increase in the HLA-B8, DR3 haplotype in Graves' patients with clinically obvious GO relative to those without GO could not be confirmed in later studies (42).

The only undisputed locus so far, both in Caucasian and in Japanese patients, seems to be the HLA-DP region, in which HLA-DPBI*201 (new nomenchature for DPB 2.1 or 8, DPw2) appears to be protective against ophthalmopathy. The protective effect is, however, weak. Polymorphisms in a number of genes which discriminate little when considered one by one, can in combination procedure an overall, more meaningful pattern (15). Again, the obtained results of combinations do not convincingly demonstrate significant associations between specific genotypes and the phenotype of Graves' ophthalmopathy in the population of patients with Graves' disease (11).

ENVIRONMENTAL FACTORS

The environment is undoubtedly and important factor in the development of Graves' disease (3). Stress, smoking, iodine intake, infections, irradiation and particular immunological treatments have all been associated with the occurrence of Graves' hyperthyroidism, although the evidence for a causal relationship is mostly circumstantial and sometimes very weak indeed. It is remarkable that stress has been studied extensively in Graves' patients, but not specifically in relation to the phenotype of Graves' ophthalmopathy. The same holds true for the other environmental factors, with the exception of smoking and internal irradiation delivered by radioiodine treatment.

Smoking

Association of Smoking and GO

The prevalence of smokers among patients with Graves' hyperthyroidism is higher than in controls (43-51) (Table 3), and the prevalence of toxic diffuse goiter is higher in smoking than in non-smoking women in a population-based study (52). The risk to develop Graves' hyperthyroidism in relation to smoking is, however, small: the reported odds ratio is 1.9 (95% CI 1.1-3.2) (49). The association between smoking and Graves' ophthalmopathy is much stronger, and invariably observed in all studies (Table 3). Reported odds ratios for the increased risk for Graves' ophthalmopathy associated with smoking relative to controls are 20.2 (2.8-144.8) for current smokers and 8.9 (1.3-60.2) for current and ex-smokers (43), and 7.7 (4.3-13.7) for current smokers including those who had stopped smoking in the last five years (49). Among patients with Graves' hyperthyroidism, reported odds ratios for the risk on GO associated with smoking are 10.1 (1.4-73) for current smokers and 4.5 (0.8-24.3) for current and ex-smokers (43), 2.4 (1.1-5.2) for current smokers (13) and 2.1 (1.1-3.9) for current and ex-smokers (47). The higher risk in current smokers than in former smokers indicates a direct and immediate effect of smoking (42,51). In a prospective study of newly diagnosed patients with Graves' hyperthyroidism who were followed for one year during antithyroid drug treatment, smoking was associated with a 1.3-fold increase in the overall incidence of GO; the incidence of proptosis and diplopia increased 2.6 and 3.1-fold respectively (51).

Several studies indicate that among the patients with Graves' ophthalmopathy, smokers have more severe eye disease than nonsmokers as evident from a significant increase in the odds ratios in patients with more severe eye disease (Figure 1) (44,47,49). A dose-response relationship between smoking an severity of GO is not unequivocally established, as some studies found no association between the number of cigarettes per day or the duration of smoking and the severity of the ophthalmopathy (48,49). In contrast, other studies did observe a dose-response effect: patients with moderate to severe GO were more often heavy smokers (>10 pack-years) than patients with slight GO (44), and in a prospective study the relative risk of developing GO increased in parallel with the current number of cigarettes smoked per day whereas lifetime tobacco use was not an independent risk factor (51). Likewise, in a cross-sectional study the number of cigarettes smoked daily was higher in patients with GO than in patients without GO, but duration of smoking and pack-years were not different between both groups (50).

Mechanisms explaining the association between smoking and GO

The association between smoking and GO is for real, but is it a causal relationship? If so, which biologic mechanisms explain a putative cause-and-effect relationship? Satisfactory answers to these questions have so far not been obtained. Smoking has been associated with other autoimmune disease like

Crohn's disease (53), rheumatoid arthritis (54) and Goodpasture's syndrome (55), but an association is conspiciously absent with chronic autoimmune thyroiditis causing primary hypothyroidism (44,49). In subjects genetically predisposed to autoimmune thyroid disease, smoking is apparently not related to Hashimoto's disease but confers a specific risk to Graves' disease. Neither thyroid hormone excess itself nor the presence of a goiter are likely the causal link by which smoking increases the risk of Graves' hyperthyroidism, because other causes of hyperthyroidism (toxic nodular goiter) or of goiter (sporadic nontoxic goiter) are not associated with smoking (44,49). Thus, it is doubtful if the goitrogenic effect of thiocynanate in cigarette smoke is large enough to cause release of thyroidal antigens which theoretically may crossreact with orbital tissues (56). Equally doubtful in this respect is the biologic significance of the slight rise of serum T4 and fall of serum TSH observed in smokers relative to nonsmokers, possibly mediated via stimulation of the sympathetic nervous system by cigarette smoke and benzpyrene - another constituent of tobacco (56). Indeed, the serum concentrations of TSH receptor autoantibodies are not different between smokers and nonsmokers in most studies (7,47,56), except in one which reports slightly higher levels in smokers (48).

Table 3. Prevalence of Smokers† Among Patients with Graves' Hyperthyroidism (GH) in the Presence or Absence of Clinically Apparent Graves' Ophthalmopathy (GO) and in Controls.

GH with GO		GH without GO		Controls		Reference
n	smokers	n	smokers	n	smokers	
12	83%	24	46%	42	31%	43
307	64%	167	48%	486	28%	44
85	62%	62	23%	81	14%	45
39	95%	45	22%			46
52	71%	103	42%			13
62	63%	142	45%	372	42%	47
24	79%	147	48%		(34%)	48
100	81%	100	56%	200	39%	49
34	64%	49	46%	168	35%	50
151	47%	102	32%			51
865	65%	941	43%	1349	34%	

† defined as current smokers (ref. 45, 51), current smokers and smokers who had stopped smoking in the past year (ref. 43, 13, 48, 50), current smokers and ex-smokers (ref. 44, 47, 49) or not stated (ref. 46)

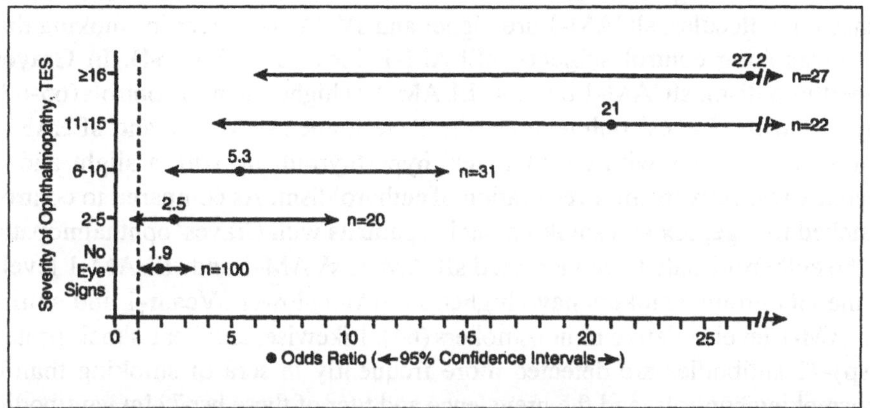

Figure 1. Increase in the prevalence of smokers (represented by the odds ratio with 95% confidence intervals) in relation to the severity of the eye disease (assessed by the total eye score, TES) in patients with Graves' hyperthyroidism. Reproduced with permission (49).

The mechanisms by which cigarette smoking enhances autoimmunity, remain largely enigmatic. Local and/or systemic effects of smoking on the immune system may be involved. Locally, physical damage precipitated by smoke upon the target tissue of the autoimmune attack, might activate the immune system, like in Goodpasture's syndrome (55). Applied to Graves' ophthalmopathy, does smoke really gets into the eyes? In this respect it is interesting to note that orbital fibroblasts produce more glycosaminoglycans (GAGs) when cultured under hypoxic conditions; tobacco glycoprotein enhances the production of IL-1, which also stimulates the secretion of GAGs (57). Systemic effects of smoking include promotion of B and T cell polyclonal activation with the resultant production of co-stimulatory cytokines (55). Nevertheless, serum cytokine concentrations of healthy subjects are not different between smokers and nonsmokers, with the exception of higher IL-6R levels in smokers (58). In patients with Graves' hyperthyroidism serum levels of sIL-2R, IL-6, IL-6R, and sCD30 are higher then in controls, with (apart from IL-6) a return to normal levels after restoration of the euthyroid state (59-63). Serum levels of IL-1RA and IL-6 are similar but IL-6R higher in patients with active Graves' ophthalmopathy than in patients with Graves' hyperthyroidism and no or inactive ophthalmopathy (61,53). Patients with Graves' ophthalmopathy who had been rendered euthyroid, still have higher serum levels of sIL-2R, IL-6, IL-6R, TNFαRI, TNFαRII and sCD-30 (but not of IL-1RA) than controls matched for age, sex and smoking habits; serum cytokines were not different between smokers and nonsmokers in this group of moderately severe untreated GO patients except higher IL-1RA levels in smokers (58). With respect to serum adhesion molecules, sICAM-1 are higher and sVCAM-1 lower in smoking than in nonsmoking control subjects; sELAM-1 does not differ (64). In Graves' hyperthyroidism, sICAM-1 but not sELAM-1 is higher than in controls (65-67). Patients with Graves' ophthalmopathy have higher sICAM-1 and sELAM-1 levels than patients with only Graves' hyperthyroidism, with a slight and no decrease respectively after restoration of euthyroidism. As compared to controls matched for age, sex and smoking habits, patients with Graves' ophthalmopathy in the euthyroid state have increased sICAM-1, sVAM-1 and sELAM-1 levels; in the GO group, smokers have higher sICAM-1, lower sVcam-1 and similar sELAM-1 levels relative to nonsmokers (64). Likewise, anti heat-shock-protein (hsp)-72 antibodies are detected more frequently in sera of smoking than of nonsmoking controls, and the prevalence and titer of these hsp72 IgG antibodies is higher in Graves' disease patients than in controls (68). Cytokines, adhesion molecules and hsp-72 are all involved in the immunopathogenesis of GO, and it is likely that the serum concentrations of these molecules reflect to a certain extent what is going on in the orbit. The observed differences at the serum level between smokers and nonsmokers may just indicate more severe ophthalmopathy in smokers.

Discontinuation of smoking

The association between smoking and Graves' ophthalmopathy - although incompletely understood in terms of biologic mechanisms - leads understandable to the advice to quit smoking in subjects susceptible to Graves' disease and in patients with already established Graves' disease. The advice is sound in view of the manifold ill-effects of smoking on health, but is the advice evidence-based in case of Graves' disease? In other words, should stop smoking prevent the development of Graves' disease and improve outcome in already established Graves' disease? The answer to both questions is in all likelihood yes. Graves' ophthalmopathy seems to be a preventable disease to a certain extent (69). In an European survey, 43% of respondents (mainly from Western European countries) thought the incidence of GO was decreasing (in line with the general fall in cigarette smoking over the last decades), whereas 12% thought it to be increasing (strikingly, reported by all respondents from Hungary and Poland, where the number of smokers has risen considerably since 1990) (70). Also, the development of Graves' ophthalmopathy after the onset of Graves' hyperthyroidism is higher in smokers than in nonsmokers (51), and likewise cigarette smoking increases the risk for progression of GO after radioiodine therapy four-fold (71). In Graves' hyperthyroidism, smokers have a shorter duration of remission following cessation of antithyroid drug treatment and more relapses than nonsmokers (72). The outcome of Graves' ophthalmopathy is also worse in smokers, in whom improvement of eye changes after orbital irradiation and glucocorticoids is less frequent than in nonsmokers (71). The early report that smokers and nonresponders to immunosuppression in GO have lower IL-1RA serum concentrations (73), has not been confirmed in two subsequent studies (58,74).

IRRADIATION

External irradiation

External irradiation of the neck for malignant tumors is followed by thyroid disease in about half of the exposed patients, hypothyroidism being the most prevalent. In patients with Hodgkin's disease who had received irradiation therapy, the actuarial risk of Graves' hyperthyroidism was 3.1% at 20 years; the median time to occurrence was 4.8 yr (range 0.1-17.6 yr) (75). The relative risk of Graves' disease after treatment for Hodgkin's disease ranges from 7.2 to 20.4, as estimated from population-based incidence rates. Age, sex, radiation dose, and exposure to chemotherapy were not significant risk factors. A high proportion (about two-thirds) of Graves' patients had Graves' ophthalmopathy.

Internal irradiation

Internal irradiation of thyroid follicular epithelial cells delivered by treatment with radioiodine poses a small risk for developing or worsening of ophthalmopathy. Although this adverse effect of ^{131}I therapy has been much disputed, two large randomized clinical trials have provided rather good evidence in this respect (76). In patients with Graves' hyperthyroidism and no or slight ophthalmopathy before treatment the relative risk of developing or worsening of GO was 3.2 (95% CI 1.1-8.8) after ^{131}I therapy vs 1.0 after antithyroid drug treatment (77). The study results have been criticised because thyroxine was routinely given to the medical group but not until hypothyroidism had developed in the radioiodine group. Subsequent studes indeed demonstrated an association between high TSH levels and the development of eye changes after ^{131}I therapy (78,79). Nevertheless, the results of another trial in which the confounding factor of an increased TSH was absent, were essentially similar: eye changes occurred more often in the radioiodine than in the methimazole group (Table 4) (80). A causal relationship between radioiodine treatment and eye changes is plausible in view of the release of thyroid antigens following radiation injury; the resulting T-cell activation and prolonged increase in the concentration and activity of TSH receptor antibodies may trigger autoimmune reactions in the orbit (81). Indeed, radioiodine treatment induces a transient increase in the production of both proinflammatory and antiinflammatory cytokines (82), and the serum concentration of TSH receptor antibodies significantly increase after radioiodine but steadily decline upon antithyroid drug treatment (83). Fortunately, the radioiodine-induced eye changes are mostly transient and mild in nature; they occur especially in patients who smoke and have high pre-treatment serum T3 levels (≥5 nmol/l) (77,80).

Table 4. Randomized Clinical Trial on Eye Changes Upon Treatment of Graves' Hyperthyroidism in Patients with no or Mild Prior Ophthalmopathy (80).

Randomization	Number of	Eye changes		
groups	patients	Improvement	No change	Worsening
methimazole	148	2%	95%	3%
^{131}I	150	0%	85%	15%
^{131}I+prednisone	145	35%	65%	0%

IMMUNOLOGICAL INTERVENTIONS

Patients treated with interferon-α for malignancy or hepatitis C and patients treated with interferon-β1b for multiple sclerosis develop thyrotoxicosis in 1-2% (84,85). The induced thyroid hormone excess is mostly transient and associated with a low radioiodine thyroidal uptake, reflecting the inflammatory type of thyrotoxicosis. Only in a few cases the thyrotoxicosis resembles Graves' disease, with an elevated radioiodine uptake and the emergence of TSH receptor antibodies; Graves' ophthalmopathy in this setting has not been described.

In contrast, treatment of multiple sclerosis with the humanised anti-CD52 monoclonal antibody Campath-1H was followed by Graves' hyperthyroidism (increased thyroidal uptake of technetium-99, positive TSH receptor antibodies) in 9 out of 27 patients (33%), of whom two also developed Graves' ophthalmopathy (86). It was hypothesized that Campath-1H treatment causes a breakdown in self-tolerance mechanisms after the induced lymphocyte depletion by a quicker recovery of CD8 T cells (inplicated in the pathogenesis of thyroid autoimmunity) and a low production of memory CD4 cells (which suppress autoimmunity after lymphopenia in experimental animals) (86)

CONCLUDING REMARKS

Clinical manifestations of Graves' ophthalmopathy occur in about 40% of all patients with Graves' hyperthyroidism, and it is likely that genetic and environmental factors determine whether or not the phenotype of Graves' ophthalmopathy will be expressed in Graves' disease patients. Genetic epidemiological studies have so far not convincingly identified significant differences in polymorphism frequencies of a number of candidate genes of Graves' disease between patients with and without clinically apparent Graves' ophthalmopathy. Possible exceptions are the CTLA-4 A/G genotype and the HLA-DPB1*201 locus, which confer susceptibility and protection to GO respectively; the effects are, however, weak.

More progress has been made in the delineation of environmental factors. Smoking is definitely an important risk factor for Graves' ophthalmopathy. Smokers have more severe eye disease than nonsmokers. A dose-response relationship has been observed in some but not all studies on the association between smoking and Graves' ophthalmopathy; the biologic mechanism responsible for the observed association remains incompletely understood. The outcome of immunosuppression is less favourable in smokers than in nonsmokers with Graves' ophthalmopathy. Radioiodine treatment carries a small risk for devloping - mostly transient and mild - eye changes, especially in smokers.

It follows that Graves' ophthalmopathy to a certain extent is a preventable disease: smoking should be strongly discouraged in subjects susceptible to Graves' disease and in patients with already established Graves' disease, and radioiodine treatment should be applied cautiously (not at all or in conjunction with glucocorticoids) in hyperthyroid patients at risk for development or worsening of eye changes (i.e. in smokers, in pre-existent active eye disease, and at pretreatment T3 levels greater than 5 nmol/l).

REFERENCES

1. Vanderpump PJ, Tunbridge WMG. The epidemiology of autoimmune thyroid disease. In Volpe P (ed): Autoimmune endocrinopathies. Towata, NY, Humana Press, 1999, p 141.
2. Tellez M, Cooper J, Edmonds C. Graves' ophthalmopathy in relation to cigarette smoking and ethnic origin. Clin Endocrinol 1992; 36: 291-294
3. Burch HB, Wartofsky L. Graves' ophthalmopathy: current concepts regarding pathogenesis and management. Endocr Rev 1993; 14: 747-793.
4. Bartley GB, Fatourechi V, Kadrmas EF et al. The incidence of Graves' ophthalmopathy in Olmsted County, Minnesota. Am J Ophthalmol 1995; 120: 511-517.
5. Burch HB, Gorman CA, Bahn RS, Garrity JA. Ophthalmopathy. In Braverman LE, Utiger RD (ed): Werner & Ingbar's The Thyroid, 8th edition. Philadelphia, PA, Lippincott, Williams & Wilkins, 2000, p 531-548.
6. Fatourechi V. Localized myxedema and acropachy. In Braverman LE, Utiger RD (ed): Werner & Ingbar's The Thyroid, 8th edition. Philadelphia, PA, Lippincott, Williams & Wilkins, 2000, p 548-555.
7. Gerding MN, Meer JWC van der, Broenink M, Bakker O, Wiersinga WM, Prummel MF. Association of thyrotropin receptor antibodies with activity rather than severity of Graves' ophthalmopathy. Clin Endocrinol 2000; 52: 267-271.
8. Kendler DL, Lippa J, Rootman J. The initial characteristics of Graves' ophthalmopathy vary with age and sex. Arch Ophthalmol 1993; 111: 197-201.
9. Perros P, Cromble AL, Matthews JNS, Kendall-Taylor P. Age and gender influence the severity of thyroid-associated ophthalmopathy: a study of 101 patients attending a combined thyroid-eye clinic. Clin Endocrinol 1993; 38: 367-372.
10. McLachlan SM, Rapoport B. Genetic factors in thyroid disease. In: Braverman LE, Utiger RD (ed); Werner & Ingbar's The Thyroid, 8th edition. Philadelphia, PA Lippincott, Williams & Wilkins, 2000, p 474-487.
11. Gough S. The immunogenetics of Graves' disease. Curr Op Endocrinol Diab 1999; 6: 270-276.
12. Heward JM, Allahabadia A, Daykin J, et al.Linkage disequilibrium between the human leukocyte antigen class II region of the major histocompatibility complex and Graves' disease: replication using a population case control and family-based study. J Clin Endocrinol Metab 1998; 83: 3394-3397.
13. Tellez M, Cooper J, Edmonds C. Graves' ophthalmopathy in relation to cigarette smoking and ethnic origin. Clin Endocrinol 1992; 36: 291-294.
14. Bech K, Lumholtz B, Nerup J, et al. HLA antigens in Graves' disease. Acta Endocrinol 1977; 86: 510-516.
15. Kendall-Taylor P, Stephenson A, Stratton A, Papiha SS, Perros P, Roberts DF. Differentiation of autoimmune ophthalmopathy from Graves' hyperthyroidism by analysis of genetic markers. Clin Endocrinol 1988; 28: 601-610.
16. Inoue D, Sato K, Maeda M, et al. Genetic differences shown by HLA typing among Japanese patients with euthyroid Graves' ophthalmopathy, Graves' disease and Hashimoto's thyroiditis: genetic characteristics of euthyroid Graves' ophthalmopathy. Clin Endocrinol 1991; 24: 57-62.
17. Inoue D, Sato K, Enomoto T, et al. Correlation of HLA types and clinical findings in Japanese patients with hyperthyroid Graves' disease: evidence indicating the existence of four subpopulations. Clin Endocrinol 1992; 36: 75-82.

18. Ohtsuka K, Nakamura Y. Human leucocyte antigens associated with hyperthyroid Graves' ophthalmopathy in Japanese patients. Am J Ophthalmol 1998; 126: 805-810.
19. Schleusener H, Schernthaner G, Mayr WR, et al. HLA-DR and HLA-DR5 associated thyrotoxicosis - two different types of toxic diffuse goiter. J Clin Endocrinol Metab 1983; 56: 781-785.
20. Stensky V, Balazs C, Kozma L, Rochlitz S, Bear JI, Farid NR. Identification of subsets of patients with Graves' disease by cluster analysis. Clin Endocrinol 1983; 18: 335-345.
21. Frecker M, Stenszky V, Balazs C, Kozma L, Kraszits E, Faria NR. Genetic factors in Graves' ophthalmopathy. Clin Endocrinol 1986; 25: 479-485.
22. Farid NR, Balazs C. The genetics of thyroid-associated ophthalmopathy. Thyroid 1988; 8: 407-409.
23. Weetman AP, Zhang L, Webb S, Shine B. Analysis of HLA-DQB and HLA-DPB alleles in Graves' disease by oligonucleotide probing of enzymatically amplified DNA. Clin Endocrinol 1990; 33: 65-71.
24. Boehm BO, Kühol P, Manfras BJ, et al. HLA-DRB3 gene alleles in Caucasian patients with Graves' disease. Clin Investig 1992; 70: 956-960.
25. Badenhoop K, Schwarz G, Schleusener H, et al. Tumor necrosis factor β gene polymorphisms in Graves' disease. J Clin Endocrinol Metab 1992; 74: 287-291.
26. Frecker M, Mercer G, Skanes VM, Farid NR. Major histocompatibility complex (MHC) factors predisposing to and protecting against Graves' eye disease. Autoimmunity 1988; 1: 307-315.
27. Payami H, Joe S, Farid NR, et al. Relative predispositional effects (RPEs) of marker allele with disease: HLA-DR alleles and Graves' disease. Am J Hum Genet 1989; 45: 541-546.
28. Weetman AP, So AK, Warner CA, Foroni L, Fells P, Shine B. Immunogenetics of Graves' ophthalmopathy. Clin Endocrinol 1988; 28: 619-628.
29. Gaag R vd, Wiersinga WM, Koornneef L, et al. HLA-DR4 associated response to corticosteroids in Graves' ophthalmopathy patients. J Endocrinol Invest 1990; 13: 489-492.
30. Kamizono S, Hiromatsu Y, Seki N, et al. A polymorphism of the 5'-flanking region of tumour necrosis factor α gene is associated with thyroid-associated ophthalmopathy. Clin Endocrinol 2000; 52: 759-764.
31. Weetman AP, Poole J. Failure to find an association of blood group P1 with thyroid-associated ophthalmopathy. Clin Endocrinol 1992; 37: 423-425.
32. Kotsa K, Watson PF, Weetman AP. A CTLA-4 gene polymorphism is associated with both Graves' disease and autoimmune hypothyroidism. Clin Endocrinol 1997; 46: 551-554.
33. Donner H, Rau H, Walfish PG, et al. CTLA4 alanine-17 confers genetic susceptibility to Graves disease and to type 1 diabetes mellitus. J Clin Endocrinol Metab 1997; 82: 143-146.
34. Watson PF, French A, Pickerill AP, McIntosh RS, Weetman AP. Lack of association between a polymorphism in the coding region of the thyrotropin receptor gene and Graves' disease. J Clin Endocrinol Metab 1995; 80: 1032-1035.
35. Allahabadia A, Heward JM, Mijovic C, et al. Lack of association between polymorphism of the thyrotropin receptor gene and Graves' disease in United Kingdom and Hong Kong Chinese patients: case control and family-based studies. Thyroid 1998; 8: 777-780.
36. Bahn RS, Dutton CM, Heufelder AE, Sarkar G. A genomic point mutation in the extracellular domain of the thyrotropin receptor in patients with Graves' ophthalmopathy. J Clin Endocrinol Metab 1994; 78: 256-260.

37. Cuddily RM, Dutton CM, Bahn RS. A polymorphism in the extracellulair domain of the thyrotropin receptor is highly associated with autoimmmune thyroid disease in females. Thyroid 1995; 5: 89-95.
38. Blakemore AIF, Watson PF, Weetman AP, Duff SW. Association of Graves' disease with an allele of the interleukin-1 receptor antagonist gene. J Clin Endocrinol Metab 1995; 80: 111-115.
39. Cuddihy RM, Bahn RS. Lack of an association between alleles of interleukin-1 and interleukin-1 receptor antagonist genes and Graves' disease in a North American Caucasian population. J Clin Endocrinol Metab 1996; 81: 4476-4478.
40. Mühlberg T, Kirchberger M, Spitzweg C, Herrmann F, Heberling H-J, Heufelder AH. Lack of association of Graves' disease with the A2 allele of the interleukin-1 receptor antagonist gene in a white European population. Eur J Endocrinol 1998; 38: 686-690.
41. Siegmond T, Usadel KH, Donner H, Braun J, Walfish PG, Badenhoop K. Interferon-γ gene microsatellite polymorphisms in patients with Graves' disease. Thyroid 1998; 8: 1013-1017.
42. Heufelder AE, Weetman AP, Ludgate M, Bahn RS. Pathogenesis of Graves' ophthalmopathy. In: Prummel MF (ed). Recent developments in Graves' ophthalmopathy. Kluwer Academic Publishers, Boston 2000, p 15-37.
43. Hagg E, Asplund K. Is endocrine ophthalmopathy related to smoking? Brit Med J 1987; 295: 634-635.
44. Bartalena L, Martino E, Marcocci C. et al. More on smoking habits and Graves' ophthalmopathy. J Endocrinol Invest 1989; 12: 733-737.
45. Shine B, Fells P, Edwards OM, Weetman AP. Association between Graves' ophthalmopathy and smoking. Lancet 1990; 1: 1261-1263.
46. Balazs C, Stensky V, Farid NR. Association between Graves' ophthalmopathy and smoking (letter). Lancet 1990; 2: 754.
47. Winsa B, Mandahl A, Karlsson FA. Graves' disease, endocrine ophthalmopathy and smoking. Acta Endocrinol 1993; 128: 156-160.
48. Tallstedt L, Lundell G, Taube A. Graves' ophthalmopathy and tobacco smoking. Acta Endocrinol 1993; 129: 147-150.
49. Prummel MF, Wiersinga WM. Smoking and risk of Graves' disease. JAMA 1993; 269: 479-482.
50. O'Hare JA, Geoghegan M. Cigarettes smoking as a promotor of Graves' disease. Eur J Int Med 1993; 4: 289-292.
51. Pfeilschifter J, Ziegler R. Smoking and endocrine ophthalmopathy: impact of smoking severity and current vs lifetime cigarette consumption. Clin Endocrinol 1996; 45: 477-481.
52. Ericsson U-B, Lindgarde F. Effect of cigarette smoking on thyroid function and the prevalence of goitre, thyrotoxicosis and autoimmune thyroiditis. J Int Med 1991; 229: 67-71.
53. Calkins BM. A meta-analysis of the role of smoking in inflammatory bowel disease. Dig Dis Sci 1989; 34: 1841-1854.
54. Silman AJ. Smoking and the risk of rheumatoid arthritis. J Rheumatol 1993; 20: 1815-1816.
55. George J, Levy Y, Schoenfeld Y. Smoking and immunity: an additional player in the mosaic of autoimmunity. Scand J Immunol 1997; 45: 1-6.
56. Bertelsen JB, Hegedüs L. Cigarette smoking and the thyroid. Thyroid 1994; 4: 327-331.
57. Metcalfe RA, Weetman AP. Stimulation of extraocular muscle fibroblasts by cytokines and hypoxia: possible role in thyroid-associated ophthalmopathy. Clin Endocrinol 1994; 40: 67-72.

58. Wakelkamp IMMJ, Gerding MN, Meer JWC vd, Prummel MF, Wiersinga WM. Both Th_1 and Th_2 derived cytokines in serum are elevated in Graves' ophthalmopathy. Clin Exp Immunol 2000; in press.
59. Chow CC, Lai KN, Leung JC, Chan JC, Cockram CS. Soluble interleukin-2 receptor in hyperthyroid Graves' disease and effect of carbimazole therapy. Clin Endocrinol 1990; 33: 317-321.
60. Celik I, Akalia S, Erbas T. Serum levels of interleukin-6 and tumor necrosis factor-alpha in hyperthyroid patients before and after propylthiouracil treatment. Eur J Endocrinol 1995; 132: 668-672.
61. Salvi M, Gizasole G, Pedrazzoni M, et al. Increased serum concentrations of interleukin-6 (IL-6) and soluble IL-6 receptor in patients with Graves' disease. J Clin Endocrinol Metab 1996; 81: 2976-2979.
62. Okumara M, Hidaka Y, Kuroda S, Takeoka K, Tada H, Amino N. Increased serum concentration of soluble CD30 in patients with Graves' disease and Hashimoto's thyroiditis. J Clin Endocrinol Metab 1997; 82: 1757-1760.
63. Salvi M, Pedrazzoni M, Girasole G, et al. Serum concentrations of proinflammatory cytokines in Graves' disease: effect of treatment, thyroid function, ophthalmopathy and cigarette smoking. Eur J Endocrinol 2000; 143: 197-202.
64. Wakelkamp IMMJ, Gerding MN, Meer JWCvd, Prummel MF, Wiersinga WM. Smoking and disease severity are independent determinants of serum adhesion molecule levels in Graves' ophthalmopathy. Clin Exp Immunol, submitted for publication.
65. Heufelder AE, Bahn RS. Soluble intercellular adhesion molecule-1 (sICAM-1) in sera of patients with Graves' ophthalmopathy and thyroid diseases. Clin Exp Immunol 1993; 92: 296-302.
66. De Bellis A, Bizzarro A, Gattoni A, et al. Behavior of soluble intercellular adhesion molecule-1 and endothelial-leucocyte adhesion molecule-1 in patients with Graves' disease with or without ophthalmopathy and in patients with toxic adenoma. J Clin Endocrinol Metab 1995; 80: 2118-2221.
67. Ozata M, Bolu E, Sengul A, et al. Soluble intercellular adhesion molecule-1 concentrations in patients with subacute thyroiditis and in patients with Graves' disease with or without ophthalmopathy. Endocrine J 1996; 43: 517-525.
68. Prummel MF, Pareeren Yv, Bakker B, Wiersinga WM. Anti-heat shock protein (hsp)72 antibodies are present in patients with Graves' disease and in smoking control subjects. Clin Exp Immunol 1997; 110: 292-295.
69. Keltner JL. Is Graves' ophthalmopathy a preventable disease? Arch Ophthalmol 1998; 116: 1106-1107.
70. Weetman AP, Wiersinga WM. Current management of thyroid-associated ophthalmopathy in Europe. Results of an international survey. Clin Endocrinol 1998; 49: 21-28.
71. Bartalena L, Marcocci C, Tanda ML, et al. Cigarette smoking and treatment outcome in Graves' ophthalmopathy. Ann Int Med 1998; 129: 633-635.
72. Ünüvar N, Serter R, Aral Y. The effects of smoking on remission and relapse of Graves' disease (letter). Clin Endocrinol 1997; 46: 337-378.
73. Hoffbauer LC, Mühlberg T, Konig A, et al. Soluble interleukin-1 receptor antagonist serum levels in smokers and nonsmokers with Graves' ophthalmopathy undergoing orbital radiotherapy. J Clin Endocrinol Metab 1997; 82: 2244-2247.
74. Bartalena L, Monetti L, Tanda ML, et al. Soluble interleukin-1 receptor antagonist concentration in patients with Graves' ophthalmopathy is neither related to cigarette smoking nor predicitive of subsequent response to glucocorticoids. Clin Endocrinol 2000; 52: 647-651.

75. Hancock SL, Cox RS, McDougall IR. Thyroid diseases after treatment of Hodgkin's disease. New Engl J Med 1991; 325: 599-605.
76. Krogh Rasmussen Å, Nygaard B, Feldt-Rasmussen U. ^{131}I and thyroid-associated ophthalmopathy. Eur J Endocrinol 2000; 143: 155-160.
77. Tallstedt L, Lundell G, Torring O, et al. Occurrence of ophthalmopathy after treatment for Graves' hyperthyroidism. New Engl J Med 1992; 326: 1733-1738.
78. Tallstedt L, Lundell G, Blomgren H, Bring J. Does early administration of thyroxine reduce the development of Graves' ophthalmopathy after radioiodine treatment? Eur J Endocrinol 1994; 130: 494-497.
79. Kung AWC, Ysu CC, Cheng A. The incidence of ophthalmopathy after radioiodine therapy for Graves' disease: prognostic factors and the role of methimazole. J Clin Endocrinol Metab 1994; 79: 542-546.
80. Bartalena L, Marcocci C, Bogazzi F, et al. Relation between therapy for hyperthyroidism and the course of Graves' ophthalmopathy. New Engl J Med 1998; 338: 73-78.
81. Wiersinga WM. Preventing Graves' ophthalmopathy. New Engl J Med 1998; 338: 121-122.
82. Jones BM, Kwok CCH, Kung AWC. Effect of radioactive iodine therapy on cytokine production in Graves' disease: transient increases in interleukin-4 (IL-4), IL-6, IL-10, and tumor necrosis factor-α, with longer term increases in interferon-γ production. J Clin Endocrinol Metab 1999; 84: 4106-4110.
83. Törring O, Tallstedt L, Wallin G, et al. Graves' hyperthyroidism: treatment with antithyroid drugs, surgery, or radioiodine - a prospective randomized study. J Clin Endocrinol Metab 1996; 81: 2986-2993.
84. Kok LKH, Greenspan FS, Yeo PPB. Interferon-α induced thyroid dysfunction: three clinical presentations and a review of the literature. Thyroid 1997; 7: 891-896.
85. Schwid SR, Goodman AD, Mattson DH. Autoimmune hyperthyroidism in patients with multiple sclerosis treated with interferon beta-1b. Arch Neurol 1997; 54: 1169-1170.
86. Coles AJ, Wing M, Smith S, et al. Pulsed monoclonal antibody treatment and autoimmune thyroid diseases in multiple sclerosis. Lancet 1999; 354: 1691-1695.
87. Vaidya B, Imric H, Perros P, et al. Cytotoxic T lymphocyte antigen-4 (CTLA-4) gene polymorphism confers susceptibility to thyroid associated orbitopathy. Lancet 1999; 354: 743-744.

8

CLINICAL PRESENTATION AND NATURAL HISTORY OF GRAVES' OPHTHALMOPATHY

P. Perros, A.J. Dickinson, P. Kendall-Taylor
University of Newcastle on Tyne, Departments of Medicine and Ophthalmology

INTRODUCTION

Graves' ophthalmopathy (GO) is clinically apparent in about 35% patients with Graves' disease, but is subclinically present in most patients (8). The presentation of GO is highly variable. None of the clinical signs of GO are pathognomonic, yet this condition is rarely a diagnostic challenge to the experienced clinician. However delays in making the diagnosis by non-specialists is common. Clinicians managing patients with GO have to decide which aspects of a patient's presentation warrant referral to a specialist centre. The clinical course of GO through time is multiphasic and spontaneous regression occurs in most patients. The "natural history" of this disease is a concept of critical importance in prognosis, and timing of therapeutic interventions.

CLINICAL PRESENTATION

Presentation of patients with Graves' ophthalmopathy

The symptoms and signs of GO are variable and unique to each patient. Some individuals have florid symptoms and few clinical signs of GO, whilst others may be entirely uncomplaining despite severe, sight-threatening disease. It is common for patients with GO who are seen at tertiary referral centres to report several months of troublesome symptoms which have been dismissed as "conjunctivitis", "allergy" or other trivial diagnoses by their primary care physician (11).

Most patients are in their 40's or 50's at the time of onset of GO (8,28,38). The female to male ratio is approximately 2:1 (8,27,28,38). Some differences exist in the presentation between male and female patients. Male patients are more likely to be older at the time of presentation than females (28,38,50). A relationship between the severity of GO and age is also evident both in men and women, older patients being more susceptible to severe disease, particularly optic neuropathy (50). GO is uncommon in children with Graves' disease, and when it occurs it tends to be mild and usually transient (20). The mode of onset of GO is also highly variable. Some patients have an acute, almost explosive presentation, whilst others develop the disease insidiously and may not be aware of it. A significant proportion of patients with GO display no exophthalmos, yet have severe GO and are at risk of optic neuropathy ("concealed exophthalmos").

The diagnosis of GO is usually easy in patients who are known to have Graves' disease. However, in patients presenting with unilateral proptosis, or who are euthyroid (with no previous history of autoimmune thyroid disease), alternative pathologies have to be excluded. The differential diagnosis in patients presenting with unilateral proptosis includes primary and secondary orbital tumours, carotid-cavernous fistula, unilateral myopia, and inflammatory diseases (36). Myasthenia gravis may cause confusion as many myasthenic patients also have autoimmune thyroid disease (35), however ptosis is a common and early feature of myasthenia, rarely found in GO, and the diplopia of myasthenic patients is characteristically variable. The limitation of extraocular muscle movement and lower lid retraction of chronic progressive extranuclear ophthalmoplegia may rarely lead to the erroneous diagnosis of GO. Upper lid retraction can be a sign of neurological mid-brain disease. Orbital imaging (MRI, CT scanning or ultrasonography) is indicated in cases where there is doubt about the diagnosis. Enlargement of the bellies of extraocular muscles, particularly the inferior and medial recti is typical in GO, and is present in both orbits, even in cases when the disease is clinically unilateral. The tendinous insertions of muscles are radiologically spared in GO, unlike other pathologies. Biopsy of extraocular muscles may be indicated when a malignancy is suspected. Orbital myositis cannot be reliably distinguished from GO by histological examination, but a rapid and good response to modest doses of steroids supports the diagnosis of myositis (42).

Ophthalmological referral of every patient with Graves' disease is unnecessary, however, it is increasingly evident that early diagnosis and treatment of GO is associated with better outcome (5,15). Therefore, physicians who manage patients with Graves' disease should possess the skills to assess which patients have active disease, and select those who either need urgent treatment to preserve vision, or would benefit from symptomatic measures. Similarly, they should be aware of the potential for rehabilitative surgery in those whose disease is inactive.

In this section the symptoms and clinical signs that should provoke referral to a specialist centre are discussed. Patients with Graves' disease who have apparently normal eyes and no symptoms of GO do not require further ophthalmological assessment.

Symptoms

When it becomes apparent during consultation that a patient has symptoms or signs suggestive of GO, a detailed history should be taken focusing on the eyes.

- Change in the appearance of the eyes is a common feature, but may not be obvious to the examiner unless the patient produces pre-morbid photographs. Changes include eyelid/peri-orbital swelling, bulging of the eyes, redness of the periorbital tissues and the appearance of "vertical furrows" between the brows.
- Grittiness or foreign body sensation, photophobia and excessive watering all occur frequently during the active phase of the disease. They may signify corneal drying secondary to eyelid retraction, or superior limbic keratoconjunctivitis. The latter is denoted by visible evidence of inflammation between the upper eyelid and the eyeball; it is highly suggestive, although not pathognomonic, of GO (10,25).
- Double vision, particularly when tired or on waking, and pain precipitated by extremes of gaze are symptoms of impaired muscle motility.
- Orbital aching unrelated to gaze suggests venous congestion
- Blurred distant vision, inability to read small print, subjective awareness of changes in colour appreciation, and scotomas may signify optic neuropathy. Blurred vision which corrects with blinking suggests abnormality of the tear film rather than optic neuropathy as the underlying cause (1).
- Rarely, patients will report an alarming episode of sudden "popping" of their eye and complete inability to close the lids, due to subluxation of the globe.

Subjective assessment

Previous assessment protocols for GO have paid little attention to symptoms. This important aspect of patients' evaluation was acknowledged by the recommendations of the International Thyroid Associations' working group (39). The patient's own description of symptoms is a valuable resource for the clinician. It can lead to diagnosing a complication of GO, as is the case in some patients with optic neuropathy who are aware of a change in colour perception. Furthermore, the consequences of GO on the individual's quality of life is paramount in managing each patient and tailoring treatment to that person's needs which may be vastly different for a taxi driver compared to a public relations officer. The impact of GO on quality of life has recently been studied systematically and not surprisingly was found to be significant and comparable to other chronic conditions.

It is not unusual for patients with GO to have multiple symptoms. The clinician should attempt to stratify their relative importance by inviting comments on the severity of each symptom. Grading the severity on a scale of 0-10 is helpful for the physician in identifying which aspect of GO has greatest impact on the patient.

Time course of symptoms

Patients should be asked about the duration of symptoms since onset, and whether over the proceeding 1-2 months each symptom has improved, deteriorated, or remained unchanged. As a general rule, patients who are symptomatic have active disease, and will describe not only daily fluctuations, but significant changes over several months.

Objective assessment by the endocrinologist

A laborious detailed ophthalmological examination in the setting of an endocrine outpatient service is neither a realistic expectation, nor necessary. However, a focused rapid examination not requiring specialized equipment can be learnt and applied relatively easily, and will detect those patients who require referral to an ophthalmologist.

Examination of the eyes must be systematic:

- Appearance of the lids. Swelling, redness, upper and lower lid retraction should be noted (Figure 1 a,b,c). If the eyelids do not close on attempted gentle closure (lagophthalmos), it should be noted whether the cornea remains visible, and whether Bell's phenomenon is present or absent (Figure 2). If the cornea cannot be protected by the eyelids, then there is a real risk of sight-threatening corneal breakdown.

- The conjunctivae should be examined for signs of redness, and chemosis (Figure 1 d,e).

- The corneas should be examined for obvious ulcers / opacities (Figure 1f).

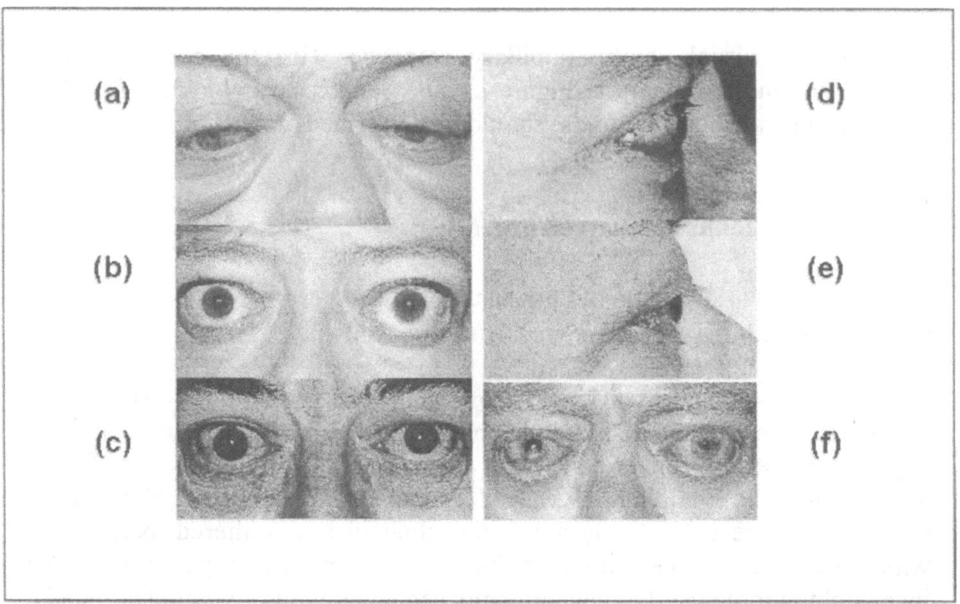

Figure 1. (a) lid swelling, (b) lid retraction, (c) lid erythema, (d) conjunctival redness, (e) conjunctival edema (chemosis), (f) corneal ulceration.

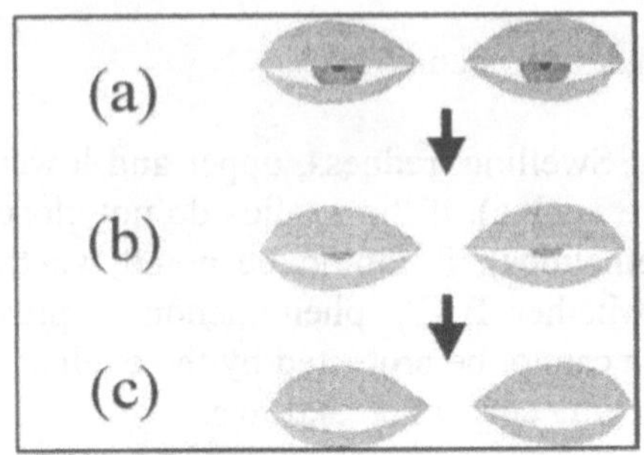

Figure 2. Lagophthalmos and Bell's phenomenon.
(a) The lids fail to meet on attempted closure
(b) & (c) Bell's phenomenon (reflex elevation of the globe on attempted lid closure) is present in this example of lagophthalmos and the cornea is thus protected.

- Eye movement should be tested for restriction, which may or may not elicit diplopia. An obvious squint, or the presence of a compensatory head posture (usually chin up) should be noted.

- Corrected visual acuity, pupillary responses (looking for a relative afferent pupillary defect, Figure 1) and fundoscopy (looking for disk swelling and choroidal folds) should be performed.

Patients who should be referred urgently

- When there is suspicion of optic neuropathy
- Patients with risk of imminent corneal breakdown

The absence of conclusive signs of optic neuropathy must not deter referral. Reduction in acuity and disk swelling can be late signs, and a relative afferent pupillary defect will never be seen in many, due to bilateral disease (Figure 3). Patients who complain of blurred vision not improved by blinking, or patients who are subjectively aware that their vision is altered, particularly with regard to colour perception or "blank spots", mandate urgent assessment by an ophthalmologist. Optic neuropathy can occur with or without proptosis, but is unusual in patients without some evidence of dysmotility.

Urgent assessment is also required for patients with an obvious corneal opacity, or with an unprotected cornea due to lagophthalmos, usually with an absent Bell's phenomenon.

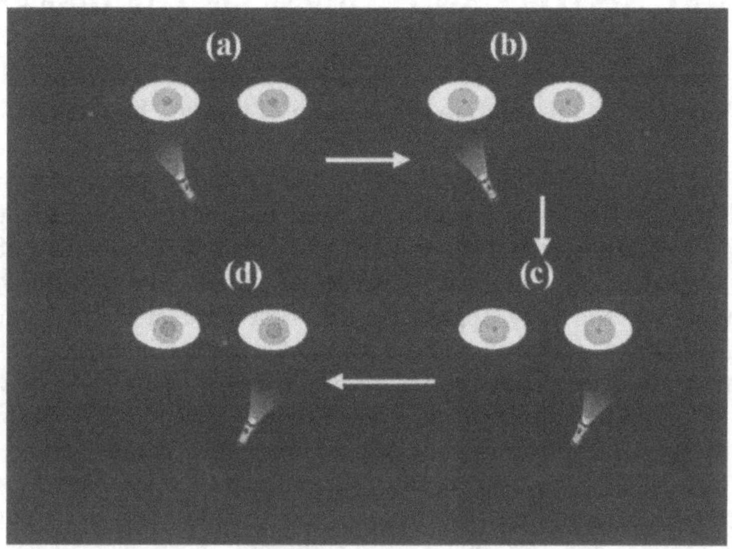

Figure 3. Relative afferent papillary defect. Example of compression of the left optic nerve. (a) a bright light is shone in the right (normal) eye. (b) a normal consensual papillary response is observed in both eyes. (c) the light source is shone on the left eye d) The pupils fail to constrict and may dilate

Patients who should be referred, but not urgently

- Those with a history of globe subluxation.
- Patients with foreign body sensation, which fails to resolve quickly despite regular use of artificial tears and lubricant ointment at night.
- Patients with a compensatory head posture, or with diplopia apparent during normal activities, particularly if primary gaze or reading is affected (13).
- Any patient who is psychologically and socially affected by the appearance of their eyes.
- Patients whose history suggests progressive deterioration of symptoms. Such patients are likely to have active disease, and should be taken seriously whether clinical signs are few or many, as early intervention is likely to result in better outcome (55).

NATURAL HISTORY AND COURSE OF THE DISEASE

Time of onset of GO in relation to the onset of Graves' hyperthyroidism

There is a close temporal relationship between the development of GO and that of Graves' hyperthyroidism in the majority of patients, both conditions occurring within 18 months of each other in 60% to 85% of patients (8,19,28,33). GO may precede or follow the development of hyperthyroidism and may appear for the first time after the patient has received treatment. GO may also be associated with other types of thyroid dysfunction: in an incidence cohort, Bartley et al (6) found that of 120 cases of GO, 90% had hyperthyroidism, 0.8% hypothyroidism, 3.3% Hashimoto's thyroiditis and 5.8% were euthyroid; in the much larger series of 557 consecutive patients, Kendler et al (28) found that 61% were hyperthyroid at or before the onset of GO, 20% females and 11% males were hypothyroid, and 34% females and 16% males were euthyroid; those over 50 years were more likely to be hypo- or euthyroid than hyperthyroid.

Natural History of GO when untreated

The majority of affected patients have only mild disease, which does not require any disease-modifying treatment (7). Although there are few reports of the natural history of GO in the untreated patient, the observations of Rundle (22,41) several decades ago still appear to offer a true, if general, picture of the likely course (Figure 4). The early phase of the disease is one of progressive deterioration; after reaching a plateau, which may last for months or even years, there is then a slow improvement.

The critical question is whether eventual return to the pre-morbid normal state is to be expected. In Rundle's curve the line depicting severity does not return to its baseline. In an early study (22) 104 patients were traced 15 or more years after the initial presentation and reassessed: in 75 exophthalmos was unchanged and in 2/3 the extraocular muscle involvement was unchanged. In a study conducted in our own clinic (38) 59 patients were assessed every 3 months for 1 year or more, maintained euthyroid, but without any therapeutic intervention for their GO.

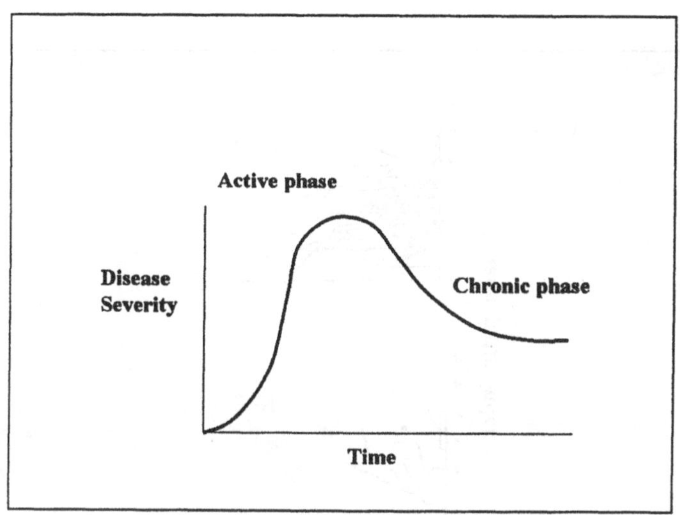

Figure 4. Rundle's curve, showing the early active phase of development and deterioration, followed by a plateau and then by slow improvement

Individual measures of disease severity included soft tissue involvement, diplopia, proptosis and differential intraocular pressure; in addition a cumulative score, or ophthalmopathy index (OI), was calculated. 22% showed no change in OI and 64.4% showed modest improvement, whereas 13.5% deteriorated and required disease-modifying treatment (Figure 5); the individual parameters also improved in most cases, with the least obvious change being in proptosis. Several other studies have used serial exophthalmometry, with rather variable results, but in general a poor incidence of improvement (43,44). These data are consistent with both Rundle's original observation, that although there is frequently some improvement this is by no means complete, and also with the clinical impression that proptosis shows less tendency to resolution than other features.

The likely explanation for this sequence of events relates to the underlying pathology. The ascending section of the curve reflects the period during which the autoimmune process is evolving – when there is inflammation of retrobulbar tissues, lymphocytic infiltration, production of glycosaminoglycans (GAGs) and edema. As this subsides a plateau is reached; but with regression of the inflammatory process, fibrosis may develop, so that the affected tissues do not return to their healthy state and the patient may still have some increase in retrobulbar pressure (hence the continuing proptosis) and chronic dysfunction of extraocular muscles.

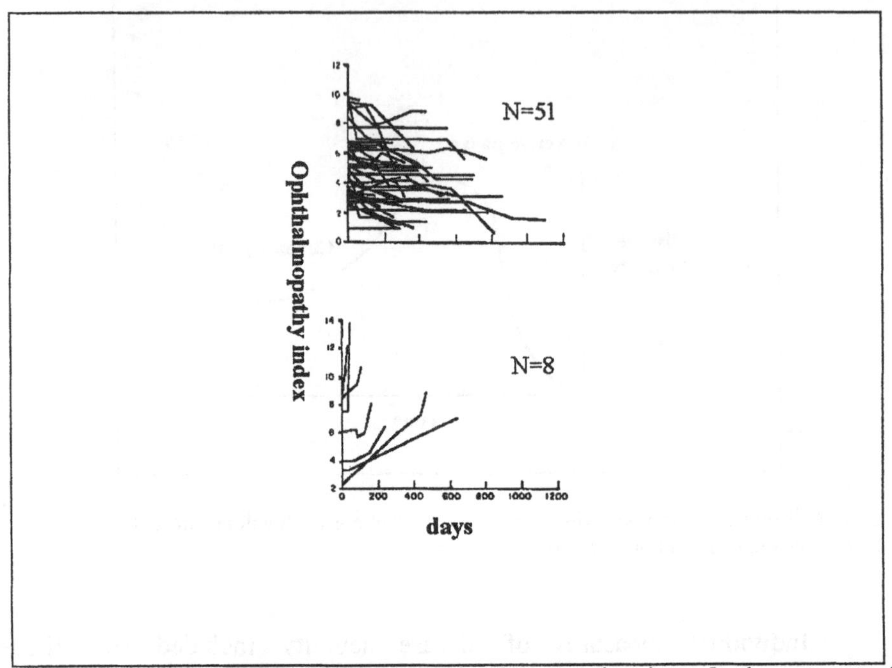

Figure 5. The natural history of GO history in 59 untreated patients. In the upper panel, patients showed either spontaneous improvement or no change, whereas the lower panel shows those who deteriorated and required disease-modifying treatment (38).

Understanding this process of development has important clinical implications, and also explains why the results of therapeutic studies can be difficult to interpret. At the time a patient is seen in the clinic, the doctor must determine whether the condition is in the steep ascending part of the curve, or at the same level but on the other side of the plateau. What might be interpreted as therapy-induced improvement may be due to spontaneous change; or the apparent absence of response may indicate that progression of the active disease has been delayed. A distinction therefore needs to be made between activity and severity.

Effects of treatment of Graves' disease on the course of GO

Although most patients develop thyrotoxicosis and GO at approximately the same time, these two manifestations of Graves' disease may run different courses. The endocrinologist faces two common dilemmas:

i) if the patient displays signs of GO, which treatment modality for the hyperthyroidism is best? ii) when GO has become manifest after initiation of treatment for hyperthyroidism, what role if any has the treatment for thyrotoxicosis played in triggering the onset of GO? The effect (if any) of the treatment modalities of thyrotoxicosis on the natural history of GO has been a subject which has generated debate and controversy for decades (12,47,30,53,34).

Early publications were merely reports of individual centres' experience. Valuable as they are, they are subject to bias in selecting patients and reporting effects (17). The last decade has seen the publication of a number of prospective studies that have attempted to address these important questions. Notable among them are a series of studies from the Pisa group and from Sweden. In a prospective randomized study, Bartalena et al (3) reported on the course of eye disease in patients treated with radioiodine with and without steroid cover. Most patients became hypothyroid after radioiodine. There was a striking difference in ophthalmological outcome in the two groups. Patients who received radioiodine alone had progressive GO and many required specific ophthalmological treatment. Those who in addition had prophylactic steroids fared well in terms of their eye disease. The authors concluded that steroid cover prevented the exacerbation of the eye disease associated with radioiodine therapy. This study however, did not incorporate a control group of patients treated with antithyroid drugs for comparison. It can be argued that all included patients were destined to develop progressive GO (if for instance they happened to be at the ascending limb of Rundle's curve) (Figure 4). Tallstedt et al (46) initiated a large prospective randomized study comparing the effects of antithyroid drugs, radioiodine and subtotal thyroidectomy on the development and progression of GO. Patients treated with radioiodine almost invariably developed hypothyroidism. Radioiodine was also significantly associated with a risk of developing or exacerbating GO. This group proceeded to show that prophylactic thyroxine replacement therapy after radioiodine (45) reduced the risk of development or progression of GO.

The Pisa group (2) reported on a large prospective, randomized study comparing the effects of radioiodine ablation with antithyroid drug treatment on the progression of GO. The objective was to answer conclusively the question of whether radioiodine made the eyes worse. Significant differences were found between the groups and indeed radioiodine seemed to be detrimental to the eyes (though an alternative interpretation could be that antithyroid drugs had a beneficial effect). However, some questions still remain (18). Hypothyroidism may still have had confounding effects on the outcome; although hypothyroidism was promptly corrected, its incidence in the radioiodine treated group of patients was threefold greater than in the methimazole treated group. The apparent detrimental effect of radioiodine on the eyes was not nearly as great in magnitude as the authors' earlier published study (3), despite similar inclusion criteria, and the appearance of GO after radioiodine was frequently transient. A less well known prospective, randomized (though smaller) controlled study by Manso et al (32) found no detrimental effect of radioiodine on the eyes of patients, but in this study no patient developed hypothyroidism after radioiodine, the confounding effects of smoking were eliminated and the ophthalmological assessments were possibly more objective as they were based on serial CT scans of the orbits.

Taken together these data are suggestive of a possible detrimental effect, albeit small, of radioiodine on the eyes compared to antithyroid drug treatment or thyroidectomy. From a practical point of view it would seem reasonable to avoid radioiodine in patients with active, severe GO; if radioiodine is inevitable early thyroxine replacement is recommended. Prophylactic steroids may also be considered.

The effects of thyroidectomy have been studied by the Swedish group (46) and by the Pisa group (34). Despite early work suggesting that total thyroidectomy may be beneficial (9) it would appear that the effects of thyroidectomy on GO are neutral.

The available treatments of hyperthyroidism do not appear to have a major effect on the course of GO. Of far more importance it seems, is maintenance of euthyroidism by whatever means.

Effects of hypothyroidism on the course of GO

It has for some time been the impression of clinicians that hypothyroidism has an adverse effect on GO. Several studies now appear to substantiate this: treatment-induced hypothyroidism led to worsening of GO (26,40), and elevated TSH levels after ^{131}I were also associated with exacerbation of the GO (29). In the large series from Sweden referred to above, the introduction of T4 treatment early after ^{131}I therapy, before hypothyroidism developed, caused a significant reduction in this worsening (45).

Effects of treatment of the GO on the long-term outcome

The questions of interest here are: 1) to what extent do disease-modifying treatments or surgery alter the course of the disease? 2) do the eyes eventually go back to normal?

Mild cases of GO will more or less regress spontaneously; but for the more severely affected patient, it needs to be stated here that no currently available treatment entirely suppresses the disease process so, not surprisingly, the features do not fully regress. Although high dose steroids result in significant improvement in some 60% of cases (5), in 20 to 40% cases there is little or no response to steroids and/or radiotherapy (5). Even those patients who do respond are unlikely to revert to normal. Surgery does of course alter the natural history: decompression is often effective, but is not without complications (14,48). The best chance of reversing the course of the disease in the severely affected case is often with a combination of disease-modifying treatment, surgical decompression, corrective muscle and lid surgery.

Despite the use of all available treatments, many patients feel that their eyes are still abnormal years later. Bartley et al (6) undertook a long term follow up study (median 9.8 years) of their incidence cohort of 120 patients using a patient self-assessment questionnaire. Of 92 respondents, 61% felt that their appearance had not returned to its former level, and 52% still thought their eyes appeared abnormal; this was despite the availability of surgical and medical treatment. Terwee et al (49) found that, in 158 patients studied 11.7 years (mean) after treatment with orbital radiotherapy and/or steroids, the quality of life was less than expected with respect to appearance of the eyes and visual function.

Environmental and genetic factors which may influence the course of the disease

Although there are as yet no direct data demonstrating either environmental or genetic effects on the course of GO, there is evidence to show that the disease severity is greater in association with certain of these factors. Thus indirectly it could be surmised that these factors have an adverse effect on the course of the disease.

CTLA-4: Understanding of the genetic basis underlying Graves' disease is at a rather early stage, but several candidate genes and loci have been identified by association and linkage studies. The CTLA-4 gene encodes a transcription factor that is a negative regulator for T-lymphocytes; case control studies suggest that the CTLA-4 gene may be a susceptibility locus for Graves' disease (24) and positive linkage of CTLA-4 to Graves' disease has been demonstrated (52); interestingly the association appeared to be particularly strong in those patients who also had GO (Figure 6) (51).

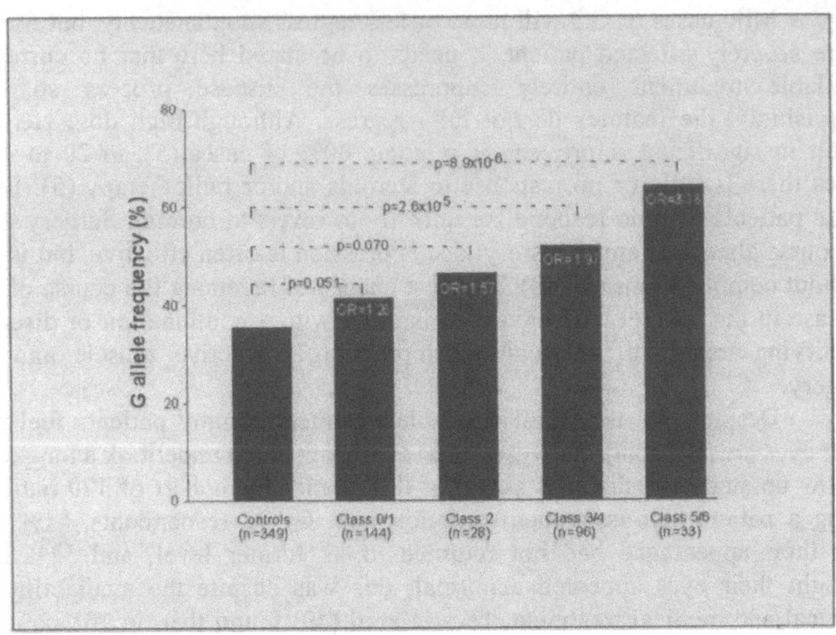

Figure 6. The *CTLA-4A/G* polymorphism in Graves' disease probands with varying severity of GO. The frequencies of the T allele at *CTLA-4C/T* (the y-axis) is shown for the controls and Graves' probands with different NOSPECS classes of GO. The association of the G allele correlates with the severity of GO manifestations, and is most marked in the subgroup of Graves' patients with the class 5 and 6 GO ($p=8.9x10^{-6}$, OR 3.18). (Courtesy of Dr. B. Vaidya)

Cigarette smoking markedly increases the risk of developing GO, and in several studies 70 to 80% of patients were cigarette smokers compared to a level in the control population of about 30% or less (4,21); cigarette smoking also increases the severity of the GO (5). Mann (31) calculated an increased risk of developing GO with an odds ratio of 7.7, and furthermore found that the number of cigarettes smoked per day was a significant determinant for the incidence of diplopia and proptosis. Smokers appear to respond less well to treatment with steroids or radiotherapy than non-smokers (5). The mechanism for these effects of cigarette smoking are as yet unknown, but it seems clear that smoking influences the risk, the severity and the response to treatment.

The severity of the hyperthyroidism, defined by a very high serum T3 (46), and of the autoimmune process, with a very high titre of TSHRAb (16,26), are also associated with more severe GO. In addition TSHRAbs correlated with the clinical activity score and with proptosis, but not with duration of the disease (16). These features may reflect not so much an 'environmental effect', but may rather be indicative of a particularly active form of the autoimmune condition.

CONCLUSIONS

Patients with GO may present in numerous ways, but the diagnosis is rarely difficult. Early, appropriate referral to specialist centres depends on careful evaluation of patients' symptoms and clinical signs. The knowledge that most patients with moderately severe GO do not attain full recovery should be an incentive to the specialist to seek to improve methods of assessment and treatment.

REFERENCES

1. Bahn RS, Bartley GB, Gorman CA. Emergency treatment of Graves' ophthalmopathy. Baillieres Clin Endocrinol Metab. 1992; 6:95-105.
2. Bartalena L, Marcocci C, Bogazzi F, Manetti L, Tanda ML, Dell'Unto E, et al. Relation between therapy for hyperthyroidism and the course of Graves' ophthalmopathy. N Engl J Med 1998; 338:73-78.
3. Bartalena L, Marcocci C, Bogazzi F, Panicucci M, Lepri A, Pinchera A. Use of corticosteroids to prevent progression of Graves' ophthalmopathy after radioiodine therapy for hyperthyroidism. N Engl J Med. 1989; 321:1349-52
4. Bartalena L, Martino E, Marcocci C, Bogazzi E, Panicucci M, Velluzzi F et al. More on smoking habits and Graves' ophthalmopathy. Journal of Endocrinological Investigation 1989; 12:733-737.
5. Bartalena L, Pinchera A, Marcocci C. Management of Graves' ophthalmopathy: reality and perspectives. Endocr Rev. 2000; 21:168-99.
6. Bartley GB, Fatourechi V, Kadrmas EF, Jacobsen SJ, Ilstrup DM, Garrity JA, Gorman CA. Long term follow-up of Graves' ophthalmopathy in an incidence cohort. Ophthalmology 1996; 103:958-962.
7. Bartley GB, Fatourechi V, Kadrmas EF, Jacobsen SJ, Ilstrup DM, Garrity JA *et al.*Clinical features of Graves' ophthalmopathy in an incidence cohort. Am J Ophthalmol 1996; 121:284-290.
8. Burch HB, Wartofsky L. Graves' ophthalmopathy: current concepts regarding pathogenesis and management. Endocr Rev 1993; 14:747-793.
9. Catz B & Pernik SL. Total thyroidectomy in the management of thyrotoxic and euthyroid Graves' disease . Am J Surg. 1969. 118. 434-439
10. Char I. Superior limbic keratoconjunctivitis: multifactorial mechanical pathogenesis. Clin Experiment Ophthalmol. 2000; 28:181-4.
11. Cole M, Mitchell S, Paisey R, Yeldham D. Recognising and treating thyroid-associated ophthalmopathy. Practitioner. 1995; 239:261-3.
12. DeGroot LJ, Gorman CA, Pinchera A, Bartalena L, Marcocci C, Wiersinga WM, Prummel MF, Wartofsky L, Marocci C. Therapeutic controversies. Retro-orbital radiation and radioactive iodide ablation of the thyroid may be good for Graves' ophthalmopathy. J Clin Endocrinol Metab. 1995; 80:339-40.
13. Fells P, Kousoulides L, Pappa A, Munro P, Lawson J. Extraocular muscle problems in thyroid eye disease. Eye. 1994; 8:497-505.

14. Garrity JA, Fatourechi V, Bergstrahl EJ, Bartley GB, Beatty CW, DeSanto LW *et al.* Results of transantral orbital decompression in 428 patients with severe Graves' ophthalmopathy. Am J Ophthalmol 1993; 116:533-547.
15. Gerding MN, Prummel MF, Wiersinga WM. Assessment of disease activity in Graves' ophthalmopathy by orbital ultrasonography and clinical parameters. Clin Endocrinol (Oxf). 2000; 52:641-6.
16. Gerding MN, van der Meer JW, Broenink M, Bakker O, Wiersinga WM, Prummel MF. Association of thyrotrophin receptor antibodies with the clinical features of Graves' ophthalmopathy. Clin Endocrinol 2000; 52:267-71
17. Gorman C. Radioiodine therapy does not aggravate Graves' ophthalmopathy. J Clin Endocrinol Metab 1995; 80:340-2.
18. Gorman CA, Offord K. Therapy for hyperthyroidism and Graves' Ophthalmopathy. N Eng J Med. 1998; 338:1546.
19. Gorman CA. Temporal relationship between onset of Graves' ophthalmopathy and diagnosis of thyrotoxicosis. Mayo Clin Proc. 1983; 58:515-9.
20. Gruters A. Ocular manifestations in children and adolescents with thyrotoxicosis. Exp Clin Endocrinol Diabetes 1999; 107:S172-4.
21. Hagg E, Asplund K. Is endocrine opthalmopathy related to smoking? Br Med J 1987; 295:634-635.
22. Hales IB and Rundle FF. Ocular changes in Graves' Disease. Quart J Med 1960; 29:113-126.
23. Heufelder AE, Spitzweg C. Immunology of Graves' ophthalmopathy. Dev Ophthalmol. 1999; 30:24-38.
24. Heward JM, Allahabadia A, Armitage M, Hattersley A, Dodson PM, Macleod K, Carr-Smith J, Daykin J, Daly A, Sheppard MC, Holder RL, Barnett AH, Franklyn JA, Gough SC The development of Graves' disease and the CTLA-4 gene on chromosome 2q33. J Clin Endocrinol Metab 1999; 84:2398-401
25. Kadrmas EF, Bartley GB. Superior limbic keratoconjunctivitis. A prognostic sign for severe Graves ophthalmopathy. Ophthalmology. 1995;102:1472-5.
26. Karlsson AF, Westermark K, Dahlberg PA, Jansson R, Enoksson P. Ophthalmopathy and thyroid stimulation. Lancet.1989; 2:691
27. Kendall-Taylor P, Perros P. Clinical presentation of thyroid associated orbitopathy. Thyroid. 1998; 8(5):427-8.
28. Kendler DL, Lippa J, Rootman J. The initial clinical shatacteristics of Graves' orbitopathy with age and sex. Arch Ophthalmol. 1993. 111: 197-201
29. Kung AEC, Yau CC Cheng A. The incidence of ophthalmopathy after radioiodine therapy for Graves' disease: prognostic factors and the role of methimazole. J Clin Endocrinol. Metab. 1994. 79. 542-546
30. Lazarus JH. Relation between thyroid eye disease and type of treatment of Graves' hyperthyroidism. Thyroid. 1998; 8:437.
31. Mann K. Risk of smoking in thyroid-associated orbitopathy Exp Clin Endocrinol Diabetes 1999; 107 Suppl 5:S164-7
32. Manso PG, Furlanetto RP, Wolosker AMB, Paiva ER, de Abreu MT, Maciel RMB. Prospective and controlled study of ophthalmopathy after radioiodine therapy for Graves' hyperthyroidism. Thyroid 1998; 8:49-52.
33. Marcocci C, Bartalena L, Bogazzi F, Panicucci M, Pinchera A. Studies on the occurrence of ophthalmopathy in Graves' disease. Acta Endocrinol (Copenh). 1989; 120:473-8.

34. Marcocci C, Bruno-Bossio G, Manetti L, Tanda ML, Miccoli P, Iacconi P, Bartolomei MP, Nardi M, Pinchera A, Bartalena L. The course of Graves' ophthalmopathy is not influenced by near total thyroidectomy: a case-control study. Clin Endocrinol (Oxf). 1999; 51:503-8.
35. Marino M, Barbesino G, Pinchera A, Manetti L, Ricciardi R, Rossi B, Muratorio A, Braverman LE, Mariotti S, Chiovato L. Increased frequency of euthyroid ophthalmopathy in patients with Graves' disease associated with myasthenia gravis. Thyroid. 2000; 10(9):799-802.
36. McKinnon SG, Gentry LR. Systemic diseases involving the orbit. Semin Ultrasound CT MR. 1998; 19(3):292-308.
37. Mourits MP, Prummel MF, Wiersinga WM, Koornneef L. Clinical activity score as a guide in the management of patients with Graves' ophthalmopathy. Clin Endocrinol 1997; 47:9-14.
38. Perros P, Crombie AL, Kendall-Taylor P. Natural history of thyroid associated ophthalmopathy. Clin Endocrinol 1995; 42:45-50.
39. Pinchera A, Wiersinga W, Glinoer D, Kendall-Taylor P, Koornneef L, Marcocci C *et al.* Classification of eye changes of Graves' disease. Thyroid 1992; 2:235-236.
40. Prummel MF, Wiersinga WM, Mourits MPh, Koorneef L, Berghout A & van der Gaag R. Effects of abnormal thyroid function on the severity of Graves' ophthalmopathy. Arch Int Med. 1990 150 1098-1011
41. Rundle FF. Development and course of exophthalmos in Graves' disease with special reference to the effect of thyroidectomy. Clinical Science 1945; 5: 177
42. Scott IU, Siatkowski MR. Thyroid eye disease. Semin Ophthalmol. 1999; 14(2):52-61.
43. Solem JH, Segaard E and Ytteborg J. The course of endocrine ophthalmopathy during antithyroid therapy in a prospective study. Acta Med Scand 1979; 205:111-114.
44. Streeten DHP, Anderson GH, Reed GF and Woo P. Prevalence, natural history and surgical treatment of exophthalmos. Clin Endocrin 1987; 27:125-133.
45. Tallstedt L, Lundell G, Blomgren H, Bring J. Does early administration of thyroxine reduce the development of Graves' ophthalmopathy after radioiodine treatment? Eur J Endocrinol. 1994; 130:494-7.
46. Tallstedt L, Lundell G, Torring O, Wallin G, Ljunggren JG, Blomgren H, Taube A. Occurrence of ophthalmopathy after treatment for Graves' hyperthyroidism. The Thyroid Study Group. N Engl J Med. 1992; 326:1733-8.
47. Tallstedt L, Lundell G. Radioiodine treatment, ablation, and ophthalmopathy: a balanced perspective. Thyroid. 1997; 7:241-5.
48. Tallstedt L. Surgical treatment of thyroid eye disease. Thyroid 1998; 8:447-452.
49. Terwee CB, Wakelkamp IMMJ, Tan HS, Dekker FW, Prummel MF, Wiersinga WM. Long-term effects of Graves' ophthalmopathy on health-related quality of life. 2001. Submitted
50. Trobe JD, Glaser JS, Laflamme P. Dysthyroid optic neuropathy. Clinical profile and rationale for management. Arch Ophthalmol. 1978; 96(7):1199-1209.
51. Vaidya B, Imrie H, Perros P, Dickinson J, McCarthy MI, Kendall-Taylor P *et al.*Cytotoxic T-lymphocyte antigen-4 (CTLA-4) gene polymorphism confers susceptibility to thyroid associated orbitopathy. Lancet 1999; 354:743-744.
52. Vaidya B, Imrie H, Perros P, Young ET, Kelly WF, Carr D *et al.* The cytotoxic T lymphocyte antigen-4 is a major Graves' disease locus. Hum Mol Genet 1999; 8:1195-1199.

53. Weetman AP, Harrison BJ. Ablative or non-ablative therapy for Graves' hyperthyroidism in patients with ophthalmopathy? J Endocrinol Invest. 1998; 21:472-5.
54. Weetman AP. Medical Progress: Graves' Disease. N Engl J Med. 2000; 343:1236-1248.
55. Wiersinga WM, Prummel MF. An evidence-based approach to the treatment of Graves' ophthalmopathy. Endocrinol Metab Clin North Am. 2000; 29:297-319.

9

IMAGING IN GRAVES' OPHTHALMOPATHY

George J. Kahaly, *Wibke Müller - Forell, °Gregor J. Förster, 'Susanne Pitz, "Hans Peter Rösler, and **Wolf J. Mann
*Departments of Endocrinology / Metabolism, *Neuroradiology, °Nuclear Medicine, 'Ophthalmology, "Therapeutic Radiology, and **ENT; Gutenberg - University Hospital, Mainz, Germany*

INTRODUCTION

Graves' ophthalmopathy (GO) is an autoimmune condition of the orbit which is closely associated with Graves' hyperthyroidism, though either condition may exist without the other. It may antedate, coincide with or follow hyperthyroidism (1-5). Assessment of the frequency of the association depends on the method used for detecting GO; with sensitive methods sub clinical GO can be demonstrated in 60-70% of patients with hyperthyroidism, whereas it is clinically apparent and moderately severe in about 10%. The clinical features of the disorder vary from a mild grittiness of the eyes to severe diplopia, loss of vision and disfiguring proptosis. The pathogenesis is poorly understood, and the available methods for prevention and treatment are far from ideal. The most obvious pathological change within the orbit is the enlargement of extra ocular muscles (6). In most cases microscopy reveals that the muscle fibers are preserved and the increase in muscle bulk reflects changes in the connective tissue: fibroblasts are very numerous, there is lymphocyte infiltration (8-12), an excessive deposition of collagen and of glycosaminoglycans (GAG) which lead to interstitial edema. A role for cytokines in GO (13) seems likely: it may be that the autoimmune response evokes the local production within the orbit of cytokines which cause fibroblast stimulation and hence the production of collagen and GAGs (14-18). The muscles most frequently affected are the medial and inferior recti. Functionally the effect is of tightness or contraction of the muscles, and thus the patient may experience difficulty with upward or lateral gaze. The increased bulk of the muscles and of orbital connective tissue leads to an increase in pressure within the orbit, which results in some cases in proptosis, and in other cases, where the tissues at the apex of the orbit are involved, in optic neuropathy and disc edema.

There is a natural tendency towards spontaneous improvement: the spontaneous course depicts an active phase, which slowly abates after which an inactive phase ensues (19), which may still be associated with ophthalmic abnormalities. Although sparse, there are histology data to support this idea of active and inactive disease phases. The orbital tissues are edematous in patients with early disease, whereas patients with longstanding GO have fibrous tissues. On histological examination, early disease was associated with a mononuclear cell infiltrate, while in the late stages only dense collagen scar tissue was found. In addition to macrophages, T- and B-lymphocytes, granulated mast cells may be present. Thus, there seems to be consensus that edema with a lymphocyte infiltrate of the orbital tissues characterize the active stage, whereas fibrosis can be seen during all stages, but is much more abundant in inactive eye disease (20-24). This natural course of GO has been the basis for the initiation of immunomodulatory therapies. They are aimed at the edematous, lymphocyte infiltration and the activated fibroblasts. Medical treatment will only be effective during the active phase and should not be given to patients with inactive eye disease. In contrast, it is generally recommended that rehabilitative surgery (as opposed to acute decompression because of sight loss) should only be done on patients with inactive disease (25,26). If this kind of surgery were to be performed during the active stages, the result might be lost due to an ongoing disease process. Thus, the main reasons to use medical therapies are to alleviate the eye features during the active stage of the disease and hopefully obliterate the need for surgery, as well as to inactivate the disease in order to submit the patient safely to rehabilitative surgery.

IMAGING PROCEDURES IN GO

Differential diagnosis of GO include lymphoma, metastasis, tumors of the nasal cavity or sinuses, and fistula of the carotid sinus cavernous. However, the major differential diagnosis of GO is myositis, a local form of the orbital pseudotumor. This nonspecific, inflammatory condition may involve every orbital structure to a different extent. Enlargement of the muscle including the tendon is characteristic for this inflammation of a single muscle; the isolated orbital pseudotumor shows no preference for a muscle group. With respect to diagnostic procedures as well as follow-up after specific conservative and/or surgical treatment, imaging with computed tomography (CT), magnetic resonance imaging (MRI), orbital ultrasound (US), and somatostatin receptor scintigraphy with the radio labeled somatostatin analog (Octreotide, octreoscan) plays an important role in the interdisciplinary management of subjects with GO (27). Especially CT and MRI show the actual objective morphological findings (28), quantitative MRI giving additional information concerning the acuteness or chronicity of the disease. Major morphological diagnostic criteria include a spindle like spreading of the rectus muscles (> 4 mm) without involvement of the tendon, a compression of the optic nerve in the orbital apex (crowded orbital apex syndrome) and the absence of any space occupying intraorbital process. A longer lasting course of the disease may lead to a corresponding impression of the lamina papyracae, the normally parallel configured medial wall of the orbit, similar to a spontaneous decompression.

Recently, members of the European Thyroid Association (ETA) were invited to answer a questionnaire to determine how expert thyroidologists assess and treat GO (29). Eighty-four responses were received from 19 European countries, representing approximately 60% of the clinically active ETA members. Marked geographical variation was noted, particularly in the treatment of GO. Observed consensus was nation-wide rather than Europe-wide. For imaging of GO, major differences in investigation usage between European countries were registered. CT scans were used by 32% of German centers, which conducted the most MRI scans (50%). In Denmark and the Netherlands, 88 and 100%, respectively used CT scans compared to 13 and 0% for MRI scans. Octreoscans were performed only in Austria, Belgium, Germany, Italy, the Netherlands, and Poland. Eighteen centers used US plus either CT or MRI, 5 used CT and MRI and 5 used octreoscan plus either CT or MRI. All in all, CT scans; MRI, US, and octreoscans were used in 65, 34, 28, and 7%, respectively. In the following, detailed description of the different modern imaging techniques and their clinical applications will be discussed.

COMPUTED TOMOGRAPHY (CT)

Technique

CT can distinguish normal and abnormal structures of different tissue density on the basis of differential x-ray absorption's. Orbital fat absorbs x-rays to a lesser degree than water; it is imaged in CT as a black, low-density area that contrasts with the higher-density image of extra ocular muscles and the optic nerve (30). CT's ability to differentiate these tissues is due to relative contrast differences greater than 14%; modern scanners can distinguish tissues with less than 1% contrast difference. The presence of orbital fat allows high spatial and density resolution of orbital structures. Inherent tissue differences in the orbit obviate the need for intravenous contrast unless a patient present with visual loss. The common principle of CT is the digital recording of data and a complicated arithmetic procedure (Fourier transformation) in order to convert the data into different gray scales. In comparison to (the so-called isodense) brain tissue such as bone or extra vascular fresh blood with high absorption values are called hyper dense, while low absorbing tissue such as water or fat are hypo dense. In most institutions, orbital CT scans are routinely performed using 1- to 2-mm thick sections at 2-mm intervals in the axial plane. Individual volume elements (voxels) obtained from these axial slices can be reformatted in any plane to produce coronal, sagittal, paraxial, or parasagittal oblique images. In contrast to direct coronal scans, sagittal and coronal reformations avoid high spatial frequency artifacts from dental appliances and other metal implants. Multiplan reformations enable to view a lesion in the optimum anatomic plane and assess its location relative to contiguous orbital, bone, sinus, and central nervous system structures. Axial CT examination of the orbit should be prepared in a line parallel to the infraorbital-meatal line, a line between the upper part of the external acoustic meatus and the orbital floor, which guarantees images parallel to the orbital axis and a common visualization of the intraorbital course of the optic nerve with the medial (lateral) external muscles in one slice. In case of a positive tilt artifacts of the petrous bone will disturb the image, while a negative tilt will miss the target of a single slice for visualization of the optic nerve. Modern CT equipment enables a routine application of spiral technique (simultaneous x-ray exposition and defined table movement) of 2/3 mm slice-thickness and distance respectively. A coronary projection perpendicular to the skull base is necessary in order to define the involvement of the inferior and/or superior rectus muscles. As in every x-ray application one should recognize the lens during CT examination of the orbit as being one of the most sensitive organs. In axial examination parallel to the axis of the orbit the lens is in the center and the radiation dosage is comparable to a carotid angiography's or a conventional tomography of the orbit. Depending on the slice thickness and table movement the total lens dose may be from 40.3 mSv (2 mm slice thickness and table movement respectively) to 41.5 mSv (3 mm slice thickness and table movement) per slice. The threshold dose for a cataract is known to be the equivalent of an exposure dose of 0.5 Sv for a single exposure, keeping in mind a latency of up to 25 years after x-ray exposition, but cumulative effect of the radiation.

Clinical applications

In GO the imaging pattern is relatively characteristic (Figures 1 and 2): the extra ocular muscles appear to be the primary area of orbital involvement in GO, while others suggest that fat and muscle volume are increased (31-34). The lacrimal gland can occasionally be enlarged. Among patients with GO, fat volumes as high as 22 ml and muscle volumes as great as 21.5

ml were recorded. The error rate in these measurements was 1 to 7% depending on the relative size of the volume measured. Forbes et al. (35-37) found the mean volume of normal extra ocular muscles to be 4.69 ml (range 3.66-6.2 ml) in females and 4.79 ml (3.07-6.18 ml) in males. For orbital fat the figures were 10.1 ml (8.2-12.2 ml) in females and 11.19 (8.6-14 ml) in males. Extra ocular muscle enlargement can be asymmetric in as many as 30% of the cases. In a series of 116 patients with Graves' disease, definite enlargement of extraocular muscles in 85% was noted (38). The inferior rectus was enlarged in 77%, the superior in 51%, and the lateral rectus in 80%. In another series of 80 CT examinations of GO patients, the inferior rectus was enlarged in 60%, the medial in 50%, the superior in 40%, and the lateral in 22%. In Japanese CT scan study on 349 thyroid patients (39) the inferior rectus was enlarged in 43%, the medial in 38%, the superior in 29%, and the lateral in 16%. One muscle was enlarged in 31%, two muscles in 25%, three muscles in 24%, and all four recti in 21% of patients with ocular involvement. In most studies, CT findings have correlated with clinical impressions of the severity of extra ocular muscle enlargement (Table 1). Bilateral orbital involvement on CT scans is noted in approximately 50-75% of patients presenting with unilateral eye findings. Unlike patients with orbital myositis or orbital pseudotumor, evidence of muscle involvement on CT of GO is usually limited to the non-tendinous portion of the muscle. Often several muscles are enlarged, especially at the orbital apex. The use of reformation improves delineation of the recti muscle involvement. In GO patients, there is no evidence of an orbital mass, nevertheless, in a few GO patients; axial CT may demonstrate an enlarged inferior rectus muscle than can simulate an apical neoplasm. CT is also useful in GO subjects to delineate the etiology of decreased vision. Several investigators have noted that increased extra ocular muscle volume or area on CT correlates with compressive optic neuropathy (40). Increased muscle volume on CT was associated with optic nerve compression (41-42) and the area of the medial rectus muscle on a mid-axial scan correlated with total muscle volume (r = 0.88) and can be used to predict possible optic nerve compression. Other findings that may be noted on CT are a dilated superior ophthalmic vein and abrupt angulations of the posterior muscle belly. An additional sign of nerve compression is fat prolapsed into the CNS (43). Nevertheless, MR scans show the optic nerve compression better than CT evaluation.

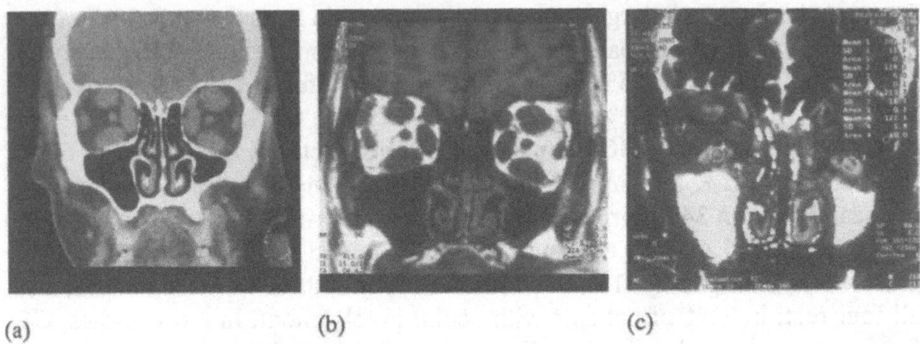

(a) (b) (c)

Figure 1. Coronal CT scans with involvement of all external muscles, especially both oblique (panel a). Coronal reformation demonstrates degree of recti muscle involvement at different levels of the orbit. Corresponding MRI with T1 weighted images (panel b), and corresponding coronal T2-time image, where the most edema is detectable in both inferior, superior and oblique recti muscles. T2 measurements detected a difference of more than 0.1 sec in contrast to the not inflammatory involved lateral muscles (panel c).

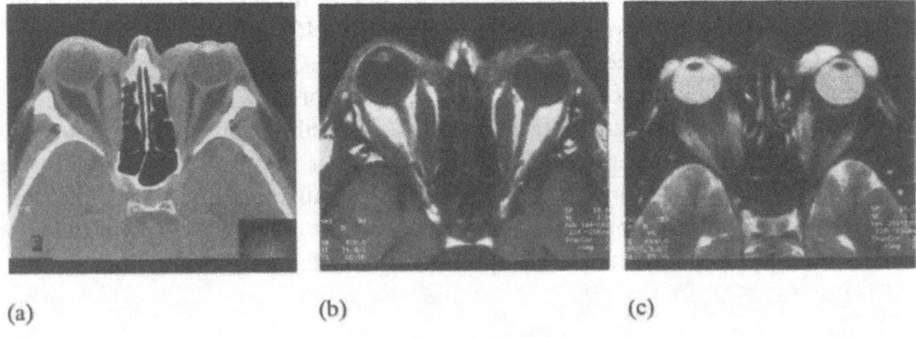

(a) (b) (c)

Figure 2. Axial CT demonstrating bilateral proptosis, thickening of the medial and lateral recti muscles, and a slight impression of the right lamina papyracae (panel a). Tendons of the recti muscles are not enlarged. Note the thickening of both conjunctivas. Corresponding MRI with T1 weighted images (panel b). Corresponding coronal T2-weighted (fat suppressed) MRI with signal enhancement of both the enlarged rectus muscles, as well as edema of the involved conjunctiva of both eyes (panel c).

Table 1. Computed Tomography (CT)

Advantages
- Highly available (routinely performed in most institutions)
- Short investigation time (15 min.)
- Moderate costs (500 German Mark)
- Precise imaging of orbital apex, bony structures, sinus
- Accurate determination of area or volume of orbital tissue ("region of interest technique").
- Increased extra ocular muscle volume / area correlates with compressive optic neuropathy
- Accuracy: investigator independent

Disadvantages
- Less helpful for evaluation of disease activity
- Radiation exposure (0.5 mSv/2 mm thick sections)

Indications
- Mandatory pre- (and post?) orbital decompression surgery
- Uncertain diagnosis and if MRI is not available! Soft-tissue spatial resolution obtainable with MRI is greater than that obtained with CT and shows greater tissue contrast.

CT (and MRI) findings suggestive of GO
- Enlarged extra ocular muscles; tendons insertion often spared
- Absence of orbital masses, vascular engorgement, sinus involvement
- Occasional slight bowing of medial orbital wall ("Coca-Cola sign")
- Occasional inferior rectus enlargement on axial scan; simulates an orbital tumor
- Occasional compression of the optic nerve by enlarged extra ocular muscles
- Intracranial fat prolapsed with optic nerve compression
- Rare lacrimal gland enlargement

MAGNETIC RESONANCE IMAGING (MRI)

Technique

MRI is a diagnostic imaging technique that does not use ionizing radiation (5,45,46). It is based on the principle that hydrogen nuclei with an odd number of nucleons (protons and neutrons) behave as small magnets or dipoles. Protons are ubiquitous, and their resonance is the basis of clinical MRI techniques. Imaging with MR represents free moving protons of a given tissue, producing energy (read as signals) while returning into their primary position in a high magnetic field after deflection by a high frequency pulse.

On principle bright signals were defined as hyper intensity, while low signal areas were defined as hypo intensity to signal void of complete loss of signal. When the orbit is placed in a magnetic field there is a net alignment of protons. When exposed to radio-frequency (RF) excitation there is a reversal of polarity of some of these hydrogen nuclei, and they are raised to a higher energy level. When the RF is terminated, the protons return to the baseline polarity, and the emitted energy can be measured. This is called Tl relaxation (Tl) and is best measured immediately after RF termination. Exposure to RF excitation also initiates a uniform synchronous precession, or spin, among the protons. When the RF is terminated, this precession diminishes at differing rates for protons in different molecular environments. The energy emission measured from this event is called T2 relaxation time (T2). Since the RF-initiated events depend on the frequency and magnetic field strength, the location of these events in three-dimensional space can be determined by imposing a gradient (approximately 0.1 tesla [T] per centimeter on the magnetic field and varying the RF). Optimal current strength for clinical imaging is 1.5 T, currently used scanners range from 0.15-4.5 T. Orbital anatomic detail is obtained with surface coils and thin section scans. Signal-to-noise ratio improves with increasing field strength. The components of the MR signal that form an image reflect proton density, Tl/T2 relaxation, and vascular flow, if present. In MR, relative rates of demagnetization and loss of processional frequency and proton density are responsible for signal intensity differences. Imaging techniques, field strength, and tissue magnetic susceptibility influences these MR parameters. The time lapse of the so-called resonance signal is characterized by the two parameters Tl and T2 which are specific for a given tissue and defined by the biochemical environment (Table 2) A basic rule for MRI is that Tl weighted (Tlw) images are best for anatomic structure, while T2w sequences give more information about the different tissue composition (Table 3). Concerning the examination protocol, no differences should be made in the strategy of orientation compared with CT. The advantage of MRI is the ability to view several (axial, coronal, sagittal) angles without movement of the patient. Tlw axial and coronal sequences give an overview of the extent of the disease, concerning globe proptosis and involvement of the different recti muscles. In some cases application of Gadolinium, the MR-contrast agent may help in better delineation of fatty degeneration, when applied with fat suppressed (FS) sequences. FS enables the differentiation of the intense signal enhancement of the recti muscles, which otherwise would look as intense as fat tissue. T2w sequences show the proton content of the pathology. Due to a worsening of the signal to noise ratio, slice thickness of routine examinations should not be less than 3 mm. T2 measurement with fat suppression (STIR sequence - short time inversion recovery), performed in the coronal view increases sensitivity of MRI for different proton concentrations. Orbital fat that has a short Tl and medium T2 relaxation will produce a relatively strong signal. Muscle is intermediate in signal intensity; vitreous has long T1 and T2, cortical bone is displayed as black (signal void) as there is no mobile hydrogen and therefore no MR signal. Soft-tissue spatial resolution obtainable with proton MRI is greater than that obtained with high-resolution CT and shows greater tissue contrast. In some disease processes, MRI is more sensitive to alterations in water content or hydrogen concentration than is CT or other conventional imaging techniques.

Table 2. Magnetic Resonance Imaging (MRI)

Advantages
- Tissue differentiation
- Lack of ionizing radiation
- Capability of Multiplan (high quality!) imaging: optimal orbital anatomic detail obtained with surface coils and thin section scans.
- T2 relaxation time: sensitive for demonstrating interstitial edema within rectus eye muscles and edema in orbital fat. Compared to CT, MRI is more sensitive to alterations in water content or hydrogen concentration processes
- Accuracy: investigator independent
- High negative predictive value

Disadvantages
- Less helpful for evaluation of bony structures
- Expensive (800 German Mark)
- Investigation time 45-60 min.
- "Claustrophobia"

Indications
- Uncertain diagnosis (thyroid vs. other cause of orbital disease)
- Patient with thyroid disease and decreased vision: MR scans with fat saturation and gadolinium (contrast agent) are indicated. MRI can detect compressive optic nerve changes and differentiate them from no compressive neuropathy. Sensitivity of MR to detect and delineate the etiology of visual loss in these patients surpasses that possible with CT
- GO in which it is uncertain whether medical, irradiation, or surgical intervention is appropriate: better delineation of inflammatory from fibrotic disease than clinical evaluation.

Table 3. MRI: Signal intensities of different orbital tissues

	T1W	T1W (FS)	T2W (pw)	T2W
Fat tissue	↑↑	↓↓	↑	↗ To →
Globe	↓	↓	→	↑
Rectus muscles	↓	↑↑ (After G)	↗	↘
Bone	O	O	O	O
Marrow	↑	↓	↑	↘
Gray matter	↓	↓	→	↗ To ↑
White matter	↗	↗	→	↓
CSF	↓	↓	→	↑ To ↑↑
Vessels	O	O	O	O

FS: fat suppression; T1: T1 relaxation time, T1w: T1 weighted, PW: proton-weighted; G: Gadolinium
→: Intermediate signal (gray)
↗: Moderate hyper intense (light gray)
↑: Hyper intense (white)
↘: Moderate hypointens (middle gray)
↓: Hypo intense (dark gray)
O: no signal (black)

Clinical applications

MRI offers the potential of being able to estimate disease activity although cost and availability are current limitations of this modality. Pulse sequences that examine T2 can estimate the water content of tissues. Quantitative MRI allows noninvasive detection of edematous changes in orbital tissue: when examining the extra ocular muscles, normal T2 might imply burned out, fibrotic disease with normal or low water content, whereas prolonged T2 might suggest ongoing inflammation with tissue edema possibly amenable to immunosuppression or radiotherapy. Using a .28 Tesla magnet, some reports noted a correlation between T2 and response to treatment. STIR is another MRI pulse sequence that can be used to estimate water content of tissues.

Comparing the extra ocular muscle signal to control tissues, two studies found that a high STIR was associated with disease activity (46,47). Significant enlargement of one or more extra ocular muscles was observed in 86% of patients with GO, and STIR of eye muscles was increased compared to control values. STIR of eye muscles and orbital connective tissue in the patients giving favorable responses to steroids were greater than those in patients who did not respond. Furthermore, a significant correlation between STIR of eye muscle and that of orbital connective tissue was demonstrated, indicating that a common mechanism may be involved in the pathogenesis of the muscle and connective tissue components of GO. MRI of optic nerves also demonstrates compression better than CT, and delineation of compressive optic neuropathy is easier with MR than CT (48).

Infiltration of orbital tissue by lymphocytes leads to fibroblast stimulation and consequently increased GAG production. By binding large amounts of water, GAG cause edema, resulting in an increased volume. Therefore, increased water content of thickened extra ocular muscles is most likely the cause of elevated T1/T2. Reversibility of thickness and relaxation times in muscles with primarily elevated T1/T2 can be explained as a therapy-induced decrease of water content. In numerous studies, GO patients with primarily elevated T1/T2 of extra ocular muscles showed better response to steroid- and/or radiotherapy with respect to change in muscle thickening, than those with primarily normal T1/T2 (49). In a controlled study, muscles with primarily elevated T2 showed marked reduction of T2 by 30%, and muscle area by 32% after immunosuppressive therapy (44). At the end of therapy, a reduction of more than 30%, or normalization of muscle area occurred in 50% of muscles with primarily elevated T2. In contrast thickened muscles with primarily normal T2 only exhibited a slight decrease of muscle area. The predicted probability of response to treatment increased with increased mean T2 of extra ocular muscles prior to therapy (50). Of the subjects undergoing treatment with glucocorticoids and irradiation, only those with markedly prolonged T2 showed an impressive response. Recently, long-term follow-up data of a large number of patients with severe GO who were monitored by MRI before and after therapy with the immunosuppressive drug Ciclosporin were reported (51). In these patients there was a correlation between decrease in T2 of the superior, medial, and inferior rectus muscle and response to Ciclosporin treatment. In addition, the infiltrative eye signs improved in correlation with T2, muscle thickness and intraocular pressure. Thus, the major result of these studies is the relationship between response to therapy and pretherapeutic T1/T2 times. Quantitative MR allows non-invasive detection of acute inflammatory changes in extra ocular muscles. Therefore, measurement of elevated T1/T2 might play a role in the prediction of the reversibility of muscle thickening and favors the choice of anti-inflammatory therapy regimens in these patients. In previous work, T2 of the rectus eye muscles also significantly correlated with orbital accumulation of the radio labeled Octreotide (octreoscan) in untreated subjects with active GO, suggesting possible similar pathological processes in the orbital tissue with similar prognostic and therapeutic implications (52).

ULTRASOUND (US)

Technique

US is usually performed with A-scan, B-scan, or both (53-56). Immersion B-scan US is the easiest image for the nonultrasonographer to visualize; enlarged extra ocular muscles are quite clear (Figure 3). Standardized US A-scans can be used to assess certain tissue characteristics based upon reflected acoustic waves. Reflectivity in the extra ocular muscles changes as a function of tissue edema and cellular infiltration. For example, a low reflectivity on standardized A-scan may be a valid means of assessing activity of disease. Quantitative A-scan echography, using a standardized Kretz unit, is also most useful for determining if individual recti muscles are enlarged (measuring the maximum diameter of the extra ocular muscles). Maximal muscle thickness above the ninety-fifth percentile, or a variance of more than 0.5 mm between the same muscles in the two orbits, is consistent with the diagnosis of GO. The probe is directed toward the widest portion of the muscle. The width of the echographic envelope can be measured directly. In the hands of an experienced orbital ultrasonographer, the test is relatively reliable, accessible, and inexpensive. Byrne et al. (57) have completed a careful assessment with detailed statistical analysis of extra ocular muscle dimensions as measured by A and B mode echography using modern instrumentation. Healthy extra ocular muscles ranged in diameter from 2.6±0.5 mm for the inferior rectus to 5.3±0.7 mm for the levator complex. Diameter of contra lateral muscles varied by as much as 0.8 mm. On the other hand, numerous authors have reported a wide range of values representing normal values for the different rectus muscles. Furthermore, high resolution MRI with surface coils was compared to standardized US in the determination of maximum transverse extra ocular muscle diameters, and was low. The source of this discrepancy is uncertain, since both techniques are subject to imaging artifacts. In the high-resolution MR images, the muscles had a teardrop shape; perhaps the widest part of the extra ocular muscle is not consistently imaged with the US technique. Thus, operators experienced in the performance and interpretation of the study best do US examinations. The relative rarity of experienced ultrasonographers also limits the utility of this method. Finally, although orbital US has many advantages, it cannot effectively display the muscles at the apex of the orbit where compression of the optic nerve commonly occurs.

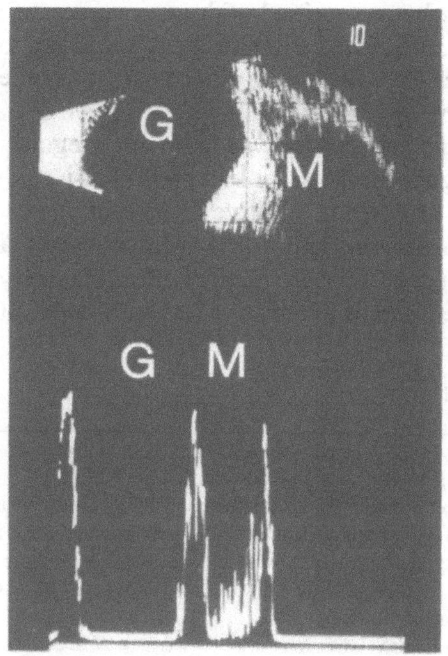

Figure 3. Ultrasound of the orbit: A- (lower panel) and B-scan (upper panel) showing enlarged extroocular rectus muscle (M), G: globe.

Clinical applications

US is a cost-effective screening test for the evaluation of GO patients (Table 4). The detection of extra ocular muscle defects with US is more sensitive than is clinical examination. If the patient is suspected of having GO, US may be used if an orbital scan is needed to confirm the diagnosis (57). In one study, while enlargement of extra ocular muscles was only noted clinically in 12% of patients, on US this was detected in 95% of cases. In a further study, 20 of 32 patients (63%) without clinical eye disease had B-scan evidence of muscle enlargement. Some US studies have routinely demonstrated enlarged optic nerves in GO; most studies have noted these findings rarely, usually in association with optic neuropathy. US is also an objective means to monitor anterior and midorbital therapeutic response, although it does not add sufficiently to clinical data as to be worthwhile. Erickson et al (58) have proposed serial US as a suitable method to follow the changes after radiotherapy in patients with GO. They indicated that standardized US assumes standardized instrument design and examination techniques with combined A-scan, B-scan, and Doppler techniques. With this method the authors claimed 99% accuracy in diagnosing GO and that the thickness of the medial, lateral, and inferior muscles can be ascertained with an accuracy of ± 0.75 mm. On the other hand, there is sufficient variability in A-scan data to limit its patent use to determine whether fibrosis has developed. Internal reflectivity of the sound beam was found to be low in subjects with active eye disease, presumably due to edema, whereas the reflectivity was high and irregular in inactive patients, due to fibrotic echogenic scar tissue. In a preliminary study in 16 patients (59) the method seemed promising: positive and negative predictive values of 73 (reflectivity of 40% or less) and 100%, respectively (Table 5) were noted. However, after testing US in 56 patients with moderately severe GO, the results were rather disappointing: negative PV 60%, only (60).

Table 4. Ultrasound (US)

Advantages

- Cost effective screening test (< 100 German Mark).
- Detection of extra ocular muscle defects with US is more sensitive than is clinical examination. Immersion B-scan is the easiest image to visualize enlarged extra ocular muscles, whereas quantitative A-scan is most useful for determining if individual recti muscles are enlarged
- Short investigation time (15 min.)
- No ionizing radiation
- Objective means to monitor anterior and midorbital therapeutic response

Disadvantages

- Not as effective as CT in delineating the relationship of orbital pathology to contiguous structures, nor is it reliable in imaging lesions of the posterior orbit, nor those involving the bone walls
- Accuracy of muscle measurements significantly less than MRI
- Accuracy: investigator dependent
- Does not add sufficiently to clinical data as to be worthwhile

Indications

- If a patient is suspected of having GO, orbital US may be used to confirm the diagnosis
- Follow-up by same observer (prospective clinical studies)?

Findings suggestive of GO

B-scan

- Widening of echo-free area between orbital fat and bone
- Increased delineation of extra ocular muscle margin
- Posterior scalloped/indented orbital fat secondary to muscle enlargement
- "Doubling" of optic nerve sheath in optic neuropathy
- No detectable neoplasm

A-scan

- Extra ocular muscle enlargement > 95th percentile

Table 5. Accurate prediction of outcome of immunosuppressive therapy for subjects with GO

Cut off	+ve PV (%)	-ve PV (%)	N	Ref
Orbital MRI				
• T2 > 128 ms	50	75	18	45
• Signal intensity ratio > 1.8	69	86	23	47
Orbital Ultrasound				
• Reflectivity < 40 %	73	100	16	59
• Reflectivity < 40 %	85	60	56	60
Orbital Octreoscan				
• Orbit / brain ratio > 10	88	100	40	76
• Orbit / skull ratio > 1.5	87	100	12	79
• Orbit / occipital ratio > 1.85	92	70	22	81

PV: predictive value, +ve: positive, -ve: negative, N: number of investigated patients, Ref: reference

Orbital surgeons rely primarily on CT and MRI for diagnosis of orbital tumors. While a number of authors have suggested that A-scan US measurements of muscle thickness are highly accurate and reproducible, the no geometric pattern of muscle enlargement can produce measurement errors on repeat US evaluations. US is not as effective as CT in delineating the relationship of orbital pathology to contiguous structures, nor is it reliable in imaging lesions of neither the posterior orbit, nor those involving the bone walls (61). When US measurements of muscle thickness were compared with MR data, the accuracy of US was significantly less, and this problem was worse in muscles other than the inferior rectus (62). These authors compared standardized A-mode US with MRI in 20 volunteer patients. Maximum transverse diameter of each rectus muscle was determined by each method in 39 orbits. Linear regression of individual US against MRI showed coefficients of determination moderate (0.29) for inferior recti muscles and low (0.11) for other recti muscles. Further errors in using a cross-sectional approach are derived from the oval rather than round cross section of the muscles, and because the maximum thickness occurs only over a limited anteroposterior distance in the orbit. This makes it difficult for the ultrasonographer to orient the beam so that it is exactly perpendicular to the muscle at the point of interest. These and other physical limitations of the US approach may account for the wide difference in published norms for transverse diameter of the recti. For the medial rectus muscle these range from the 95th percentile values of 6.08 to < 3.6 indicating not only the inherent variability of US measurements but also differences in technique between investigators. In a further study, orbital MRI and US were performed in 43 patients with GO with recently developed diplopia (63). MRI found no correlation between diameters of 233 extra ocular muscles measured by US and. For each of the four muscles, there was a diameter above which US was always unreliable. Neither US, nor any combination of 11 clinical and laboratory parameters provided the degree of information on muscles and connective tissue that was obtainable by MRI.

Color Doppler studies have also been performed in GO. Color Doppler imaging makes it possible to assess blood flow velocity of orbital vessels and allows detection of changes in the perfusion of orbital arteries and veins. At our institution, 23 subjects with GO were examined using color Doppler (64). Compared to controls, flow velocity in the right ophthalmic artery was markedly enhanced in subjects with clinically active GO. Furthermore, maximal blood flow velocity in the superior orbital vein was significantly decreased in GO subjects vs. controls and reduced venous outflow in the superior orbital vein correlated with the severity of GO. Thus, reduced venous outflow may contribute to proptosis by creating perivenous edema and consequent swelling of orbital fat.

OCTREOSCAN

Technique

Until recently there was no imaging technique available, which could demonstrate pathological changes in orbital tissues and could be regarded as a reliable inflammatory parameter for GO. Octreotide, a somatostatin (SM) analog labeled with indium has been used to localize tumors which possess surface or membrane receptors for SM in vivo (65-67) and to predict the inhibitory effect of Octreotide on hormone secretion by the tumors. By applying octreoscan, accumulation of the radionuclide was also detected both in the thyroid and orbit of patients with Graves' disease. If peak activity in the orbit 5 hours (hr) after injection (pi) of radio labeled octreotide is set at 100%, a decrease to 40% is found at 24 hr, significantly different from the decrease in blood pool radioactivity which is shown to be 15% at 24 hr. Accumulation of the radio nuclide is most probably due to the presence of activated SM receptors bearing lymphocytes in the orbital tissue. Alternative explanations are binding to receptors on other cell types (myoblasts, fibroblasts, endothelial cells) or local blood pooling due to venous stasis by the orbital inflammation. Wide differences exist between various studies regarding the administered dose of radio nuclide, the time interval after injection for determining the orbital uptake, the selection of orbital slices for quantification of the orbital uptake, and the method of correction for background radioactivity (68-71). Earlier studies used rather large doses and preferred to measure orbital uptake 24 hr pi, while later studies administered lower doses and measured orbital uptake only 2 hr pi arguing that the low dose decreases the radiation burden and the cost of examination. Nevertheless, a low dose might cause problems in count statistics and at 2 hr pi, 12% of the dose is still in the blood pool causing high background uptake. Furthermore, the radiation burden received from a high dose of 222 Mbq is 16 mSV, in the same order as that from chest CT or angiography. The inference is that for discrimination purposes a 4-hr time interval is preferred when a low dose is chosen. However, any remaining orbital radioactivity at 24 hr after administering a high dose might represent a greater degree specific tissue binding, possibly enhancing both the differential diagnostic and predictive value of octreoscan. Another technical problem is the selection of regions of interest (ROI), which may result in considerable intra- and interobserver variation. Single photon emission computed tomography (SPECT) images are obviously required and measuring uptake in a number of orbital slices from SPECT images is of great advantage in the quantification of the results. Using the left temporal skull area has originally performed correction for background activity. It was suggested that at least part of this radioactivity is due to uptake in the parotid gland and the authors recommended background measurements in the occipital skull area. The brain itself is used to measure background but for most investigators it seems less suitable to correct for blood pool radioactivity.

Recently, analysis of inter-/intra-observer variance and reproducibility in the evaluation of orbital SPECT images was performed (72). Transverse SPECT images were reconstructed, an optimal orbital image was selected and predetermined ROIs for both orbits were positioned by three independent observers 15 to 19 times each. In a second step, SPECT data of 8 different patients with GO were evaluated in the same manner by four independent observers 3 to 4 times each. Variance component partitioning was used to compare the order of intra- and inter-observer variation. For the right and the left orbit, the inter-observer variance proportion was 90 and 79%, whereas intra-observer variance partition was 10 and 21%, respectively. The corresponding ratios 0.11 and 0.27 summarize the comparison of sources of variance. The overall reliability was 84%, representing the patient's influence on the total variance. Intra-observer reliability for each observer was 88-98%. Using the Spearman Brown prophecy formula it follows that two replications per patient are sufficient to ensure a minimum reproducibility of 90%, which is also confirmed by the low intra-observer variation. Furthermore, intra-class correlation as a measure of observer reproducibility was 94%. Thus, due to the increased inter-observer variance proportion and the high variation in intra-observer reliability, evaluations of orbital octreoscan have to be done by the same and experienced observer leading to comparable data. Furthermore, an automatic and quantitative computerized technique for evaluation of these SPECT data could be exactly reproducible and would lead to more accurate and representative results. Therefore, standardized 3 dimensional (3-D) orbital volumes of interest (VOI) were generated on 10 MRI data sets of normal subjects (72). After position-orientation on a standard MRI data set, SPECT data were evaluated three times by automatically super-imposition with the size-adapted standardized VOIs (Figure 4). Orbital radionuclide activity was measured as uptake (%) of injected tracer activity and compared to the 2-D evaluation method. Advantages of the new, standardized, 3-D evaluation technique are both the accurate quantitative determination of the orbital uptake as well as the independence of observer variation.

Clinical applications

At our institution, both cross sectional as well as longitudinal and prospective studies in consecutive patients with Graves' disease and active GO showed that a high uptake of radio labeled Octreotide correlated with orbital inflammation and active hyperthyroidism (51, 74-76). In vivo imaging of SM receptors by the radionuclide as a sensitive nuclear medicine technique and a high positive predictive value was able to select those patients who might benefit from treatment with immunosuppressive agents. Furthermore, in the follow-up of these patients, the change in Octreotide binding during combined steroid/radiotherapy points to the fact that this type of scanning can be used to monitor the effects of treatment. Krenning et al. have also performed Octreoscan in patients with Graves' disease and controls (77). Thyroidal Octreotide accumulation was increased in thyrotoxicosis, and was almost absent after radio iodine-induced hypothyroidism. A correlation between thyroidal Octreotide accumulation and free T4 (disease expression) and thyroid binding-inhibiting immunoglobulins (disease activity) was present in untreated Graves' disease. Orbital Octreotide uptake was significantly higher in patients with active GO compared to those with slight GO, enhanced orbital radionuclide activity decreased after therapy. A correlation between orbital Octreotide uptake and the clinical score (disease activity) and total eye score (disease expression) was noted. High pre-treatment orbital uptake correlated with a response to radiotherapy in GO patients. The ability of this scintigraphic method to detect active eye involvement as compared to a purely clinical evaluation was also evaluated in subjects with GO, and a correlation between both methods was noted. All patients with highly active GO were clearly identified by both procedures. In patients with negative or intermediate clinical activity, the scan was also positive, thus disclosing a significant number of cases with active disease. Octreoscan also provided a higher number of positives as compared to MRI. Positive scans were also seen (particularly 4 hr pi) even under steroid therapy indicating persistent active disease, whereas patients with disease of long duration were negative. Successful immunoglobulin therapy significantly decreased inflammatory eye signs, clinical activity of the disease, and orbital radionuclide accumulation (78).

The long-acting synthetic SM analog Octreotide has been reported to have a beneficial effect in GO, probably by modulating lymphocyte responsiveness, and GAG production. In a placebo-controlled study, 12 GO patients received 0.3 mg Octreotide daily for 12 weeks (79). The seven patients who showed amelioration in ocular manifestation had positive orbital scans, while patients who did not respond had negative ones. None of the Graves' patients without clinical apparent GO had a positive octreoscan. Negative results in clinically highly suspected conditions might only be interpreted as absence of significant SM receptor accumulations, not as absence of disease. This may suggest that an orbital accumulation of the radiopharmacon may represent lymphocyte infiltration with inflammatory edema in the orbit and/or enhanced vascularisation, and is most probably due to the presence of SM receptor bearing active lymphocytes in these tissues. Results of octreoscan in GO patients correlated both with clinical activity scores as well as T2 of extra ocular recti muscles (80). Successful therapy with SM analogs (81) was associated with a fall in orbital uptake. Thus, octreoscan is mainly indicated in clinical practice to select GO patients who will benefit from immunomodulation. To this end one must know the predictive value of octreoscan for the outcome of immunosuppressive treatment. In one study, when a clinical improvement of GO was considered after 3 months of octreotide therapy, the positive and negative predictive values of octreoscan were 87 and 100%, respectively. When Lanreotide was used, the positive predictive value was 90% (82). In a recent paper (75), 14 of 16 GO patients, with an orbit–to–brain ratio > 10, 4 hr pi, responded to steroid-/radiotherapy, in contrast to none of 4 patients with a ratio < 10. Regarding the evaluation of GO activity, it was found that when an orbit/brain radio nuclide ratio greater than 10, 4 hr pi, was chosen as the cut-off point, a sensitivity of 94 and a specificity of 100% were given.

In conclusion, because of a favorable target to background ratio, octreoscan carries a high sensitivity and may be regarded as a semi-objective tool in the evaluation of patients with Graves' orbital and thyroidal disease, both at initial stages as well as during treatment (Table 6). A positive orbital octreoscan in GO patients indicates clinically active eye disease in which immunosuppressive treatment might be of therapeutic benefit. However, the following limitations restrict the widespread use of this technique. First, it is an expensive method with a non-negligible radiation burden. Second, it is nonspecific i.e. positive octreoscans may be obtained in patients with orbital diseases such as meningioma, myositis, lymphoma, granulomatosis, sarcoidosis, Wegener's, as well as sinusitis and infections of the nasal mucous. Last, octreoscan does not permit detailed orbital imaging or evaluation of eye muscle swelling. Thus, it remains to be seen if orbital octreoscan will become a widely available tool in the management of GO patients.

Table 6. Octreoscan

Advantages
- Favorable target to background ratio
- Highly sensitive for inflammation of orbital tissue
- Activity parameter for GO
- High positive predictive value for response to medical treatment
- Somatostatin receptor binding
- Thyroid imaging

Disadvantages
- Does not permit morphological orbital imaging
- Expensive (1200 German Mark)
- Interobserver variability
- Radiation burden: whole body dose equivalent (16 mSv for administered doses of 220 MBq)

Indications
- Evaluation of disease activity if clinical signs unclear, and if MRI is not available
- Prior to medical (immunosuppressive or octreotide) therapy?

SUMMARY

Orbital US, CT, as well as MRI are commonly used as imaging techniques to demonstrate pathological changes in ocular adnexa of patients with GO. Low cost, short time of investigation and lack of radiation characterize orbital US, a technique which ought to be more widely used. Thus, where available, orbital US may be useful diagnostically and also to evaluate the severity of eye muscle involvement. Nevertheless, although interesting data have been recently reported, neither a clear differentiation regarding disease activity is possible, nor is an evaluation of retro bulbar tissue precise enough. The more generally available techniques CT or MRI are particularly useful for diagnostic purposes where other orbital pathology, for example tumor, may need to be excluded; they also usefully demonstrate optic nerve compression at the apex of the orbit. When performing CT, radiation exposure is relatively high and differentiation between active and inactive GO is not possible. On the other hand, short investigation time, precise imaging of the orbital apex and moderate costs, are some advantages of this procedure. Furthermore, with the help of a computerized program (region of interest technique), the orbital adipose/connective volume can be accurately determined. CT delivers a significant radiation dose to the lens, which if repeated constitutes a risk for cataract development. For this reason MRI is preferable, particularly if repeat scans are required to assess response to treatment. The possibility of tissue differentiation, lack of ionizing radiation, and capability of Multiplan imaging uniquely suit MRI for eye studies. Although sensitive in demonstrating interstitial edema within the rectus muscles in patients with active disease, as well as providing a good predictive value with respect to immunosuppressive therapy, quantitative MRI with T1/T2 measurement is also an expensive method and non-specific for the orbital changes in GO. Furthermore, the time of investigation, 45 minutes, is long.

Until recently in nuclear medicine, there had not been any comparable inflammatory parameter in GO. Orbital octreoscan is a non-specific diagnostic method but has high sensitivity because of a favorable target to background ratio. This technique visualizes SM receptors in Graves' disease: radionuclide uptake is detected in both the thyroid and orbit of these patients. Accumulation of the radionuclide is most probably due to the presence in the orbital tissue of activated lymphocytes bearing SM receptors. Alternative explanations are binding to receptors on other cell types or local blood pooling due to venous stasis by the autoimmune orbital inflammation. A SPECT scan is necessary to properly quantify the orbital uptake. Although orbital octreotide uptake is shown to be a sensitive method with respect to the clinical differentiation between active and inactive GO, further studies with a large number of GO patients as well as patients with orbital tumors, myositis and orbital pseudotumor are needed to define the role and specificity of this scan. Furthermore, since octreoscan studies are expensive, they may be less readily available to clinicians. Radiation exposure is another disadvantage. To conclude, in unclear cases of proptosis or recently developed diplopia, prior to orbital decompression surgery, in the case of non-response to a conservative anti-inflammatory treatment or if, for any other reason, imaging is needed in subjects with GO, actually MRI is the imaging method of choice.

REFERENCES

1. Bahn RS, Garrity JA, Gorman CA. Diagnosis and management of Graves'ophthalmopathy. J Clin Endocrinol Metab 1990; 71: 559-563.
2. Riley FC. Orbital pathology in Graves'disease. Mayo Clin Proc 1972; 47: 975-979.
3. Bartley GB, Gorman CA. Diagnostic criteria for Graves'ophthalmopathy. Am J Ophthalmol 1996; 119: 792-795.
4. Kahaly G (Ed). Endocrine Ophthalmopathy. Molecular, immunological and clinical aspects. Karger publishers, Basel, 1993.
5. Kahaly GJ, Böckmann, Beyer J, Bischoff S. Longterm observation of endocrine ophthalmopathy and retrospective appraisal of therapeutic measures. J Endocrinol Invest 1990; 13: 287-293.
6. Char DH. Thyroid eye disease. Butterworth-Heinemann publishers, Boston, 1999, 3rd edition.
7. Kahaly G, Hansen C, Felke B, Dienes HP. Immunohistochemical staining of retrobulbar adipose tissue in Graves' ophthalmopathy. Clin Immunol Immunopathol 1994; 73: 53-62.
8. Otto E, Ochs K, Leyendecker E, Gentsch A, Kahaly GJ. Autoimmune endocrine ophthalmopathy and retrobulbar antigens. Horm Metab Res 1995; 27: 533-538.
9. Otto E, Förster G, Kuhlemann, Hansen C, Kahaly GJ. TSH receptor in endocrine autoimmunity. Clin Exp Rheumatol 1996; 14: 77-84.
10. Otto EA, Ochs K, Hansen C, Wall JR, Kahaly GJ. Orbital tissue-derived T lymphocytes from patients with Graves'ophthalmopathy recognize autologous orbital antigens. J Clin Endocrinol Metab 1996; 81: 3045-3050.
11. Kahaly GJ, Otto E, Förster G, et al. T cells and orbital connective tissue in endocrine orbitopathy. Exp Clin Endocrinol Diabetes 1996; 104: 79-83.
12. Förster G, Otto E, Hansen C, Ochs K, Kahaly GJ. Analysis of orbital T cells in thyroid-associated ophthalmopathy. Clin Exp immunol 1998; 112: 427-434.
13. Natt N, Bahn RS. Cytokines in the evolution of Graves'ophthalmopathy. Autoimmunity 1997; 26: 129-136.
14. Kahaly G, Schuler M, Sewell AC, Bernard G, Beyer J & Krause U. Urinary glycosaminoglycans in Graves' ophthalmopathy. Clin Endocrinol 1990; 33: 35-44.
15. Hansen C, Otto E, Kuhlemann K, Förster G, Kahaly GJ. Glycosaminoglycans in autoimmunity. Clin Exp Rheumatol 1996; 14: 59-68.
16. Hansen C, Fraiture B, Rouhi R, Otto E, Förster G, Kahaly GJ. HPLC glycosaminoglycan analysis in patients with Graves'disease. Clin Sci 1997; 92: 511-517.
17. Kahaly GJ, Förster G, Hansen C. Glycosaminoglycans in thyroid eye disease. Thyroid 1998; 8: 429-432.
18. Hansen C, Rouhi R, Förster G, Kahaly GJ. Increased sulfatation of orbital glycosaminoglycans in Graves'ophthalmopathy. J Clin Endocrinol Metab 1999; 84: 1409-1413.
19. Hales IB & Rundle FF. Ocular changes in Graves' disease. A long-term follow-up study. Quart J Med 1960; 29: 113-126.
20. Kahaly GJ, Schrezenmeir J, Krause U, et al. Ciclosporin and prednisone vs prednisone in treatment of Graves' ophthalmopathy: a controlled, randomized and prospective study. Eur J Clin Invest 1986; 16: 415-422.
21. Kahaly GJ, Pitz S, Müller-Forell W, Hommel G. Randomized trial of intravenous immunoglobulins vs prednisolone in Graves'ophthalmopathy. Clin Exp Immunol 1996; 106: 197-202.
22. Kahaly GJ, Roesler HP, Kutzner J, et al. Radiotherapy for thyroid-associated orbitopathy. Exp Clin Endocrinol Diabetes 1999; 107: 201-207.

23. Kahaly GJ, Roesler HP, Pitz S, Hommel G. Low vs high-dose radiotherapy for Graves' ophthalmopathy: A randomized, single-blind trial. J Clin Endocrinol Metab 2000; 85: 102-108.
24. Kahaly GJ, Gorman CA, Kal KB, et al. Radiotherapy for Graves' ophthalmopathy. In Prummel MF (ed): recent developments in Graves' ophthalmopathy. Kluwer publishers 2000, pp 115-131.
25. Mann WJ, Kahaly GJ, Lieb W, Amedee RG. Orbital decompression for endocrine ophthalmopathy: the endonasal approach. Am J Rhinol 1994; 8: 123-7.
26. Mann WJ, Kahaly GJ, Pitz S, et al. Decompression surgery for thyroid-associated orbitopathy – A ten year experience. Exp Clin Endocrinol Diabetes 1999; 107: 212-213.
27. Flanders AE, Mafee MF, Rao VM, Choi KH. CT characteristics of orbital pseudotumor and other orbital inflammatory processes. J Comput Assist Tomogr 1989; 13: 40-47.
28. Flanders AE, Mafee MF, Rao VM, Choi KH. CT characteristics of orbital pseudotumor and other orbital inflammatory processes. J Comput Assist Tomogr 1989; 13: 40-47.
29. Weetman AP, Wiersinga WM. Current management of thyroid-associated ophthalmopathy in Europe. Results of an international survey. Clin Endocrinol 1998; 49: 21-28.
30. Kahaly GJ. New imaging procedures in thyroid-associated ophthalmopathy. Orbit 1996; 15: 165-175.
31. Müller-Forell W, Pitz S, Mann W, Kahaly GJ. Neuroradiological diagnosis of thyroid-associated orbitopathy. Exp Clin Endocrinol Diabetes 1999; 107: 177-183.
32. Gorman CA. The measurement of change in Graves'ophthalmopathy. Thyroid 1998; 8: 539-543.
33. Trokel L, Jacobiec FA. Correlation of CT scanning and pathologic features of opthalmic Graves'disease. Ophthalmology 1981; 88: 553-564.
34. Neigel JM, Rootman J, Belkin RI, et al. Dysthyroid optic neuropathy. Ophthalmology 1988; 95: 1515-1521.
35. Nugent RA, Belkin RI, Neigel JM, et al. Graves' orbitopathy: correlation of CT and clinical findings. Radiology 1990; 177: 675-682.
36. Forbes G, Gorman CA, Gehring D, Baker HL Jr. Computer analysis of orbital fat and muscle volumes in Graves'ophthalmopathy. Am J Neuroradiol 1983; 4: 737-742.
37. Forbes G, Gehring DG, Gorman CA, Brennan MD, Jackson IT. Volume measurements of normal orbital structures by computed tomographic analysis. Am J Neuroradiol 1985; 6: 419-424.
38. Forbes G, Gorman CA, Brennan MD, et al. Ophthalmopathy of Graves'disease : Computerized volume measurements of orbital fat and muscle. Am J Neuroradiol 1986; 7: 651-656.
39. Enzmann DR, Donaldson SS, Kriss JP. Appearance of Graves'disease on orbital computed tomography. J Comput Assist Tomogr 1979; 3: 815-819.
40. Yoshikawa K, Higashide T, Nakase Y, et al. Role of rectus muscle enlargement in clinical profile of dysthyroid ophthalmopathy. Jpn J Ophthalmol 1991; 35: 175-181.
41. Barret L, Glatt HJ, Burde RM, Gado MH. Optic nerve dysfunction in thyroid eye disease: CT. Radiology 1988; 167: 503-508.
42. Feldon SE, Celina P, Saudra K, et al. Quantitative computer tomography of Graves'ophthalmopathy. Arch Ophthalmol 1985; 103: 213-215.
43. Hallin ES & Feldon SE. Graves' ophthalmopathy: II. Correlation of clinical signs with measures derived from computed tomography. Br J Ophthalmol 1988; 72: 678-682.

44. Hosten N, Sander B, Cordes M, et al. Graves' ophthalmopathy: MR imaging of the orbits. Radiology 1989; 172: 759-762.
45. Just M, Kahaly GJ, Higer HP, et al. Graves' ophthalmopathy: role of MR imaging in radiation therapy. Radiology 1991; 179: 187-190.
46. Hiromatsu Y, Kojima K, Ishisaka N, et al. Role of magnetic resonance imaging in thyroid-associated ophthalmopathy: Its predictive value for therapeutic outcome of immunosuppressive therapy. Thyroid 1992; 2: 299-305.
47. Pauleit D, Schuller H, Textor J, et al. MR relaxation time measurements with and without selective fat suppression (SPIR) in endocrine orbitopathy. Röfö 1997; 176: 557-564.
48. Nianiaris N, Hurwitz JJ, Chen JC, Wortzman G. Correlation between computed tomography and magnetic resonance imaging in Graves'orbitopathy. Can J Opthalmol 1994; 29: 9-12.
49. Nishikawa M, Yoshimura M, Toyoda N, et al. Correlation of orbital muscle changes evaluated by magnetic resonance imaging and thyroid stimulating antibody in patients with Graves'ophthalmopathy. Endocrinol 1993; 129: 213-219.
50. Ohnishi T, Noguchi S, Murakami N, et al. Extraocular Muscles in Graves' opthalmopathy: Usefulness of T2 relaxation time measurements. Radiology 1994; 190: 857-862.
51. Utech CI, Khatibnia U, Winter Pf, Wulle KG. MR T2 relaxation time for the assessment of retrobulbar inflammation in Graves' ophthalmopathy. Thyroid 1995; 5: 185-193.
52. Kahaly G, Diaz M, Just M, Beyer J & Lieb N. Role of octreoscan and correlation with MR imaging in Graves' ophthalmopathy. Thyroid 1995; 5:107-111.
53. Werner SC, Coleman DJ, Franzen LA. Ultrasonographic evidence of a consistano orbital involvement in Graves' disease. N Engl J Med 1974; 290: 1447-1450.
54. Willinsky RA, Arenson AM, Hurwitz J, Szalai J. Ultrasonic B scan measurement of the extraocular muscles in Graves'orbitopathy. J Can Assoc Radiol 1984; 35: 171-173.
55. Holt JE, O'connor PS, Douglas JP, Byrne B. Extraocular muscle size comparison using standardized A-scan echography and computed tomography scan measurements. Ophthalmology 1985; 92: 1351-1356.
56. Delint PJ, Mourits MP, Kerlen CH, et al. B-scan ultrasonography in Graves'orbitopathy. Documenta Ophthalmol 1993 ; 85 : 1-4.
57. Byrne FS, Gendron E, Glaser J, et al. Diameter of normal extraocular muscles with echography. Am J Ophthalmol 1991; 112: 706-712.
58. Erickson BA, Harris GJ, Lewandowski MF, Murray KJ, & Massaro BM. Echographic monitoring of response of extraocular muscles to irradiation in Graves' ophthalmopathy. Int J Radiat Oncol Biol Phys 1995; 31: 651-660.
59. Prummel MF, Suttorp-Schulten MSA, Wiersinga WM, et al. A new ultrasonographic method to detect disease activity and predict response to immunosuppressive treatment in Graves' ophthalmopathy. Ophthalmology 1993; 100: 556-561.
60. Prummel MF (ed): recent developments in Graves' ophthalmopathy. Kluwer publishers 2000.
61. Given-Wilson R, Pope RM, Michell MJ, Cannon R & McGregor AM. The use of real/time orbital ultrasound in Graves' ophthalmopathy: a comparison with computer tomography. Br J Radiol 1989; 62: 705-709.
62. Demer JL, Kerman BM. Comparison of standardized echography with magnetic resonance imaging to measure extraocular muscle size. Am J Ophthalmol 1994; 118: 351-361.
63. Nagy EV, Toth J, Kaldi I, et al. Graves'ophthalmopathy: eye muscle involvement in patients with diplopia. Eur J Endocrinol 2000; 142: 591-597.

64. Benning H, Lieb W, Kahaly GJ, Grehn F. Color Doppler ultrasound findings in patients with thyroid ophthalmopathy. Ophthalmologe 1994; 91: 20-25.
65. Krenning EP, Bakker, WH, Kooij PPM,et al.: Somatostatin receptor scintigraphy with (111-In-DTPA-D-Phe1)-octreotide in man: metabolism, dosimetry, and comparison with 123-I-Tyr-3)-octreotide. J Nucl Med 1992; 33: 652-658.
66. Krenning EP, Kwekkeboom DJ, Bakker WH, et al. Somatostatin receptor scintigraphy with (III-In-DTAP-D-Phe1) and (123 I-Tyr3) – octreotide: the Rotterdam experience with more than 1000 patients. Eur J Nucl Med 1993; 20: 716-731.
67. Krassas GE, Kahaly GJ. The role of octreoscan in thyroid eye disease. Eur J Endocrinol 1999; 140: 373-375.
68. Wiersinga WM, Gerding MN, Prummel MF & Krenning EP. Octreotide scintigraphy in thyroidal and orbital Graves' disease. Thyroid 1998; 8: 433-436.
69. Durak I, Durak H, Ergin M, Yurekli Y & Kaynak S. Somatostatin receptors in the orbit. Clin Nucl Med 1995; 20: 237-242.
70. Bohuslavizki KH, Oberwohrmann S, Brenner W, & al. 111-In-Octreotide imaging in patients with longstanding Graves' ophthalmopathy. Nucl Med Commun 1995; 16: 912-916.
71. Krassas GE, Dumas A & Moncayo R. Octreoscan in Graves' ophthalmopathy (letter). Thyroid. 1997; 7: 805-806.
72. Förster GJ, Krummenauer F, Nickel O, & Kahaly GJ. Somatostatin-receptor scintigraphy in Graves'disease: Reproducibility and inter-/intra-observer variability. Cancer Biotherap Radiol (in press).
73. Förster GJ, Nickel O, Raab D, Andreas J, Kahaly GJ. Somatostatin-receptor scintigraphy in Graves'ophthalmopathy. A new, standardized method for assessement of orbital disease activity. J Nucl Med 1999; 40: 207 (abstract).
74. Kahaly G, Diaz M, Hahn K, Beyer J & Bockisch A. Indium 111- Pentetreotide scintigraphy in Graves' ophthalmopathy. J Nucl Med 1995; 36: 550-554.
75. Kahaly G, Görges R, Diaz M, Hommel G & Bockisch A. Indium –111- Pentetreotide in Graves' Disease. J Nucl Med 1998; 39: 533-536.
76. Kahaly GJ, Förster GJ. Somatostatin receptor scintigraphy in thyroid eye disease. Thyroid 1998; 8: 549-552.
77. Postema PTE, Krenning EP, Wijngaarde R, et al. (111-In-DTPA-D-Phe1) octreotide scintigraphy in thyroidal and orbital Graves' disease: A parameter for disease activity? J Clin Endocrinol Metab 1994; 79: 1845-1851.
78. Moncayo R, Baldnisera I, Decristoforo C, Kendler D, & Donnemiller E. Evaluation of immunological mechanisms mediating thyroid – associated ophthalmopathy by radionuclide imaging using somatostatin analog 111-In-octreotide. Thyroid 1997; 7: 21-29.
79. Krassas GE, Dumas A, Pontikides N & Kaltsas Th. Somatostatin receptor scintigraphy and octreotide treatment in patients with thyroid eye disease. Clin Endocrinol 1995; 42: 571-580.
80. Krassas GE, Dumas A, Kaltsas Th, Halkias A, Pontikides N. Somatostatin receptor scintigraphy before and after treatment with somatostin analogues in patients with thyroid eye disease. Thyroid 1999; 9: 47-52.
81. Gerding MN, van der Zant FM, van Royen EA, et al. Octreotide-scintigraphy is a disease-activity parameter in Graves'ophthalmopathy. Clin Endocrinol 1999; 50: 373-379.
82. Krassas GE, Kaltsas Th, Dumas A, Pontikides N & Tolis G. Lanreotide in the treatment of patients with thyroid eye disease. Eur J Endocrinol 1999; 136: 416-422.

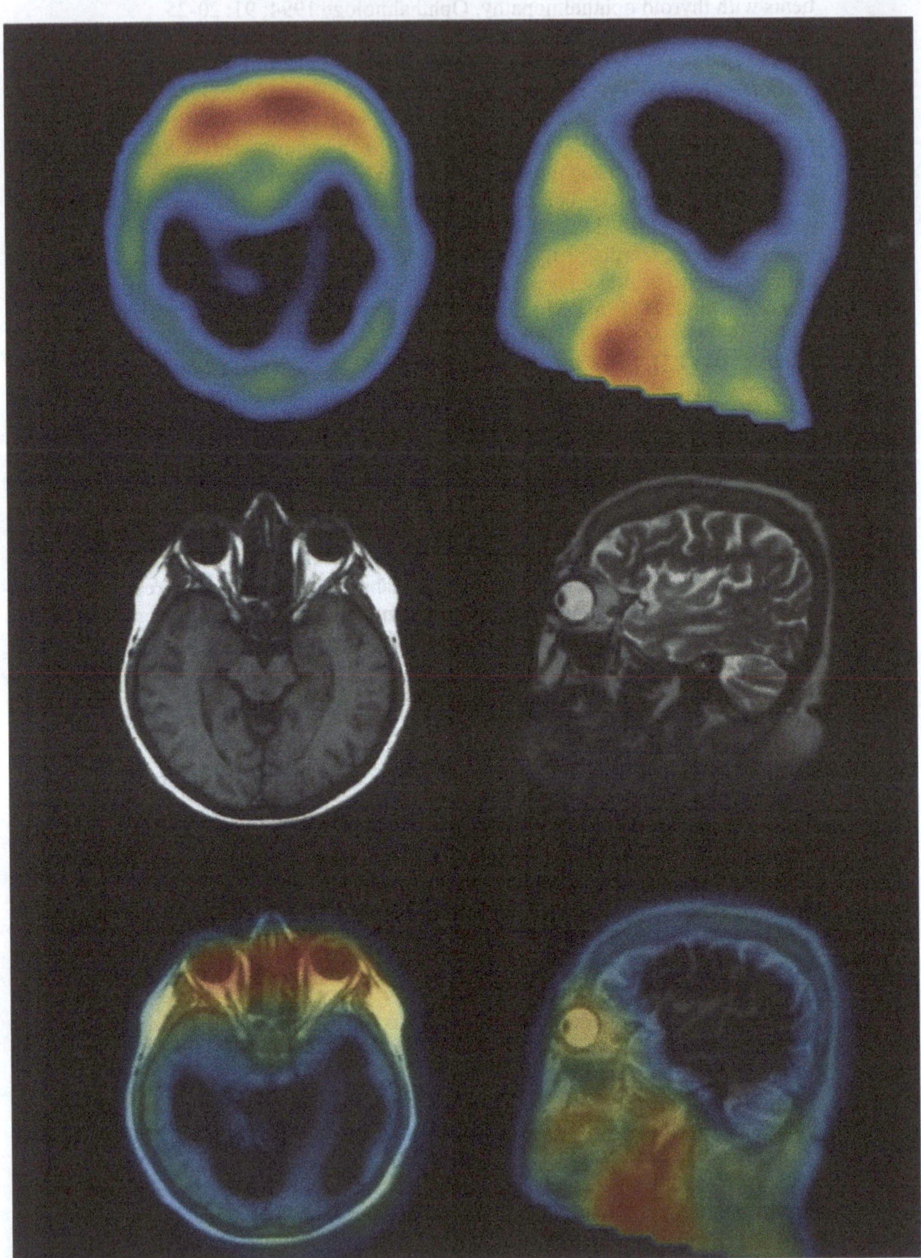

Figure 4. Somatostatin receptor scintigraphy (octreoscan) of a patient with active GO (upper level), corresponding MRI (middle), and super-imposition of both techniques with size-adapted, standardized volumes of interest demonstrating radio nuclide uptake in the orbital (retro bulbar) tissue (lower level).

10

QUALITY OF LIFE MEASUREMENT IN PATIENTS WITH GRAVES' OPHTHALMOPATHY

C. B. Terwee and Professor Martin Gerding
Clinical, Epidemiology and Biostatistics and the University of Amsterdam, Academic Medical Center, Meibergdreef 9, NL-1105 AZ Amsterdam, The Netherlands

INTRODUCTION

The measurement of the effects of Graves' ophthalmopathy (GO) and its treatments on the quality of life of these patients is a new and challenging research area. In this chapter an introduction is given to the methodology of (health-related) quality of life measurement in general and the application of these methods in GO research specifically. Special attention is given to the recently developed GO-specific quality of life questionnaire, the GO-QOL. This questionnaire was specifically developed to be used as an outcome measure for GO research. The development, reliability, validity and interpretation of the GO-QOL are discussed. In the second part of this chapter a state of the art literature review is presented on the use of patient's perceptions in the description of the impact of GO on the patients' lives and in the evaluations of treatments for GO.

HOW TO MEASURE QUALITY OF LIFE IN GRAVES' OPHTHALMOPATHY?

Health-Related Quality of Life Measurement

Introduction

In 1948 the World Health Organization broadened their definition of health to include not only the absence of disease and infirmity but also the presence of physical, mental, and social well-being (1). Since then, a general agreement has emerged that perceptions of patients of how they are feeling and how they are able to function in daily life should be included in the evaluation and monitoring of the effects of disease and treatment (2,3).

Despite the growing interest in patients' perceptions of health and quality of life there is still no consensus on a single definition of the concept of "quality of life" (4-7). A certain amount of agreement has been reached on a few points however: First, most investigators consider quality of life a subjective concept, which by definition can only be judged by the patients themselves. Secondly, quality of life should be considered a multi-dimensional concept including physical, mental, and social aspects. Thirdly, most clinicians prefer to use the term health-related quality of life (HRQL) because clinicians are most interested in those aspects of quality of life that are directly related to health (2,3).

The patient's perspective versus the physician's perspective

From the patients' perspective, clinical measures like eye muscle volume or visual acuity are of limited interest; they often correlate poorly with physical, emotional and social functioning in daily life (8). For example, it has been shown that visual acuity alone correlates poorly with the patient's own perception of visual disability (9,10). In a clinical trial on radiotherapy versus prednisone in GO patients it was found that a clinical success rate of about 50% was associated with only a modest mean benefit on the subjective eye judgement by the patient (11). In another study it

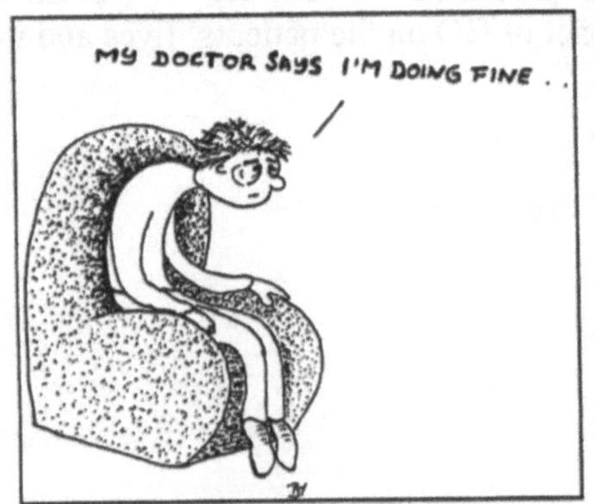

was found that after many years of treatment few GO patients experienced long-term functional impairments, but more than one third of patients were still dissatisfied with their appearance (12).

These discrepancies between clinical measures and patients' experiences can be explained by the fact that the degree of daily functioning and well-being as perceived by the patient is not only determined by the severity of signs and symptoms, but also by characteristics of the individual and the environment such as coping ability, motivation, social support, the physician-patient relationship etc.. These relationships are illustrated in a model of patient outcomes, introduced by Wilson and Cleary (13), which is closely related to the WHO classification of impairments, disabilities and handicaps (14) (Figure 1).

Different measures of disease status can be thought of as existing on a continuum of outcome levels with increasing complexity. Clinical (biological or physiological) measures like proptosis or eye muscle motility are on the left side of the model. The perception of these clinical findings by the patient are expressed in perceived symptoms such as pain or diplopia. These symptoms can lead to functional limitations in daily activities such as driving or reading, which influences the experienced health (general health perceptions) and overall quality of life, the latter also including other aspects of life besides health, such as financial situation, job satisfaction etc (13).

The different levels of outcome are causally related but are influenced by personal factors and characteristics of the environment. The more you move to the right of the model, the larger the influence of these factors. As a consequence the correlation with clinical measures becomes weaker the more you move to the right in the model. This model explains why two people with the same clinical disease status (based on physiological measures) can have a very different perception of their daily functioning and general health (2).

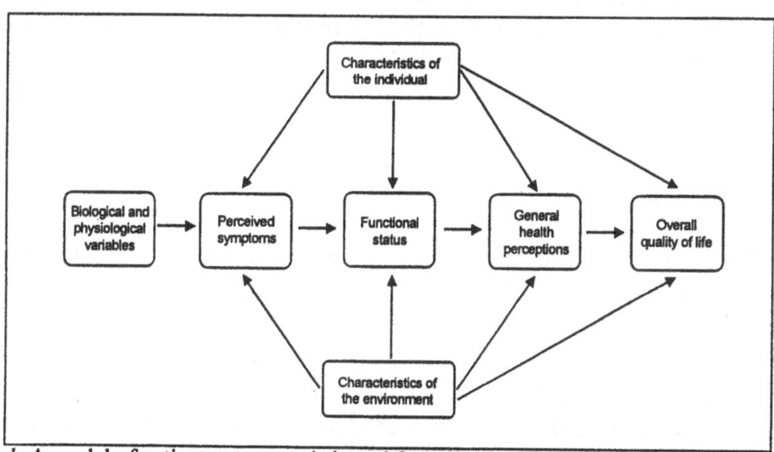

Figure 1. A model of patient outcomes (adapted from Wilson & Cleary, 1995) (13)

When do physicians need to measure HRQL in GO patients?

From the model described above, it follows that HRQL measures can be of important additional value in the description of disease severity of a patient population because they highlight a different outcome level of interest than the clinical measures of disease status.

HRQL measures can also be important indicators of treatment success. For example, patients' perceptions of (changes in) HRQL measures are especially useful in the evaluation of treatments that induce side effects like prednisone or involve risks like surgery. Patients weigh these side effects and risks against the benefits of treatment in their perception of the net effect on their HRQL.

It has been argued that, because of weak correlations between clinical measures and patients' experiences of HRQL, HRQL measures should be considered the most important indicators of treatment success in cases where the primary goal of treatment is to improve daily functioning and general health rather than to prolong life (3). This is actually always the case in the treatment of GO.

Finally, for society as a whole, HRQL measures are often the most important outcomes of medical care. In general, HRQL measures are among the best predictors of the use of general medical and mental health services, as well as strong predictors of mortality, even after controlling for clinical measures (15,16).

In summary, for studies on GO, HRQL assessment is important in the following kind of studies:

1. Cross-sectional studies aimed at describing the severity of GO on multiple outcome levels, including the impact of GO on patients' daily functioning and perception of health in general.
2. Longitudinal studies aimed at the evaluation of treatment efficacy or compare different treatments on HRQL.
3. Studies aimed at predicting future health or future use of medical care.

Instruments to measure HRQL in GO patients

When HRQL is considered a subjective concept, only the patients involved can judge the quality of their lives and therefore, the only approach to measuring HRQL is to ask the patients themselves (17). This can be done either by interview techniques, but mostly self-assessment questionnaires are being used, to be filled in by the patients themselves.

Several short and simple validated self-assessment questionnaires are internationally used. A distinction should be made between general and disease-specific questionnaires (18). General HRQL questionnaires are mostly multi-dimensional and designed to measure the most important aspects of HRQL that apply to many different impairments, patients and populations. These questionnaires are therefore useful to compare the HRQL of GO patients with that of other patient populations or "healthy" people to estimate the relative impact of GO on patients' lives. Some of these questionnaires have been cross-culturally validated in many languages. Examples are the Medical Outcomes Study short-form health surveys (SF-36 or MOS-24) (19-21) and the Sickness Impact Profile (SIP) (22).

However, general HRQL questionnaires are often very broadly based and may contain items of little or no relevance for a specific disease. For example, a question about problems with carrying groceries is not relevant for patients with GO. In addition, they may miss certain relevant items for a specific disease, such as questions about the consequences of diplopia or a changed appearance in GO. Therefore, disease-specific questionnaires are often developed that are specifically tailored to a particular disease or intervention. These are better useful in clinical trials which request outcome measures that can detect small but clinically important changes over time or discriminate between groups of patients with different disease severity (18). In the next section a disease-specific quality of life questionnaire for patients with GO (the GO-QOL) is described.

The GO-QOL

Description of the questionnaire

The Graves' Ophthalmopathy Quality Of Life questionnaire (GO-QOL) is the first instrument available to measure HRQL in patients with GO (23). The GO-QOL was specifically developed for patients with GO, and is meant to be used as an outcome measure in clinical studies evaluating (new) treatments for GO. The questionnaire was developed in cooperation with GO patients, and includes 16 questions that are focused on functional limitations in daily life caused by GO that are important to patients and influence their quality of life. The questionnaire is composed of two parts: The first eight questions concern limitations in visual functioning as a consequence of diplopia and/or decreased visual acuity; the second eight questions concern limitations in psychosocial functioning as a consequence of a changed appearance (see appendix).

Scoring system

All questions are scored as "severely limited" (1 point), "a little limited" (2 points), or "not limited at all" (3 points). The answering options "no drivers' license" or "never learned to ride a bike" are scored as missing values. The first eight questions can be summarized into one total score (also called subscale) called "visual functioning", and the second eight questions can be summarized into one total score or subscale called "appearance". Total scores should only be calculated when at least half of the items in the scale are completed. Otherwise, the total score should be assigned a missing value. Both subscales range from 8 to 24 points when there are no missing values (raw score). Higher scores indicating better health. Finally, the total scores can be transformed to a score ranging from 0 to 100 which is comparable to other HRQL questionnaires. The transformation formula is given below:

$$\text{Final score} = \frac{\text{raw score} - \text{minimum score}}{\text{maximum score} - \text{minimum score}} \times 100$$

Examples- suppose each question is scores 2 points:

1. No missing values: the raw score of 16 points. The minimum and maximum scores are 8 and 24 points respectively, so the final score is (16-8)/(24-8) x 100 = 50 points.
2. One missing value: the raw score is now 14 points. The minimum and maximum scores are now 7 and 21 points respectively, so the final score is (14-7)/(21-7) x 100 = 50 points.

Reliability and validity

All measurement instruments should be evaluated for their reliability and validity. Reliability refers to the accuracy (amount of measurement error) and consistency (internal consistency and reproducibility) of the measure. Validity refers to the extent to which the instrument measures what it is supposed to measure (24).

Reliability and validity of the GO-QOL was assessed in three different patient populations: The calculation of two different total scores as described above was based on the assumption that questions within subscales are highly correlated with each other, while questions between subscales are less correlated or not at all. This assumption was checked and found to be justified in two samples of 70 and 93 patients respectively (23,25). Correlations of the GO-QOL total scores with demographic and clinical variables and with total scores from general HRQL questionnaires (MOS-24 and SIP) were in accordance with expected ideas about their interrelationships. For example, it was expected that older patients and patients with more severe eye motility disturbances or diplopia would experience more problems with visual functioning, while females and patients with more proptosis would experience more problems with appearance (23,25). Expected results were also found for correlations between changes in GO-QOL scores and changes in clinical and general HRQL variables (26). These analyses confirmed that the GO-QOL subscales are really measuring the concepts that they are supposed to measure.

A high coherence was found between the individual questions within a subscale, which confirms the internal consistency of the subscales (23, 25). The reproducibility of the GO-QOL scores was found to be acceptable for group comparisons in clinical studies (25). The use of the GO-QOL for individual patient monitoring should be further studied.

Translation and cross-cultural validation

The GO-QOL was developed and validated in the Netherlands. For the application of the GO-QOL in English-speaking countries the GO-QOL was translated into UK English according to general guidelines proposed for the translation and cross-cultural validation of HRQL instruments (27,28), The translation was performed by three native English speakers with excellent knowledge of Dutch and three native Dutch speakers with excellent knowledge of English. A method of forward and backward translation was used. Attention was given to the conceptual equivalence of the questions. It is important that the translated questions are similar in meaning to the questions in the original language. The final English translation is presented in the appendix. However, it was noticed that the question about limitations with bicycling may not be relevant in English speaking countries. This question will be omitted or replaced by an equivalent question in a future version of the GO-QOL. In addition, the English version should yet be pilot-tested in English patients.

Interpretation and sample size calculation

Interpretation of HRQL scores is often difficult because HRQL measures have no direct biological meaning and general standards for interpretation are lacking (29-32). For the GO-QOL a specific longitudinal study was performed to define a minimal amount of change in score that can be considered an important improvement in HRQL for patients (26). This "minimal clinically important difference" (MCID) is an essential ingredient for sample size calculations as well as for the interpretation of treatment effects (33). Pre- and post-treatment GO-QOL scores were obtained from a sample of 164 patients who underwent either radiotherapy, orbital decompression, eye muscle surgery, eyelid lengthening or blepharoplasty. The MCID was defined based on the amount of change in GO-QOL scores that was observed in patients who subjectively reported to be improved from their treatment. It was concluded from this study that a mean change of 6 points could be considered an important change in daily functioning for patients. For more invasive therapies which involve larger treatment burden like radiotherapy or orbital decompression, a change of at least 10 points was recommended as the MCID. Standard deviations of change were about 14-25 points and were smaller for visual functioning than for appearance (26). However, when the GO-QOL is going to be used in clinical studies several issues should be taken into account when interpreting treatment effects. The smallest amount of change that can be considered an important change in HRQL for patients will depend on possible side effects and costs of the treatment and the availability and efficacy of alternative treatment options. Therefore, it was stated that the MCID should not be considered a fixed property of an instrument, but will vary from study to study. Also, the MCID used in sample size calculations will vary, depending on aspects like placebo effects and heterogeneity of the patient population. Mean GO-QOL changes of about 5 points were found in clinically unchanged patients over a three- to six-month period (26). In another study, GO-QOL changes of 2.5 and 4 points (with standard deviations of 13.6 and 13.7 points) were found in clinically stable patients over a two-week period (25). These figures could be used as indicators of changes in untreated patients. Placebo effects might be at least this large. Sample size calculations should be based on the expected difference in score changes between patients in the treatment versus placebo group and the pooled standard deviation of change. With a mean difference between the groups of 6-10 points, and with pooled standard deviations of about 14-20 points, sample sizes would be required of between 40 and 200 patients per arm. Sample sizes can be considerably reduced by using repeated measurements over time. In that case, more sophisticated statistical analysis are required.

GRAVES' OPHTHALMOPATHY THROUGH THE EYES OF THE PATIENT: STATE OF THE ART

As stated before, patients' experiences in terms of functional limitations and perceived health have hardly been studied in GO research. In this paragraph an overview is presented of studies providing information regarding the effects of GO or GO-related symptoms on the HRQL of these patients. The studies are categorized according to the three kinds of studies mentioned before in which HRQL assessment is important: (1) cross-sectional studies aimed at describing the impact of having GO or GO-related symptoms on patients' HRQL; and (2) longitudinal studies aimed at evaluating the effects of treatment on patients' HRQL. We did not find any studies who used HRQL measure to predict future health or future use of medical care of GO patients.

The Impact of Graves' Ophthalmopathy on Patients' Lives

Only a few studies have measured the effects of GO on HRQL directly. In a cross-sectional study of 70 newly diagnosed GO patients, Gerding et al. found that all scores of the MOS-24, except for the score for bodily pain, were markedly decreased compared to the scores of a comparison group of patients without any chronic condition. The HRQL scores of GO patients were on average 8% to 36% lower than the HRQL scores of the comparison population (34). Comparable results were found by Terwee et al. in a group of 206 GO patients who completed the SF-36 shortly before treatment with radiotherapy or surgery (Figure 2) (26). Also comparable results were found by Kahaly et al. in 100 consecutive GO patients with varying degrees of GO severity (Figure 2) (35).

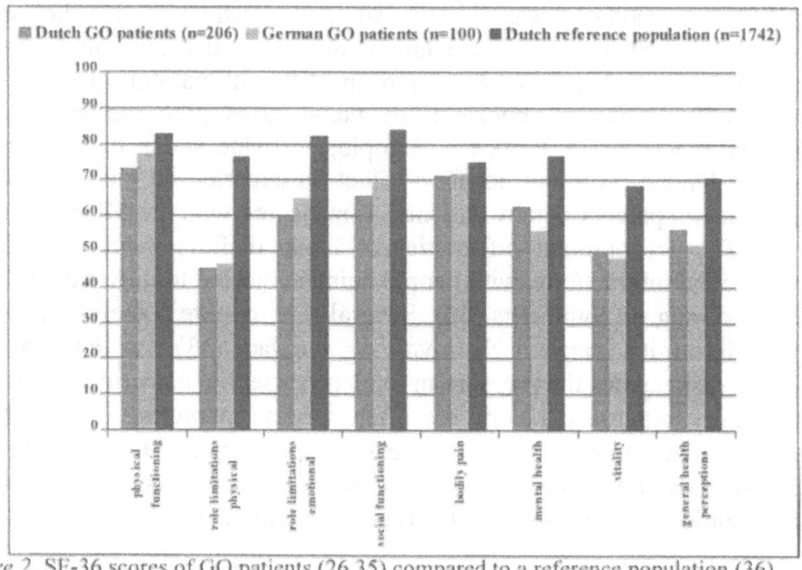

Figure 2. SF-36 scores of GO patients (26,35) compared to a reference population (36)

The HRQL of GO patients seems to be mostly affected by physical and emotional problems with work or other daily activities (role limitations), problems with social functioning, mental health, vitality and general health perceptions.

Bartley et al. used a follow-up questionnaire to describe the long-term effects of GO in an incidence cohort of 120 patients with newly diagnosed GO (12). After a median follow-up of 10 years, 61% of the patients reported that their eyes had not returned to what it was before the development of thyroid disease, 52% of the patients reported that their eyes did not appear normal at that time, and 38% of he patients were not satisfied with the appearance of their eyes (12).

Some understanding of the impact of the visual limitations and facial disfigurement associated with GO can be obtained from literature in related research areas. It has been shown that difficulties with vision in general have profound effects on daily functioning and overall quality of life in elders (37,38). Salive et al. showed that patients with severe visual impairment had a three-fold higher risk of limitations in mobility and activities of daily living than those with a visual acuity of 20/40 or better (38). Several investigators have demonstrated significant decreases in daily functioning and well-being as experienced by a mixed sample of ophthalmic patients and by patients from a general population who had trouble seeing, using validated HRQL measures such as the vision-specific SIP or SF-36 (39-42). Trouble seeing was found to be associated with problems with work or other daily activities, worse general health perceptions and decreased mental health (40,41). Lee et al. found that blurred vision had a more negative effect on functional status and well-being than indigestion, trouble urinating, or having headaches (41).

From another research area some understanding can be obtained about the psychosocial consequences of facial disfigurement. Negative experiences have been demonstrated in different patient groups, e.g. in patients with congenital abnormalities, facial burns, portwine stains, or head and neck cancer (43-47). As an example, portwine stains in the face were shown to have a profound negative effect on experienced mental health and general health perceptions by patients, as measured with the MOS-24 (48).

The predominant difficulties of facial disfigurement lie within the area of social interactions, with people being subjected to unwanted intrusions such as staring or comments (46). Several reports note society's aversion to visible deformity, particularly involving the face (43). At the root of the patient's distress lies the pressure in modern society to confirm to an idealized appearance. Image and beauty are often used as marketing tools portraying the look of super models as the desired appearance. This obsession with appearance devalues those who do not match the perceived ideal and leads to stigmatization of those with visible disfigurement (49).

Because GO is closely related to Graves thyroid disease, the impact of having thyroid disease could also influence the HRQL of GO patients. Bianchi et al. assessed HRQL in patients with a variety of thyroid diseases. This study showed significantly impairments in all HRQL aspects measured with the SF-36, in comparison to a normative population. The most important effects were problems with work or other daily activities, worse general health perceptions and limitations in social functioning(50). Ljunggren et al. reported several results from an extensive questionnaire completed by 179 patients with Graves' hyperthyroidism who entered a clinical trial. Sixty percent of these patients reported severe discomfort prior to treatment. Sixty-five percent reported that they could manage their professional work, although often only during part of the work time. Sixty-six percent reported impaired social relations. Of the 25% who had endocrine ophthalmopathy, 20% reported that their eye problems seriously restricted their professional work, and social activities were seriously affected in 19%. Thirty-four percent reported their eye problems to be more troublesome than their thyroid disease (51).

Evaluation of Treatments for Graves' Ophthalmopathy from the Patient's Perspective

In 1992 a joint committee of thyroid associations recommended the inclusion of self-assessment of the eye condition by the patient in the evaluation of treatment effects for GO (52). A review of the literature since 1992 yielded the following efforts of measuring patient's experiences in the evaluation of treatment effects:

Treatment of thyroid disease

Berg et al. used one question about perceived general health, extracted from the SF-36, to study the subjective outcome of radioiodine treatment in 236 hyperthyroid patients1-5 years after therapy. A significant lower rating of health was found in these patients compared to a reference population of women with a comparable age range. A larger number of patients with Graves' disease (43%) experienced eye discomfort. The authors concluded that although therapy had been successfully in eliminating the hyperfunction of the thyroid, other health problems, like ophthalmopathy, may still be present which necessitate a long-term follow-up in these patients (53).

Ljunggren et al. randomly compared antithyroid drugs with subtotal thyroidectomy and iodine-131 therapy in 179 patients with Graves' hyperthyroidism. A follow-up questionnaire was send to the patients three years after treatment. In all three groups, 95-98% of the patients were satisfied with the treatment alternative. In the medical group, 38% of the patients relapsed and 90% of them felt very disappointed at the time of relapse. Around 20% of the patients in the surgical group reported unexpected problems or complaints. Patients in the iodine group reported significantly more eye problems than patients in the other groups. The authors concluded that the ophthalmopathy seriously affected the quality of life of the patients in their study (51,54).

Linos et al. studied the results of surgery for hyperthyroidism in 400 patients, of which 49 patients had some degree of exophthalmos. In a follow-up questionnaire, about 90% of the patients reported considerable subjective improvement in their preoperative symptoms. Also 90% of the patients were satisfied with the aesthetic results of their incision. The authors concluded that surgery has minimal psychological cost and allows easy return to usual daily activities (55).

In a recent randomized clinical trial comparing radioiodine therapy, radioiodine therapy plus prednisone, and methimazole therapy, patients were asked to describe their eye disease as improved, unchanged, or worsened, compared to their last visit. These subjective ratings were included in the primary outcome measure as a minor criterion, but no results on patient's assessment were described in the paper (56).

Immunosuppression

In 1989 Prummel and coworkers introduced the Subjective Eye Score as a secondary outcome measure in their clinical trial of prednisone versus cyclosporine, by asking patients to rate their eye condition on a scale from 1 to 10 before and after treatment. They concluded that prednisone was more effective than cyclosporine, but the improvement in the subjective eye score was considered small (57). Although never validated, this rating scale has been used in several studies thereafter (11, 57-59). Baschieri et al. found a mean reduction of about 3.5 points in the Subjective Eye Score (ranging from 1 to 9 in this study) after intravenous immunoglobulin as well as after corticosteroid in 30 and 35 untreated, moderately severe GO patients respectively (58). Kung and coworkers found subjective improvements after somatostatin in appearance in 12.5 % of the patients, in eye discomfort in 75%, in diplopia in 25%, and in visual acuity in 50%, on a scale of best, improved, no change, or worse (scored 2,1,0,-1) The same subjective improvements after corticosteroid were found in 40%, 70%, 60% and 60% of the patients respectively, but their study included only 18 patients (60). In another small study subjective improvements were found in 7/8 patients who received intravenous methylprednisolone pulse therapy in self-assessment of appearance, visual acuity, eye discomfort and diplopia, but it was not reported how this was measured (61).

Seegenschmiedt et al. used a linear scale from 0 to 100% to measure the subjective degree of improvement in 60 patients after radiotherapy. Patients reached a mean subjective improvement of 70% (SD 25%) The authors concluded that radiotherapy was effective for severe, progressive GO after pretreatment (62). Prummel et al. found a significant improvement in the Subjective Eye Score of about 1 point after radiotherapy, which was comparable to the improvement after prednisone. They concluded that radiotherapy should be the first choice of therapy in patients with moderately severe GO because of its better tolerability (11).

Mourits et al. included the Subjective Eye Score as a secondary outcome measure in their randomized clinical trial comparing radiotherapy with sham-irradiation in 60 moderately severe GO patients. A mean improvement of 1.5 points in the Subjective Eye Score was found after radiotherapy and 1.3 points after sham-irradiation. Judgment of treatment efficacy was based on clinical characteristics only (59).

Surgery

In a small study of 13 patients who underwent decompression, patients were asked to rate their relief or reduction in orbital discomfort after orbital decompression on a Visual Analog Scale, stretching from “no relief” (0 points) to “complete relief” (10 points). The mean amount of relief was 9.2 points (SD 0.9) However, the authors argued that their study population represented a highly selected group of Graves' disease patients evaluated on the basis of their recollections of preoperative discomfort. Less invasive therapies like radiotherapy might have resulted in the same amount of relief from discomfort (63).

A group from the Mayo Clinic evaluated 491 patients who underwent orbital decompression by questionnaire including questions about eye comfort, satisfaction with the appearance of the eyes and overall satisfaction with status of the eyes at a median of 9.5 years postoperatively (64-67). Most patients had reasonably comfortable eyes (81%), good vision (71%), and a satisfactory or acceptable appearance (89%). Most patients were satisfied with the overall status of their eyes (76%). A comparable questionnaire was used in 34 patients who underwent orbital decompression primarily for cosmetic indications. The authors argued that patient satisfaction is the most important criterion of success for cosmetic operations. Based on the results of this study the authors concluded that in most patients, optimal cosmetic results may require multiple eye muscle and lid procedures (65).

In a study of Tjon et al. 48/75 (76%) patients were satisfied with the results of their orbital decompression, while 15/75 (24%) considered the results of surgery unsatisfactory (68).

In a longitudina validation study, GO-QOL scores were obtained from 164 patients before and 3 to 6 months after treatment, depending on the performed procedure (26). Twenty-three patients underwent radiotherapy, 48 orbital decompression (10 for sight loss, 38 for exophthalmos), 31 eye muscle surgery, 43 eyelid lengthening, and 19 blepharoplasty. The results are presented in Table 1. If a change of 6 to 10 points in GO-QOL scores is considered an important change in HRQL for patients, it seems that on average, radiotherapy, orbital decompression and blepharoplasty led to an important improvement in HRQL in these patients. GO-QOL changes after eye muscle surgery or eyelid lengthening were rather small. One explanation is that only 50% of patients clinically improved in diplopia from their eye muscle surgery. Score changes in the group of responders only were higher. Another possible explanation could be that both eye muscle surgery and eyelid lengthening are often part of a larger treatment strategy, in which more surgeries are necessary to achieve success for the patient. Therefore, there may be a "technical" success after one surgery, recognized by the physician and the patient (in their overall judgement), that does yet result in a change in visual functioning or appearance that exceeds the minimal clinically important difference.

Table 1. Mean (SD) GO-QOL scores before and after different treatments (26)

		before treatment	after treatment	difference	
		mean (SD)	mean (SD)	mean (SD)	p-value
Radiotherapy	Visual functioning	37.0 (20.7)	45.1 (26.9)	**8.1** (18.6)	0.05
	Appearance	72.0 (18.6)	73.6 (22.7)	2.0 (17.9)	0.61
Orbital decompression					
sight loss	Visual functioning	27.1 (22.4)	47.4 (28.3)	**20.3** (19.5)	0.01
	Appearance	51.0 (19.8)	55.0 (15.0)	4.0 (9.3)	0.21
exophthalmos	Visual functioning	64.8 (23.9)	68.0 (22.8)	3.2 (23.9)	0.42
	Appearance	44.7 (24.4)	55.8 (26.7)	**11.0** (15.5)	<0.001
Eye muscle surgery	Visual functioning	50.5 (23.3)	53.3 (28.9)	**2.8** (25.4)	0.55
	Appearance	65.1 (20.7)	67.7 (24.2)	2.6 (22.2)	0.52
Eyelid lengthening	Visual functioning	66.7 (26.9)	70.4 (26.1)	3.7 (15.0)	0.11
	Appearance	63.4 (22.9)	67.6 (21.9)	**4.2** (13.9)	0.05
Blepharoplasty	Visual functioning	64.7 (29.7)	64.9 (27.4)	0.2 (19.7)	0.97
	Appearance	58.6 (29.6)	68.8 (24.1)	**10.2** (17.5)	0.02

In bold print are those scales on which treatment was expected to have the most effect

However, these data do not provide evidence for the efficacy of the treatments in terms of HRQL, because no placebo group was included in this study and the patients were not consecutively included. The benefit of these treatments on HRQL should be established in randomized clinical trials.

Other treatments

Olver et al. described the results of botulism toxin A treatment in 14 patients with thyroid eye disease. The subjective results were assessed by questionnaire, including questions on discomfort, the rapidity of onset of the effect, the effect of treatment on appearance and side effects. All patients reported a subjective improvement in appearance and the authors concluded that the treatment was effective and acceptable (69).

Methodological Considerations

Although several authors have included some form of patient assessment in their evaluation of treatment success, patient assessment was often performed on an ad hoc basis without the development of appropriate, reliable, and valid HRQL instruments.

In many of the above described studies some sort of follow-up questionnaire was used to assess satisfaction with the perceived treatment retrospectively. Although treatment satisfaction is often used as a measure of HRQL and can be an important determinant of it, it is not a measure of (changes in) the amount of symptoms, nor a measure of functional impairments, nor a measure of perceived health in general. In fact, it might often be more an indication of the willingness to please the doctor. In addition, because treatment satisfaction does not include any of the above mentioned aspects of health, it offers little indications for future direction of treatment. Finally, it has been shown that retrospective measurement of treatment satisfaction with care is more influenced by the present health state than by the extent of improvement by treatment (70). Therefore, measures of treatment satisfaction are often not valid measures of HRQL changes in terms of the effects of treatment on daily functioning and perceived health in general.

For most of the other used measures it was never tested if the measures were really measuring what they were supposed to measure. In fact, this could be doubtful in some cases. For example, the Subjective Eye Score was often assessed by the physician in the consultation room, which may have resulted in a measure of willingness-to-please-the-doctor instead of a measure of overall perceived eye condition.

A lot of these studies measured change directly after treatment instead of estimating change from the difference between a pre- and post-treatment measurement. It has been shown that asking patients directly about the amount of change can lead to biased estimates because patients don't really remember their initial state and as a consequence tend to overestimate their treatment effect (71). Finally, the inter-observer and/or test-retest reliability of most measures was never described and probably never tested.

To date, the GO-QOL is the only validated disease-specific instrument to measure changes in HRQL after treatment. Validity and reliability of the GO-QOL have been assessed in a cross-sectional and a longitudinal design. Another important advantage of the GO-QOL is the emphasis on the *functional* consequences of GO in terms of limitations in daily activities and psychosocial functioning. These functional aspects seem to have been neglected altogether in previous measures.

SUMMARY

HRQL measurement in GO is important to describe the severity of GO on patients' daily functioning and perception of health in general, to evaluate or compare treatment effects on HRQL, and to predict future health or future use of medical care of GO patients. General HRQL instruments like the SF-36 can be used to describe the impact of having GO on patients' HRQL and to compare the HRQL of GO patients with patients with other diseases or with comparison populations without any (chronic) diseases. The GO-QOL is at present the only validated disease-specific instrument to be used as an outcome measure in clinical studies evaluating the effects of treatment on HRQL. This questionnaire needs to be translated and cross-culturally validated into multiple languages.

Clinical investigators should pay more attention to the development and use of validated HRQL instruments in studies on GO.

REFERENCES

1. World Health Organization. WHO Constitution. WHO, Geneva, 1948.
2. Testa, M.A., and D.C. Simonson. Assessment of quality of life outcomes. New England Journal of Medicine 1996; 334:835-840.
3. Guyatt, G.H., D. Naylor, E. Juniper, D.K. Heyland, R. Jaeschke, and D.J. Cook. Users' guides to the medical literature. XII How to use articles about health-related quality of life. JAMA 1997; 277:1232-1237.

4. Gill, T.M., and A.R. Feinstein. A critical appraisal of the quality of life measurements. JAMA 1994; 272(8):619-631.
5. Leplège, A., and S. Hunt. The problem of quality of life in medicine. JAMA 1997; 278:47-50.
6. Hunt SM. The problem of quality of life. Quality of Life Research 1997; 6:205-212.
7. Wood-Dauphine, S. Assessing quality of life in clinical research: From where have we come and where are we going? Journal of Clinical Epidemiology 1999; 52:355-363.
8. Guyatt, G.H., D.H. Feeny, and D.L. Patrick. Measuring health related quality of life. Annals of Internal Medicine 1993; 118:622-629.
9. Elliot, D.B., M.A. Hurst, and J. Weatherill. Comparing clinical tests of visual function in cataract with the patient's perceived visual disability. Eye 1990; 4:712-717.
10. Carta, A., L. Braccio, M. Belpoliti, L. Soliani, F. Sartore, S.A. Gandolfi, and G. Maraini. Self-assessment of the quality of vision: Association of questionnaire score with objective clinical tests. Current Eye Research 1998; 17:506-512.
11. Prummel, M.F., M.P. Mourits, L. Blank, A. Berghout, L. Koornneef, and W.M. Wiersinga. Randomized double-blind trial of prednisone versus radiotherapy in Graves' ophthalmopathy. Lancet 1993; 342:949-954.
12. Bartley, G.B., V. Fatourechi, E.F. Kadrmas, S.J. Jacobsen, D.M. Ilstrup, J.A. Garrity, and C.A. Gorman. Long-term follow-up of Graves Ophthalmopathy in an incidence cohort. Ophthalmology 1996; 103:958-962.
13. Wilson, I.B., and P.D. Cleary. Linking clinical variables with health-related quality of life. JAMA 1995; 273:59-65.
14. World Health Organization. International Classification of Impairments, Disabilities, and Handicaps. World Health Organization, Geneva, Switzerland, 1980.
15. Connelly, J.E., J.T. Philbrick, G.R. Smith, Jr., D.L. Kaiser, and A. Wymer. Health perceptions of primary care patients and the influence on health care utilization. Medical Care 1989; 27:S99-109.
16. Kaplan, G.A., and T. Camacho. Perceived health and mortality: a nine-year follow-up of the human population laboratory cohort. American Journal of Epidemiology 1983; 117:292-304.
17. Dijkers, M. Measuring quality of life. Am J Phys Med Rehabil 1999; 78:286-300.
18. Partick, D.L., and R.A. Deyo. Generic and disease-specific measures in assessing health status and quality of life. Medical Care 1989; 27:S217-S232.
19. Stewart, A.L., R.D. Hays, and J.E. Ware. The MOS Short-form General Health Survey: Reliability and validity in a patient population. Medical Care 1988; 26:724-735.
20. Ware, J.E., and C.D. Sherbourne. The MOS 36-item Short-Form Health Survey (SF-36).I. Conceptual framework and item selection. Medical Care 1992; 30:473-483.
21. Aaronson, N.K., C. Acquadro, J. Alonso, G. Apolone, D. Bucquet, M. Bullinger, K. Bungay, S. Fukuhara, B. Gandek, S. Keller, D. Razavi, R. Sanson-Fisher, M. Sullivan, S. Wood-Dauphine, A. Wagner, and J.E. Ware. International quality of life assessment (IQOLA) project. Quality of Life Research. 1:349-351, 1992.
22. Bergner, M., R.A. Bobbitt, S. Kressel, W.E. Pollard, B.S. Gilson, and J.R. Morris. The Sickness Impact Profile: Conceptual formulation and methodology for the development of a health status measure. International Journal of Health Services 1976; 6:393-415.
23. Terwee, C.B., M.N. Gerding, F.W. Dekker, M.F. Prummel, and W.M. Wiersinga. Development of a disease-specific quality of life questionnaire for patients with Graves' ophthalmopathy: The GO-QOL. British Journal of Ophthalmology 1998; 82:773-779.

24. Hays, R.D., R.T. Anderson, and D. Revicki. Assessing reliability and validity of measurement in clinical trials. In Quality of life assessment in clinical trials. Methods and practice. M.J. Staquet, R.D. Hays, and P.M. Fayers, editors. Oxford University Press, Oxford 1998; 169-182.
25. Terwee, C.B., M.N. Gerding, F.W. Dekker, M.F. Prummel, J.P. van der Pol, and W.M. Wiersinga. Test-retest reliability of the GO-QOL: A disease-specific quality of life questionnaire for patients with Graves' ophthalmopathy. Journal of Clinical Epidemiology 1999; 52:875-884.
26. Terwee, C.B., F.W. Dekker, M.P. Mourits, M.N. Gerding, L. Baldeschi, R. Kalmann, M.F. Prummel, and W.M. Wiersinga. Interpretation and validity of changes in scores on the Graves' Ophthalmopathy Quality Of Life questionnaire (GO-QOL) after different treatments. Accepted for publication in Clinical Endocrinology, 2000.
27. Guillemin, F., C. Bombardier, and D. Beaton. Cross-cultural adaptation of health-related quality of life measures: literature review and proposed guidelines. Journal of Clinical Epidemiology 1993; 46:1417-1432.
28. Anderson RT, A.N., Leplege AP, Wilkin D. International use and application of generic health-related quality of life instruments. In Quality of life and pharmacoeconomics in clinical trials. S. B, editor. Lippincott-Raven Publishers, Philadelphia. 613-630, 1996.
29. Kazis, L.E., J.J. Anderson, and R.F. Meenan. Effect sizes for interpreting changes in health status. Medical Care 1989; 27:S178-S189.
30. Terwee, C.B., F.W. Dekker, W.M. Wiersinga, M.F. Prummel, and P.M.M. Bossuyt. On Assessing responsiveness of health-related quality of life instruments: Guidelines for instrument evaluation. submitted for publication, 2000.
31. Lohr, K.N., N.K. Aaronson, J. Alonso, M.A. Burnam, D.L. Patrick, E.B. Perrin, and J.S. Roberts. Evaluating quality of life and health status instruments: Development of scientific review criteria. Clinical Therapeutics 1996; 18:979-992.
32. Lydick, E.G., and R.S. Epstein. Clinical significance of quality of life data. In Quality of life and pharmacoeconomics in clinical trials. B. Spilker, editor. Lippincott-Raven Publishers, Philadelphia. 461-465, 1996.
33. Jaeschke, R., J. Singer, and G.H. Guyatt. Measurement of health status. Ascertaining the minimal clinically important difference. Controlled Clinical Trials 1989; 10:407-415.
34. Gerding, M.N., C.B. Terwee, F.W. Dekker, M.F. Prummel, and W.M. Wiersinga. Quality of life in patients with Graves' ophthalmopathy is markedly decreased: Measurement by the Medical Outcome Study instrument. Thyroid 1997; 7:885-889.
35. Kahaly, G.J., F. Petrak, J. Batke, J. Best, M. Rothenbacher, M. Meinhold, and U.T. Egle. Quality of life and adverse events in Graves' ophthalmopathy. In Abstract book of the VIth International Symposium on Graves' Ophthalmopathy. November 27-28, Amsterdam. 9, 1998.
36. Aaronson, N.K., M. Muller, P.D.A. Cohen, M.L. Essink-Bot, M. Fekkes, R. Sanderman, M.A.G. Sprangers, A. Velde, and E. Verrips. Translation, validation, and norming of the Dutch language version of the SF-36 health survey in community and chronic disease populations. Journal of Clinical Epidemiology 1998; 51:1055-1068.
37. LaForge, R.G., W.D. Spector, and J. Sternberg. The relationship of vision and hearing impairment to one-year mortality and functional decline. J Aging Health Care 1992; 4:126-148.

38. Salive, M.E., J. Guralnik, R.J. Glynn, W. Christen, R.B. Wallace, and A.M. Ostfeld. Association of visual impairment with mobility and physical function. Journal of the American Geriatric Society 1994; 42:287-292.
39. Scott, I.U., O.D. Schein, S. West, K. Bandeen-Roche, C. Enger, and M.F. Folstein. Functional status and quality of life measurement among ophthalmic patients. Archives of Ophthalmology 1994; 112:329-335.
40. Kington, R., J. Rogowski, L. Lillard, and P.P. Lee. Functional associations of "trouble seeing". Journal of General Internal Medicine 1997; 12:125-128.
41. Lee, P.P., K. Spritzer, and R.D. Hays. The impact of blurred vision on functioning and well-being. Ophthalmology 1997; 104:390-396.
42. Scott, I.U., W.E. Smiddy, J. Schiffman, W.J. Feuer, and C.J. Pappas. Quality of life of low-vision patients and the impact of low-vision services. American Journal of Ophthalmology 1999; 128:54-62.
43. Dropkin, M.J.O., R.G. Malgady, D.W. Scott, M.T. Oberst, and E.W. Strong. Scaling disfigurement and dysfunction in postoperative head and neck patients. Head & Neck Surgery 1983; 6:559-570.
44. Ackerstaff, A.H., J.A.H. Lindeboom, A.J.M. Balm, F.H.M. Kroon, I.B. Tan, and F.J.M. Hilgers. Structured assessment of the consequences of composite resection. Clin Otolaryngol 1998; 23:339-344.
45. Macgregor, F.C. Facial disfigurement: Problems and management of social interaction and implications for mental health. Aesthetic Plastic Surgery 1999; 14:249-257.
46. Clarke, A. Psychosocial aspects of facial disfigurement: Problems, management and the role of a lay-led organization. Psychology, Health & Medicine 1999; 4:127-142.
47. Fukunishi, I. Relationship of cosmetic disfigurement to the severity of posttraumatic stress disorder in burn injury or digital amputation. Psychother Psychosom 1999; 68:82-86.
48. van der Horst, C.M., C.A. de Borgie, J.L. Knopper, and P.M. Bossuyt. Psychosocial adjustment of children and adults with port wine stains. British Journal of Plastic Surgery 1997; 50:463-467.
49. McGrouther, D.A. Facial disfigurement. The last bastion of discrimination. British Medical Journal 1997; 314:991.
50. Bianchi, G., V. Zaccheroni, R. Cerutti, E. Solaroli, F. Vescini, S. Menini, G. Rivolta, and G. Marchesini. Health-related quality of life in patients with thyroid disorders. Quality of Life Research 1999; 8:631.
51. Ljunggren, J.G., O. Törring, G. Wallin, A. Taube, L. Tallstedt, B. Hamberger, and G. Lundell. Quality of life aspects and costs in treatment of Graves' hyperthyroidism with antithyroid drugs, surgery, or radioiodine: results from a prospective, randomized study. Thyroid 1998; 8:653-659.
52. Pinchera, A., W.M. Wiersinga, D. Glinoer, P. Kendall-Taylor, L. Koornneef, C. Marcocci, and H. Schleusener. Classification of eye changes of Graves' disease. Thyroid 1992; 2:235-236.
53. Berg, G., A. Michanek, and E. Nyström. Clinical outcome of radioiodine treatment of hyperthyroidism: a follow-up study. Journal of Internal Medicine 1996; 239:165-171.

54. Törring, O., L. Tallstedt, G. Wallin, G. Lundell, J.G. Ljunggren, A. Taube, M. Sääf, B. Hamberger, and the Thyroid Study Group. Graves' hyperthyroidism: treatment with antithyroid drugs, surgery, or radioiodine - a prospective, randomized study. Journal of Clinical Endocrinology and Metabolism 1996; 81:2986-2993.
55. Linos, D.A., D. Karakitos, and J. Papademetriou. Should the primary treatment of hyperthyroidism be surgical? European Journal of Surgery 1997; 163:651-657.
56. Bartelana, L., C. Marcocci, F. Bogazzi, L. Manetti, M.L. Tanda, E. Dell'Unto, G. Bruno-Bossio, M. Nardi, M.P. Bartolomei, A. Lepri, G. Rossi, E. Martino, and A. Pinchera. Relation between therapy for hyperthyroidism and the course of Graves' ophthalmopathy. New England Journal of Medicine 1998; 338:73-78.
57. Prummel MF, M.M., Berghout A, Krenning EP, van der Gaag R, Koornneef L, Wiersinga WM. Prednisone and cyclosporine in the treatment of severe Graves' ophthalmopathy. New England Journal of Medicine 1989; 16:1403-1405.
58. Baschieri, L., A. Antonelli, S. Nardi, B. Alberti, A. Lepri, R. Canapicchi, and P. Fallahi. Intravenous immunoglobulin versus corticosteroid in treatment of Graves' ophthalmopathy. Thyroid 1997; 7:579-585.
59. Mourits, M.P., M.L. van Kempen-Hartenveld, M. Begona Garcia Garcia, H.P.F. Koppeschaar, L. Tick, and C.B. Terwee. Randomized placebo-controlled study of radiotherapy for Graves' orbitopathy. Lancet 2000; 355:1505-1509.
60. Kung, A.W.C., J. Michon, K.S. Tai, and F.L. Chan. The effect of somatostatin versus corticosteroid in the treatment of Graves' ophthalmopathy. Thyroid 1996; 6:381-384.
61. Matejka, G., B. Vergès, G. Vaillant, J.M. Petit, A. Brun-Pacaud, S. Rudoni, and J.M. Brun. Intravenous methylprednisolone pulse therapy in the treatment of Graves' ophthalmopathy. Horm. Metab. Res 1997; 30:93-98.
62. Seegenschmiedt, M., I. Keilholz, G. Gusek-Schneider, S. Barth, J. Hensen, F. Wolf, G.O.H. Naumann, and R. Sauer. Endokrine orbitopathie: Vergleich der langzeitergebnisse und klassifi-kationen nach radiotherapie. Strahlentherapie und Onkologie 1998; 174:449-456.
63. Khan, J.A., J.F. Doane, and M.M. Whitacre. Does decompression diminish the discomfort of severe dysthyroid orbitopathy? Ophthalmic Plastic and Reconstructive Surgery 1995; 11:109-112.
64. Fatourechi, V., J.A. Garrity, G.B. Bartley, E.J. Bergstrahl, and C.A. Gorman. Orbital decompression in Graves' ophthalmopathy associated with pretibial myxedema. Journal of Endocrinological Investigation 1993; 16:433-437.
65. Fatourechi, V., J.A. Garrity, G.B. Bartley, E.J. Bergstralh, L.W. DeSanto, and C.A. Gorman. Results of transantral orbital decompression preformed primarily for cosmetic indications. Ophthalmology 1994; 101:938-942.
66. Fatourechi, V., E.J. Bergstralh, J.A. Garrity, G.B. Bartley, C.W. Beatty, K.P. Offord, and C.A. Gorman. Predictors of response to transantral orbital decompression in severe Graves' ophthalmopathy. Mayo Clinic Proceedings 1994; 69:841-848.
67. Garrity, J.A., V. Fatourechi, E.J. Bergstralh, G.B. Bartley, C.W. Beatty, L.W. DeSanto, and C.A. Gorman. Results of transantral orbital decompression in 428 patients with severe Graves' ophthalmopathy. American Journal of Ophthalmology 1993; 116:533-547.
68. Tjon, F., M. Sang, P. Knegt, R. Wijngaarde, R. Poublon, E. van der Schans, and E. Krenning. Transantral orbital decompression for Graves' disease. Clinical Otolaryngology 1994; 19:290-294.
69. Olver, J.M. Botulinum toxin. A treatment of overactive corrugator supercilii in thyroid eye disease. British Journal of Ophthalmology 1998; 82:528-533.

70. Kane, R.L., M. Maciejweski, and M. Finch. The relationship of patient satisfaction with care and clinical outcomes. Medical Care 1997; 35:714-730.
71. Streiner, D.L., and G.R. Norman. Health measurement scales. A practical guide to their development and use. Oxford University Press, New York, 1989.

11

ASSESSMENT OF DISEASE ACTIVITY

Maarten P. Mourits
Department of Ophthalmology (Orbital Unit), University Medical Center Utrecht, the Netherlands

WHAT IS DISEASE ACTIVITY?

"Active" disease refers to the stage in which manifestations appear, or become worse, and the patient progressively experiences the negative consequences of the disease. This in contrast to the inactive, or burnt out stage of the disease in which the disease process is stable, although the patient may still be considerably handicapped. In Graves' ophthalmopathy (GO), patients initially have red, painful, watering eyes and swollen and retracted eyelids. Their eyes start to protrude, eye movements become painful and restricted, and vision may diminish. Basedow, in one of the first descriptions (1) of Graves' disease, reported that after an initial stage of ever increasing complaints an improvement took place ("eine reelle Besserung hervor, auch der Exophthalmos verminderte sich"). This has been the experience of other clinicians as well (2). The eyes become white again, the eyelids more puffy than swollen, and pain disappears. But contrary to Basedow's observations, proptosis persists (with lid retraction, in some cases) and severe motility impairment only improves to a certain extent, leaving the patient with double vision at least in the extremes of gaze. Figure 1 illustrates these two stages of the disease.

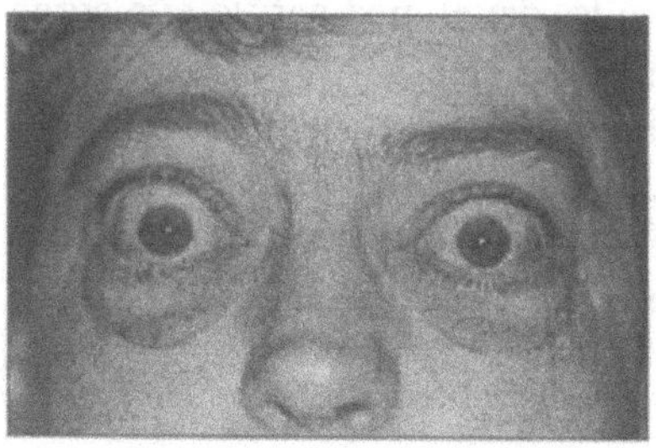

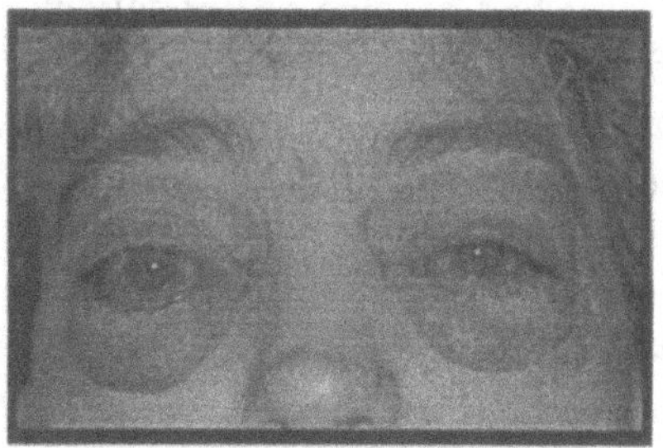

Figure 1: Patient with active GO (left) and same patient with burnt out GO (right).

Rundle did sequential measurements in patients who were not treated for their ophthalmopathy (3). He found that after a period of rapid progression, which he called the dynamic phase, the disease severity reaches a top, after which the symptoms decline although do not disappear completely and then remain unchanged (static phase). From these assessments he drafted the so called 'Rundle's curve' (Figure 2).

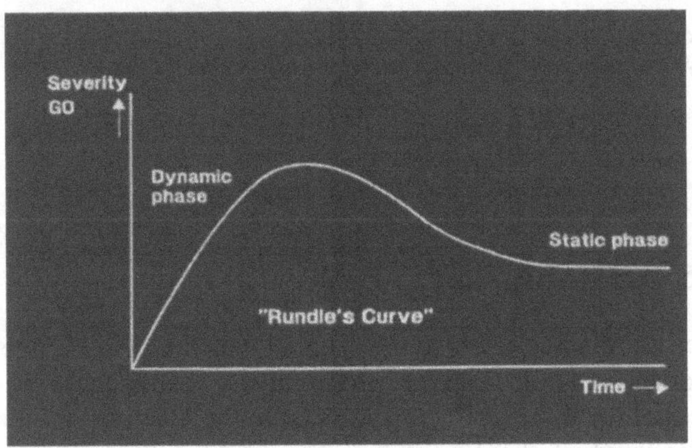

Figure 2: Rundle's curve

Rundle's curve has become generally accepted as the graphic description of the natural course of GO, although he did not define the time axis clearly. The dynamic phase was later found to last about 6-24 months (4). Conjunctival and eyelid swelling appeared to be maximal after 12 months of observation after which gradual regression occurred. Hales and Rundle, in a long-term follow-up study, noted that the general appearance of patients had improved after 15 years, but that in about 50% obvious signs of eye disease were still present (5). Eyelid retraction, soft tissue involvement and ocular motility have a tendency to improve, whereas proptosis remains stable (6,7). In most patients an end-stage is reached after about five years (8). However, we have seen a patient with moderately severe unilateral GO, who went through all the stages of 'Rundle's curve' with one eye and then, when the disease had become completely stable at that side, developed active eye signs of GO in the other orbit (9). Apparently, at least in patients with (predominantly) unilateral ophthalmopathy, there may be a second 'Rundle's curve' over time. In conclusion, after an initial stage of increasing disability lasting for about a year, a top is reached, after which the disease gradually disappears over a period of several years leaving major or minor stigmata behind.

At first, it seemed that histologic findings were consistent with 'Rundle's curve'. Naffziger found edematous eye muscles in patients with ophthalmopathy of recent onset, but fibrotic tissues in those with longer existing eye disease. Mononuclear cell infiltrates were found in the intermediate stages (10). Similar findings have been described by others (11,12). In subsequent years, much has become clear regarding the pathogenesis of GO (8). Graves' eye disease is an autoimmune disorder characterized by lymphocytic infiltrations of the peribulbar tissues. These lymphocytes produce cytokines, which stimulate glycosaminoglycan (GAG) production by orbital fibroblasts present in the extraocular muscles and orbital connective tissues. These GAG's are highly hydrophilic in nature and therefore cause edema. Lymphocytic infiltration, together with fibroblast proliferation and edema, causes swelling and proptosis, followed by orbital congestion due to venous compression, and further edema.

In later stages, these infiltrations of lymphocytes and resulting edema are replaced by another space-occupying phenomenon, e.g. the forming of fibrosis. Edema and lymphocytic infiltrations in the orbital tissues are often localised and different stages of these histologic alterations may be present at different areas of the orbit. Hufnagel et al. (13) and others (14) have found both lymphocytic infiltrations with fibrosis and collagen deposition in patients with active and inactive ophthalmopathy. Thus, although the presence of lymphocytic infiltrations and edema and the absence of fibrotic scar tissue represent early and active ophthalmopathy, and a massive deposition of fibrosis in the connective tissues with a scarcity of cells suggests burnt out disease, transition forms are found frequently.

WHAT IS THE SIGNIFICANCE OF DISEASE ACTIVITY?

The concept of disease activity is important as regards the therapeutic approach to the patient. Daicker found lymphocytic infiltration, edema and fibroblast activation in specimens of patients with ophthalmopathy of recent onset , and fibrotic changes and fat accumulation in patients with longstanding eye disease (15). He was the first to suggest that medical treatment such as corticosteroids or retrobulbar irradiation would only be effective during the early, active stage of the disease. This idea has been almost unanimously accepted, as these treatments likely act on the lymphocytic expression and edema and not on the fibrotic scars of the advanced stage of the disease. Surgery, on the other hand, deals with the increase of volumes and the presence of scar tissue. It is thus general practice to postpone surgical corrections such as rehabilitative proptosis correction, strabismus surgery and eyelid surgery till the disease has reached a quiescent stage, because ongoing active disease will annihilate good operation results. In general, three to six months of stable eye signs have to be passed before surgery will be performed. The only exception to this rule is made for patients with vision threatening optic neuropathy due to apical compression of the second cranial nerve that does not respond to medical treatment. In such a case, orbital decompression should be performed immediately.

Both the stage of the disease and its severity determines the choice of treatment. If disease activity and disease duration were identical, the choice of treatment would be obvious: patients with active GO of recent onset would be treated with immunosuppressive treatment modalities, whereas those with inactive and longstanding eye signs would be considered for surgery. However, as we have seen, the time course of GO is extremely variable and the distinction between active and burnt out disease is not always clear. Therefore, attempts have been made to create tools that are able to distinguish active from burnt out GO. The ultimate goals of such instruments are to allow prediction of the therapeutic outcome after immunosuppressive treatments and to allow successful surgery to be done as soon as possible. At the same time, such instruments should increase the proportion of successfully treated patients, by allowing only those who will benefit to be treated.

Tools that make such treatment selections possible can only be validated on their ability to predict the therapeutic outcome because a "gold standard" (i.e. histologic specimen) for disease activity does not exist. Prummel et al. have listed the drawbacks of this approach (16). In larger groups, the outcome of treatment will hardly ever be a 100% success because the efficacy of a treatment is rarely 100%. In addition, there are genetically determined factors that make patients respond differently to treatment (17). Further, a number of patients will improve, not because of the treatment given, but spontaneously as a result of the natural course of the disease. Finally, changes of amount of eyelid swelling, of redness of the eyes, of eyelid retraction, etc. are difficult to measure. However, it is on these measurements that we ground our conclusions regarding failure or success of the treatment. To overcome these difficulties, a two-by-two table can be used to calculate the sensitivity, specificity, and the positive and negative predictive value of a disease activity marker. An ideal marker would have both high positive and negative predictive value. As pointed out, these values will never be 100%. However, a high positive predictive value of a disease activity marker would select patients for immunosuppressive treatment, whereas a high negative predictive value would select patient for surgery.

PARAMETERS FOR DISEASE ACTIVITY

Duration of Ophthalmopathy

A number of investigators have found better results of immunosuppressive treatment in patients with GO of recent onset than in patients with longstanding eye disease. Donaldson et al. found that good results from retrobulbar irradiation correlate with the duration of the exacerbation of eye signs (18). In our experience, the mean duration of the ophthalmopathy did not correlate with the outcome of treatment (19,20).

The Clinical Activity Score

Already Van Dyke (21) and Sergott (22) et al. included clinical parameters in their activity score, but these were never tested for their predictive value. In 1989, we proposed a tool to measure disease activity of GO based on the classical signs of inflammation (23). During the dynamic phase of Rundle's curve, patients are complaining of a pressure feeling on their eyes and painful eye movements. Their eyes are red, the lids and conjunctiva edematous. Proptosis and lid retraction increase, eyeball movements decrease and vision may diminish. These signs show a striking resemblance to the classic manifestations of inflammation, described by Celsus and Galen centuries ago. These signs are: pain (Latin: dolor), redness (rubor), swelling (tumor) and impaired function (functio laesa). Heat (calor) is also one of the (five) classic signs, but was omitted in our score, because detection of subtle changes of temperature in the orbit would require sophisticated instruments which are beyond the scope of a simple clinical measurement tool. Thus, our proposed Clinical Activity Score (CAS) consists of 10 items. One point is given for each item present. The sum of these points is the CAS.

The CAS is fast, cheap and requires no other assessments than already done during clinical inspection of a Graves' patient. The last three items demand repetitive observations. This is not a serious draw-back, as in most Graves' patients additional information (CT-scan, thyroid functions, etc.) must be collected after their first consultation and before treatment is started and this usually requires several weeks. The CAS has gained some popularity and is frequently used as a reference for other tools to assess disease activity in GO (see below). Tested in a prospective study, we found a CAS of > 4 to have a positive predictive value of 80%, but a negative predictive value of

64% only (24). CAS values of 2 – 4 are often found, but have little significance for the prediction of the therapeutic outcome. Before rehabilitative surgery is performed, not only should the patient have a low CAS, but also a several month history of unchanging lid retraction, but several months of stable proptosis and/or consistent eye motility patterns (25).

Table 1. The Clinical Activity Score to assess disease activity in Graves' ophthalmopathy

Item	No.	Points	Description
Pain	1.	1	Painful, oppressive feeling on or behind the eyeball
	2.	1	Pain on attempted up, side or downgaze
Redness	3.	1	Redness of the eyelids
	4.	1	Diffuse redness of the conjunctiva
Swelling	5.	1	Swelling of the eyelid due to edema
	6.	1	Chemosis
	7.	1	Swollen caruncula
	8.	1	Increase of proptosis of 2 mm or more during a period between 1–3 months
Impaired function	9.	1	Decrease of eye movements in any direction of 5 degrees or more
	10.	1	Decrease of visual acuity of 1 line or more on the Snellen chart (using a pinhole) during a period of 1-3 months

For each item present one point is given. The sum of these points is the CAS (maximum is 10 points)

Echography

A- (two-) and B- (three-dimensional) scans, resulting from the recording of reflected ultrasounds passed through the eye and orbit, are widely used in ophthalmic practice for the detection of a great number of pathologic conditions ranging from detachment of the retina to intra- or extraocular tumors. Echography is cheap and harmless to the patient, but rather operator-dependent, because the technique and the interpretation are not easy to perform. A-scans, rather than B-scans, are suitable for measuring the thickness of extraocular muscles and can therefore be of help in making the diagnosis of GO. In addition, they can be used to show intramuscular structural differences and this ability has been used to make the distinction between active and burnt out ophthalmopathy. However, a prominent superior orbital rim may hinder measurment of the inferior rectus muscle, the extraocular muscle most frequently involved in GO. It was postulated that high reflectivity (caused by acoustic interfaces produced by fibrosis within the muscle) would be related to the inactive stage of the disease and low reflectivity (caused by general swelling of the muscle due to edema) to active disease. Tested in a small number of patients, this new ultrasonographic method to detect disease activity seemed very promising (26). However, in a subsequent larger study of 56 patients, the positive and negative predictive values were 85% and 60% respectively(16), making it insufficient as a test to be used on its own.

Magnetic Resonance Imaging (MRI)

MRI is a noninvasive method used to depict human (and other) structures with radiofrequency signals originating from changes in the axis of spinning protons (T1 weighted image) in the phase of those spinning protons (T2 weighted image) in a strong magnetic field (27). As the bony structures are poorly imaged, MRI is not suitable for preoperative evaluation of Graves' patients before orbital decompression is performed. However, T2 weighted MRI is used to detect edema and inflammation in the extraocular muscles. Just et al. have shown that a long T2 time is associated with a good response to retrobulbar irradiation (28), whereas the groups of Utech (29) and Nakahara (30) reported that T2 relaxation time decreases after immunosuppressive treatment. Interestingly, Hoh et al., using the Short Tau Inversion Recovery (STIR) found a correlation with the CAS and T2 times (31). Fat and water-containing tissues appear bright on both T1- and T2-weighted MRI images. The background stroma of the orbit is composed mainly of fat and has a characteristic bright signal in conventional spinning MRI. STIR, by summation of T1 and T2 and by choosing the appropriate inversion time, can selectively suppress signals from a tissue such as fat while highlighting water-containing (edema) tissues. Hiromatsu et al. were the first to use T2 times to predict the outcome of intravenous prednisone treatment. They found a positive predictive value of 69% and a negative predictive value of 86%, but their study was confined to 23 patients only (32). MRI, in particular STIR, seems to be a promising tool to assess disease activity, but larger studies must be performed to further assess this modality.

Octreotide Scintigraphy

Inflammatory changes in the orbit are thought to arise from activation of lymphocytes and orbital fibroblasts (8). These cells express somatostatin receptors on the plasma membrane, to which octreotide can bind. Octreotide is an eight-aminoacid analog of the 14-aminoacid neuropeptide somatostatin. Orbital uptake of this radiolabeled octreotide may be due to binding of this molecule to the activated cells. However, binding to receptors on other cell types, or local blood pooling due to venous stasis may be involved. Nevertheless, Postema et al. (33) showed that in patients with supposedly active GO a pronounced orbital uptake of radiolabeled octreotide (^{111}In-DTPA-D.Phe^{1}) could be demonstrated. Several studies have been performed to relate the amount of uptake to disease activity and the response to immunosuppressive treatment. A positive correlation of the octreotide uptake and the CAS and T2 relaxation time was found (33,34,35). Krassas et al., in 12 patients, found a positive and negative predictive value of octreoscans for predicting the outcome of immunosuppressive therapy of 100% and 83% respectively (36). Gerding et al., studying 22 patients and using the orbital/occipital ratio instead of the orbital/temporal ration on a scan made 4 hours after injection of approximately 111 MBq for predicting outcome of retrobulbar irradiation, found values of 92% and 70%, respectively (37). Their study showed that octreotide scintigraphy should be interpreted with caution. The intraobserver variation of interpreting octreoscans was found to differ from 6-16% and further depends on the methodology to correct for nonspecific bachground uptake (37). Considering the relatively low negative predictive value together with the facts that octreotide scintigraphy is expensive and requires a not-neglecting radioactivity burden of 100-150 MBq, the usefulness of the octreotide scan alone is limited.

Rosette Formation

Sergott et al. attempted to find immunologic distinctions that would correspond with response to corticosteroid treatment. They reported that patients with decreased T-lymphocyte levels, as assayed by spontaneous active and total rosette-forming cells, respond most favourably to corticosteroids. Further, this improvement was accompanied by a marked increase in percentages and absolute numbers of peripheral blood T-lymphocytes (22,38). Similar results were obtained by Preus et al. in 1985 (39), but to our knowledge, this test is not in use anymore.

Cytokines

Cytokines play a role in the pathogenesis of GO by inducing the expression of major histocompatibility complex class II molecules, heat-shock protein-72, involved in antigen recognition and intercellular adhesion molecule-1 involved in T-cell recruitment (40,41). Moreover, particular cytokines stimulate fibroblast to proliferate and synthesize glycoaminoglycans. These hydrophilic mucopolysaccharides attract fluid to the orbital tissues and so contribute to proptosis, eyelid and eye muscle swelling (42). A number of these cytokines have been tested for their predictive value of the outcome of immunosuppressive treatment (43,44). For this purpose, quantities in peripheral blood are measured by highly sensitive (sandwich) immunoassays. However, even if orbital cytokines are released into the bloodstream during the active stage of the eye disease, these quantities may be to small to detect and binding of these cytokines to soluble receptors, carrier proteins and autoantibodies may hinder correct measurement. Moreover, they may reflect Graves' hyperthyroidism itself, or conditions not related to GO (16). The Migration Inhibition Factor (MIF), for instance, was found in serum of patients with GO and correlated with the clinical activity score (45). Serum MIF activity, however, was also found in patients with uveitis and is thus not specific for GO. In another study, soluble interleukin-2 receptor levels were found to be increased in patients with severe GO and to correlate with disease activity (46). However, the positive and negative predictive values for treatment outcome were of limited value (71% and 54%, respectively only) (46). In contrast to Hofbauer et al. (47), Bartelena et al. found no correlation between levels of baseline soluble interleukin-1 receptor antagonist and either smoking (an important risk factor for GO) or the therapeutic response to steroids (48). No single cytokine has been found to reliably predict the outcome of immunosuppressive therapy in

GO. However, new cytokines that are discovered regularly may be worthwhile to study in this context.

Immunomodulatory Molecules

Adhesion molecules function as receptors between immunocompetent cells, connective tissue and extracellular matrix components (49), and direct circulating lymphocytes towards their target (50,51). Measurement of soluble forms of these molecules shed into the circulation has been used to assess disease activity in GO. Soluble intercellular adhesion molecule-1 (sICAM-1) was found to be increased in patients with active disease, as compared to patients with no or stable eye disease, and sICAM-1 levels declined upon prednisone treatment (52). sICAM-1 levels were also found to be increased in patients with Graves' thyroid disease without ophthalmopathy, but to a lesser extent. This could be due to expression of ICAM-1 both in orbital and thyroidal tissues (53). However, soluble endothelial-leucocyte adhesion molecule-1 (sELAM-1) appears to be more specific for Graves' eye disease and was not elevated in patients with Graves' thyroid disease without eye complaints (53). sICAM-1 levels in active GO-patients correlated well with the clinical activity score ($r=0.55$; $P<0.002$).

Autoantibodies

An attractive explanation for the close relationship of Graves' thyroid and Graves' eye disease would be the existence of cross-reacting autoantibodies with a shared antigen in the thyroid gland and in the orbit. The TSH-receptor (TSH-R) antibodies are a likely candidate as they cause Graves' hyperthyroidism, and their presence has been demonstrated in orbital tissues (54). Gerding et al., in a recent study, found a highly significant correlation between the clinical activity score and TBII (TRAK assay) ($r=0.54$; $p<0.0001$) and TSI (cAMP response of a TSH-R transfected cell line) ($r=0.50$; $p<0.0001$), the latter being used as sensitive measurements of TSH-receptor antibody levels (55). However, they found no differences in baseline TSH-R antibodies between responders (n-34) and nonresponders (n-29) to retrobulbar radiotherapy in 63 patients (56). In both responders and nonresponders, TBII and TSI decreased significantly 26 weeks after radiotherapy, and the decline was similar in both groups. Thus, TSH-R antibodies cannot be used to identify (non)responders to immunosuppressive treatment.

Glycosaminoglycans (GAGs)

The important contribution of GAGs to the development of swelling of the orbital tissues in GO has been mentioned already. GAGs are produced by activated fibroblasts and part of their metabolites (e.g. free GAG chains) are found in the circulation and are renally excreted. Urinary excretion of GAGs may, thus, mirror disease activity. Kahaly et al. found a twofold increase in urinary GAG excretion in patients with active, untreated GO as compared to controls and to Graves' patients without GO or patients with a toxic goiter (57). In addition, GAG excretions decreased when the ophthalmopathy became quiescent, whereas relapses were accompanied by increased GAG excretion (57). Using more sophisticated methods to determine urinary GAG levels and plasma GAG levels, Kahaly's group was able to confirm their previous assessments (58,59). However, these remarkable findings could not be supported by others, who found similar urinary GAG excretion in GO-patients and in controls (60,56).

COMBINATIONS OF PARAMETERS

Table 2. Positive and negative predictive values (PPV and NPV) for the outcome of immunosuppressive treatment of several parameters of disease activity

Parameter / Ref	PPV	NPV	Number
CAS 24	80	64	43
Echography 16	85	60	56
MRI 32	69	86	23
Octreoscan 37	92	70	22
sIL-2R 46	71	54	47

From Table 2 it becomes clear that no single activity parameter can predict accurately which patient will benefit from immunosuppressive treatment or in which patient surgical corrections can be performed without the risk that ongoing disease activity will adversely affect good surgical results. Prummel (16) and Gerding (56) have attempted to combine parameters of disease activity and applied a multivariate logistic regression analysis model to weigh the relative impact of each parameter on the prediction of response to immunosuppressive treatment (radiotherapy). Results were better with this approach than when only one parameter was used. Gerding made different models to select patients for immunosuppressive treatment (active disease) and for rehabilitative surgery (burnt out disease) and used ROC (Receiver-operating characteristics) curves to measure the usefulness of a test (56). The larger the area underneath the curve, the higher the AUC-value, the better the prediction value. A combination of duration of GO, soft tissue signs (including some CAS-items), bulbar elevation, echography, sIl-2r, sCD-30 and an octreoscan was found to predict the outcome of radiotherapy best (AUC = 0.89). In contrast, a combination of age, sex, duration of GO, soft tissue signs (including some CAS-items), MRI and ultrasonography appeared to be the best indicator to select patients for rehabilitative surgery (AUC = 0.94). Depending upon the cut-off point chosen, such models would increase the response rate to radiotherapy from 53% to 70% (56). A simpler method (duration of GO + severity of soft tissue involvement + bulbar elevation in degrees together with MRI) would permit acceptable results for general clinical practice. However, these models were applied to a selected group of patients, e.g. with moderately severe GO, only. In addition, disease activity was defined as response to retrobulbar irradiation. Finally, responsiveness to therapy suggests that we can reliably assess improvement, which might not always be the case, as our measurements are rather crude. Thus, Gerding's models can only be used within these margins of error and larger studies in unselected groups are warranted to test their clinical relevance.

CONCLUSION

Has progress has been made since Basedow's publication 160 years ago, and following more than a decade of intensive searching for a simple tool to discriminate active from burnt out GO? Although a number of disease activity markers have been developed, no one of these has both an acceptable positive and negative predictive value. Interestingly, the clinical activity score (CAS) was found to correlate with the STIR (31), T2 relaxation time (33,34,35), the MIF (45), sICAM-1 (53), and TBII (55). It appears that each of these parameters reflects only some of the elements comprising disease activity. The CAS is based on manifestations of inflammation such as edema and vasodilatation. Echography and MRI also detect edema. Serum levels of cytokines and immunomodulatory molecules suggest the presence of lymphocytic infiltrations. The existence of unilateral GO indicates that different stages of the disease can be present in the same patient. Histologic sections have shown different stages of the disease even within in the same orbit. Therefore, it is not that the patient is 'active', but rather, that some or more of her/his orbital tissues are inflamed. For this reason, no single, definitive answer is given by any of the various means used to assess disease parameters. Another problem is the modest efficacy of immunosuppressive treatment to which these parameters are linked. A recent placebo controlled study showed that radiotherapy was only effective in a subgroup of GO-patients (e.g. those with impaired motility) (61). As yet, no such study has been performed to test the efficacy of prednisone.

Our efforts must be directed on the development of better treatment modalities. This requires a better understanding of the etiology of Graves' disease. In the meantime, the use of a combination of the above mentioned parameters of disease activity can help us to better select appropriate treatment for GO-patients, especially those whose eye symptoms are in the grey area between very active and completely burnt out disease.

REFERENCES

1. Von Basedow CA. Exophthalmos durch Hypertrophie des Zellgewebes in der Augenhohle. Wochenschrift die Gesammte Heikunde 1840; 197-228.
2. Streeten DHP, Anderson GH, Reed GF, Woo P. Prevalence, natural history and surgical treatment of exophthalmos. Clin Endocrinol 1987; 27:125-33.
3. Rundle FF, Wilson CW. Development and course of exophthalmos and ophthalmoplegia in Graves'disease with special reference to the effect of thyroidectomy. Cli Sci 1945; 5:177-94.
4. Rundle FF. "Eye signs of Graves' disease." In *The Thyroid*, Pitt-Rivers R, Trotter WR ,eds. Washington, DC: Butterworths and Co , 1964.
5. Hales IB, Rundle FF. Ocular changes in Graves' disease. A long-term follow-up study. Q J Med 1960; 29:113-126.
6. Hamilton HE, Schultz RO, De Gowin EL. The endocrine eye lesions in hyperthyroidism. Its incidence and course in 165 patients treated for thyrotoxicosis with iodine-131. Arch Int Med 1960; 105:675-85.
7. Bartley GB. The epidemiologic characteristics and clinical course of ophthalmopathy associated with auto-immune thyroid disease in Olmsted County, Minnesota. Tr Am Ophth Soc 1994; 17;477-588.
8. Burch H, Wartofsky L. Graves' ophthalmopathy: Current concepts regarding pathogenesis and management. Endocr Rev 1993; 14:747-93.
9. Kalmann R, Mourits MP. Reactivation of unilateral Graves' orbitopathy on the contralateral side. Submitted for publication.
10. Naffziger HC. Pathologic changes in the orbit in progressive exophthalmos. Arch Ophthalmol 1933; 9:1-12.
11. Dunnington JH, Berke RN. Exophthalmos due to chronic orbital myositis. Arch Ophthalmol 1943; 30:446-66.
12. Brain RW. Exophthalmic ophthalmoplegia. Q J Med 1938; 31:293-323.

13. Hufnagel TJ, Hickey WF, Cobbs WH, Jakobiec FA, Iwamoto T, Eagle RC. Immunohistochemical and ultrastructural studies on the exenterated orbital tissues of a patient with Graves' disease. Ophthalmology 1984; 91:1411-19
14. Tallstedt L, Norberg R. Immunohistochemical staining of normal and Graves' extraocular muscle. Inv Ophthalmol Vis Sc 1988; 29:175-84.
15. Daicker B. Das gewebliche Substrat der verdickten ausseren Augenmuskuln bei der endokrinen Orbitopathie. Klin Mbl Augenheilkunde 1979; 174:843-847.
16. Prummel MF, Wiersinga WM, Mourits MP. "Assessment of disease activity of Graves' Ophthalmopathy." In *Recent developments in Graves' Ophthalmopathy,* Prummel MF, Wiersinga WM, Mourits MP, Heufelder AE, eds. Boston/Dordrecht/London : Kluwer Academic Publishers, 2000.
17. Van der Gaag R, Wiersinga WM, Koornneef L, Mourits MP, Prummel MF, Berghout A, de Vries RR, Schreuder GM, D'Amaro J. HLA-DR4 associated response to corticosteroids in Graves' ophthalmopathy patients. J endocrinol Invest 1990; 13:489-92.
18. Donaldson SS, Bagshaw MA, Kriss JP. Supervoltage orbital radiotherapy for Graves' ophthalmopathy. J Clin Endocrinol Metab 1973; 37:276-85.
19. Prummel MF, Mourits MP, Berghout A, Krenning EP, van der Gaag R, Koornneef L, Wiersinga WM. Prednisone and cyclosporine in the treatment of severe Graves' ophthalmopathy. N Engl J Med 1989; 321:1353-59.
20. Prummel MF, Mourits MP, Blank L, Berghout A, Koornneef L, Wiersinga WM. Randomised double-blind trial of prednisonr versus radiotherapy in Graves' ophthalmopathy. Lancet 1993; 342:949-54.
21. Sergott RC, Felberg NT, Savino PJ, Blizzard JJ, Schatz NJ, Graves' ophthalmopathy – immunologic parameters related to corticosteroid therapy. Invest Ophthalmol Vis Sci 1981; 20:173-82.
22. Van Dijk HJL. Orbital Graves' Disease. A modification of the "NO SPECS" classification. Ophthalmology 1981; 88:479-83.
23. Mourits MP, Koornneef L, Wiersinga WM, Prummel MF, Berghout A, van der Gaag R. Clinical criteria for the assessment of disease activity in Graves' ophthalmopathy: a novel approach. Br J Ophthalmol 1989; 73:639-44.
24. Mourits MP, Prummel MF, Wiersinga WM, Koornneef L. Clinical Activity Score as a guide in the management of patients with Graves' ophthalmopathy. Clin Endocrinol 1997; 47: 9-14.
25. Rose GE. Commentary. Clinical activity score as a guide in the management of patients with Graves' ophthalmopathy. Clin Endocrinol 1996; 47:15.
26. Prummel MF, Suttorp-Schulten MS, Wiersinga WM, Verbeek AD, Mourits MP, Koornneef L. A new ultrasonographic method to detect disease activity and predict response to immeunosuppressive treatment in Graves' Ophthalmopathy. Ophthalmology 1993; 100:556-61.
27. Armstrong P, Keevil SF. Magnetic resonance imaging-1; basic priciples of image production. Br Med J 1991; 303:35-40.
28. Just M, Kahaly G, Higer HP, Rosler HP, Kutzner J, Beyer J, et al. Graves' ophthalmopathy: role of MR imaging in radiation therapy. Radiology 1991; 179: 187-90.
29. Utech CI, Khatibnia U, Winter PF, Wulle KG. MR T2 relaxation time for the assessment of retrobulbar inflammation in Graves' ophthalmopathy. Thyroid 1995; 5:185-93.
30. Nakahara H, Noguchi S, Murakami N, Morita M, Tamaru M, Ohnishi T, et al. Graves' ophthalmopathy: MR evaluation of 10-Gy versus 24-GY irradiation combined with systemic corticosteroids. Radiology 1995; 196:857-62.

31. Hoh HB, Laitt RD, Wakeley C, Kabala J, Goddard P, Potts MJ, Harrad RA. The STIR sequence MRI in the assessment of extraocular muscles in thyroid eye disease.Eye 1994; 8:506-10.
32. Hiromatsu Y, Kojima K, Ishisaka N, Tanaka K, Sato M, Nonaka K, et al. Role of MRI in Thyroid-associated ophthalmopathy: its predictive value for therapeutic outcome of immunosuppressive therapy: Thyroid 1992; 2:299-305.
33. Postema PTE, Krenning EP, Wijngaarde R, Kooij PPM, Oei HY, van den Bosch WA, et al. ^{111}In-DPTA-D-Phe^{1}-octreotide scintigraphy in thyroidal and orbital Graves' disease: a parameter for disease activity?. J Clin Endocrinol Metab 1994; 79:1845-51.
34. Moncayo R, Baldissera I, Decistoforo C, Kendler D, Donnemiller E. Evaluation of immunological mechanisms mediating thyroid-associated ophthalmopathy by radionuclide imaging using the somatostatin anolog ^{111}In-octreotide. Thyroid 1997; 7:21-29.
35. Kahaly GJ, Diaz M, Just M, Beyer J, Lieb W. Role of octreoscan and correlation with MR imaging in Graves' ophthalmopathy. Thyroid 1995; 5:107-11.
36. Krassas GE, Dumas A, Pontikides N, Kaltsas T. Somatostatin receptor scintigraphy and octreotide treatment in patients with thyroid eye disease. Clin Endocrinol 1995; 42:571-80.
37. Gerding MN, van der Zant FM, van Royen EA, Koornneef L, Krenning EP, Wiersinga WM, Prummel MF. Octreotide-scintigraphy is a diaese-activity parameter in Graves' ophthalmopathy. Clin Endocrinol 1999; 50:373-79.
38. Sergott RC, Felberg NT, Savino PJ, Blizzard JJ, Schatz NJ. E-rosette formation in Graves' ophthalmopath. Invest Ophthalmolol Vis Sci 1979; 18:1245-51.
39. Preus M, Frecker MF, Stenszky V, Balasz C, Farid NR. A prognostic score for Graves' disease. Clin Endocrinol 1985; 23: 653-661.
40. Heufelder AE, Smith TJ, Gorman CA, Bahn RS. Increased induction of HLA-DR by interferon-gamma in cultured retroocular fibroblasts derived from patients with Graves' ophthalmopathy undergoing orbital radiotherapy.J Clin Endocrinol Metab 1991; 73:307-13.
41. Heufelder AE, Bahn RS. Modulation of intercellular adhesion molecule-1 (ICAM-1) by cytokines and Graves IjGs in cultured Graves' retroocular fibroblasts. Eur J Clin Invest. 1992; 23:10-17.
42. Smith TJ, Bahn RS, Gorman CA, Cheavens M. Stimulation of glycosaminoglycan accumulation by interfereon gamma in cultured retro-ocular fibroblasts. J Clin Endocrinol Metab 1991; 72:1162-66.
43. Balasz C, Farid NR. Soluble Interleukin-2 receptor in sera of patients with Graves' disease. J Autoimmunity 1991; 4:681-88.
44. Okumura M, Hidaka Y, Kuroda S, Takeoka K, Tada H, Amino N. Increased serum concentration of soluble CD30 in patients with Graves' disease. J clin Endocrinol Metab 1997; 82:1757-60.
45. Van der Gaag R, Broersma L, Mourits MP, Koornneef L, Wiersinga WM, Prummel MF, Berghout A. Circulating monocyte inhibitory factor in serum of Graves' ophthalmopathy patients: a parameter for disease activity? Clin Exp Immunolol 1989; 75:275-79.
46. Prummel MF, Wiersinga WM, van der Gaag R, Mourits MP, Koornneef L. Soluble IL-2 receptor levels in patients with Graves' ophthalmopathy. Clin Exp Immunol 1992; 88:405-9.
47. Hofbauer LC, Muhlberg T, Konig A, Heufelder G, Schworm H, Heufelder AE. Soluble interleukin-1 receptor antagonist serum levels in smokers and nonsmokers with Graves' ophthalmopathy undergoing orbital radiotherapy. J Clin Endocrinol Metab 1997; 82:2244-47.

48. Bartalena L, Manetti L, Tanda ML, Dell'Unto E, Mazzi B, Rocchi R, Barbesino G, Pinchera A, Marcocci C. Soluble interleukin-1 receptor antagonist concentration in patients with Graves' ophthalmopathy is neither related to cigarette smoking nor predictive of subsequent response to glucocorticoids. Clin Endocrinol 2000; 52:647-51.
49. Bahn RS, Heufelder AE. Mechanisms of disease: pathogenesis of Graves' ophthalmoathy.N Engl J Med 1993; 329:1468-75.
50. Frenette PS, Wagner DD. Molecular medicine. Adhesion molecules-Part I. N Engl J Med 1996; 334:1526-29.
51. Frenette PS, Wagner DD, Molecular medicine. Adhesion molecules- Part II. : blood vessels and blood cells. N Engl J Med 1993; 335:1468-75.
52 Heufelder AE, Bahn RS. Soluble intercellular adhesion molecule-1 (sICAM-1) in sera of patients with Graves' ophthalmopathy and thyroid disease. Clin Exp Immunol 1993; 92:296-302.
53. De Bellis A, Bizarro A, Gattoni AE. Behaviour of soluble intercellular adhesion molecule-1 and endothelial-leucocyte adhesion molecule-1 concentrations in patients with Graves' disease with or without ophthalmopathy and in patients with toxic adenoma. J Clin Endocrinol Metab 1995; 80:2118-21.
54. Heufelder AE. Involvement of the orbital fibroblast and TSH receptor in the pathogenesis of Graves' ophthalmopathy. Thyroid 1995; 4:331-40.
55. Gerding MN, van der Meer JWC, Broenink M, Bakker O, Wiersinga WM, Prummel MF. Association of thyrotrophin receptor antibodies with the clinical features of Graves' ophthalmopathy. Clin Endocrinol 2000; 52:267-71.
56. Gerding MN, van der Meer JWC, Broenink M, Bakker O, Prummel MF, Wiersinga WM. Urinary glycosaminoglycans do not correlate with disease activity in Graves' ophthalmopathy. In *Assessment of disease activity in Graves' ophthalmopathy*, Gerding MN, ed. Amsterdam, NL: L. van de Velde B.V., 1999.
57. Kahaly G, Schuler M, Sewell AC, Bernhard G, Beyer J, Krause U. Unrinary glycosaminoglycans in Graves' ophthalmopathy. Clin Endocrinolol 1990; 33:35-44.
58. Hansem Ch, Fraiture B, Rouhi R, Otto E, Forster G, Kahaly G. HPLLC glycosaminoglycan analysis in patients with Graves' disease. Clin Sci 1998; 8:429-32.
59. Kahaly G, Hansen C, Beyer J, Winand R. Plasma glycosaminoglycans in endocrine ophthalmopathy. J Endocrinol Invest 1994; 17:45-50.
60. Martinez-Bru C, Ampudia X, Castrillo P, Gonzalez-Sastre F. Urinary glycosaminoglycans in active Graves' ophthalmopathy. Clin Chem 1992; 38:2341.
61. Mourits MP, van Kempen-Harteveld ML, García-García MB, Koppeschaar HPF, Tick L, Terwee CB. Radiotherapy for Graves'orbitopathy: randomised placebo-controlled study. Lancet 2000; 355:1505-09.

12

IMMUNOSUPPRESSIVE THERAPY

Mark F. Prummel
Department of Endocrinology & Metabolism, Academic Medical Center, University of Amsterdam, The Netherlands

INTRODUCTION

On the premise that Graves' ophthalmopathy is an autoimmune disorder, immunosuppressive therapy has become the mainstay of treatment if the disease is severe enough. The pathogenesis of Graves' ophthalmopathy is not yet clear and the relative importance of cellular *versus* humoral immune responses against the orbital tissues is uncertain. This is one of the reasons that targeted immunomodulating therapies have not been used in this disease. Therefore, most patients with moderate to severe eye disease are treated with general anti-inflammatory and immunosuppressive treatments like corticosteroids and/or orbital irradiation. In the first part of this chapter the advantages and disadvantages of these and other currently used therapies will be discussed. In the second part, possible future developments involving newer forms of immunomodulation will be mentioned.

PRESENT THERAPIES

Corticosteroids

These agents have been in use for the treatment of ophthalmopathy since the early 1950's, and we now know that they a) interfere with T- and B-lymphocyte functions; b) reduce trafficking of neutrophils, monocytes, and macrophages into inflamed tissues; c) inhibit the function of immunocompetent cells; and d) suppress the release of cytokines (1). Regarding Graves' ophthalmopathy, it has been shown that corticosteroids can inhibit the synthesis and release of glycosaminoglycans (GAG's) by orbital fibroblasts *in vitro*, which is a cardinal feature in this disease because GAG's are hydrophilic molecules, attracting water and causing edematous swelling of the retro-orbital tissues (2).

Different methods of administering corticosteroids have been tried, but it has become clear that local application (e.g. subconjunctival injection) is less effective than systemic, e.g. orally or intravenously administered steroids (1,3). There are several dosage schemes, which have never been compared directly and are presumably of similar efficacy.

Table 1. Overview of available immunosuppressive regimens with commonly used doses

Treatment	Initial dose	Duration of treatment
Oral prednisone	60-100 mg / day	4-6 months
i.v. Methylprednisolone	pulses of .5-1 g for 3 days, often repeated for 1-7 weeks	followed by 20 mg of oral prednisone for total of 4-6 months
Octreotide	100 ug t.i.d.	12 weeks
Plasmapheresis	2000 ml for 4 days	high dose oral prednisone for 12 weeks
IVIG	1 g / kg for 2 days	repeated 2-5 times every 3 weeks for 4-5 months
Orbital radiotherapy	10 x 2 Gy	2 weeks
Cyclosporine	5 mg / kg + 20 mg of oral prednisone	12 weeks

The efficacy of oral prednisone is approximately 65%, meaning that 35% of the patients do not show an improvement in ocular signs or symptoms. Those who do benefit usually improve in soft-tissue involvement, eye muscle motility, and visual acuity (in cases of optic nerve involvement). However, soft-tissue signs or diplopia only rarely disappear entirely, and the net effect of glucocorticoids on proptosis is very modest, with a mean decrease in Hertel readings of only 1 mm.

Various uncontrolled studies have suggested that iv administered steroids are more effective than oral prednisone (3). This was supported by a recent study by Marcocci *et al.,* which found that iv methylprednisolone was effective in 88% of patients, as compared to 63% of those treated with oral prednisone (P=0.02) (4).

A major drawback of corticosteroid treatment is the high frequency of side-effects. In our own studies, 13% of the patients had severe, 61% moderate, and 17% minor side-effects; whereas only 9% reported no adverse events (5). It seems, that iv steroids may be associated with less frequent side-effects.

This poor tolerability should be weighted against the benefits of corticosteroid therapy. Although steroids are effective in appr. 65% (or even 88% when given intravenously), a cure is seldom achieved. In our own studies, 75% of the patients successfully treated with immunosuppression still needed subsequent major orbital surgery, such as decompressive and/or squint surgery (6,7).

Intravenous Immunoglobulins

High-dose intravenously administered immunoglobulins (IVIG) have been applied in several autoimmune diseases, including Graves' ophthalmopathy. Their mode of action is not entirely clear, but there are several mechanisms that can explain their beneficial effect. The immunoglobulins may contain anti-idiotypic antibodies that can block idiotypic epitopes. Alternatively, IVIG inhibit cytokine release, may down-regulate immunocompetent cells, or accelerate IgG catabolism (1,8). Most therapeutic IVIG preparations contain the powerful immunosuppressive cytokine TGF-Beta, which may explain (part of) the therapeutic effects (9).

IVIG has been found to be beneficial in ophthalmopathy. In a randomized clinical trial, IVIG and oral corticosteroids had similar response rates: 62 *vs* 63% respectively (10). These data were confirmed in another prospective trial (11), and both found that IVIG therapy was associated with improvements in all NO SPECS categories.

Although IVIG usually is given on an out-patient basis, the treatment is laborious and the need to travel to the clinic makes it cumbersome for the patient. It is better tolerated than prednisone, and only 10% of the patients complain about minor side-effects like headaches, or fever (10). However, in larger studies IVIG was found to cause aseptic meningitis in 11-17% of patients (12). It is also a very expensive therapy, and it carries a potential risk for transmission of infectious agents, such as the hepatitis C virus (Table 2) (13). As a precaution for severe side-effects associated with IVIG in cases of IgA deficiency, it is prudent to measure IgA before start of therapy with IVIG.

Table 2. Costs of currently used immuosupressive regimens in The Netherlands

Treatment	Dutch guilders	European euros [1]	Remarks
Oral prednisone	80	36	therapy for 5½ mo
i.v. steroids	383	174	based on 2 cycles of 3 pulses
radiotherapy	5,642	2,564	10 sessions
octreotide	5,682	2,583	based on 300 ug/d for 12 wks
cyclosporine	2,322	1,055	based on 350 mg/d for 12 wks
IVIG	29,400	13,364	based on 35 g/d of 5 cycles
plasmapheresis	3,400	1,545	based on price for acute hemodialysis

1 euro = approximately $1.00

Orbital Radiotherapy Combined With Corticosteroids

Orbital radiotherapy is also considered to be immunosuppressive and is discussed extensively in another chapter. Here we will just mention that the combination of radiotherapy with glucocorticoids is more effective than either one alone as was established in two randomized clinical trials performed by the Pisa group (14,15). However, when both trials are averaged the combination resulted in a response rate of 71%, very similar to other regimens (Table 3). One has to realize that the advantage of radiotherapy as a well tolerated treatment, is of course lost when combined with oral corticosteroids. A mayby more logical combination in this respect would consist of i.v. pulse therapy in combination with radiotherapy, but such a regimen has not been tested in a controlled trial.

Somatostatin Analogues

Indium labeled octreotide is accumulated in the orbits of patients with active eye disease, as has become clear from comparing octreoscans in active *versus* inactive ophthalmopathy patients. If the orbital uptake is corrected for background uptake in for instance the skull, this orbital/skull uptake ratio is higher in patients who subsequently respondend to orbital radiotherapy in comparison to those who did not respond (16). The reason for this uptake in the orbits of active ophthalmopathy patients is still speculative, but it is postulated that activated lymphocytes bear somatostatin receptors (17). After binding, octreotide may inhibit the release of disease modifying cytokines (1).

Octreotide was first tried in ophthalmopathy patients by Chang *et al.*, who showed improvements in NO SPECS class II and IV signs in 6 patients (18). In a prospective randomized clinical trial, Kung *et al.* found that octreotide was slightly less effective than oral prednisone (19). Krassas *et al.* have used the octreoscan to correlate the effect of somatostatin analogues with the orbital uptake of labeled octreotide. In their first study, somatostatin analogues were only useful in patients with positive octreoscans (20). After this finding, they selected their patients on the basis of the octreoscan, and found that the longer-acting compound lanreotide had a beneficial effect in 5 patients (21).

Octreotide and other somatostatin analogues are rather well tolerated, and most studies only report on mild gastrointestinal discomfort. Longer use may predispose to gallstones.

Cyclosporine

Cyclosporine is a potent immunosuppressive drug that has become the mainstay of immunosuppression (22). The drug binds to the immunophylin cyclophilin inhibiting the calcineurin phosphatase activity. Thus inhibiting the nuclear factor of activated T-cells (NF-ATc) to initiate transcription of the IL-2 gene (23). Cyclosporine does not affect the memory and suppression functions of the immune system, but it does inhibit many effector functions of T-lymphocytes. It reduces cytotoxicity and Th2 induced B-cell responses (22). Thus, cyclosporine is especially effective in inhibiting a new immune response, and we now know that it should be administered during sensitization in organ transplantation.

This latter effect, which has become clear in the last decade, is probably the reason why cyclosporine is ineffective in ophthalmopathy as monotherapy. In a prospective, randomized clinical trial we showed that this drug was inferior to oral prednisone (7). The response rate to steroids was 61% at three months after start of treatment, whereas only 22% of patients treated with cyclosporine had a response. This figure of 22% is remarkably similar to that observed in two trials using sham-irradiation. These studies showed a rate of spontaneous improvement of 28 and 31% (24,25).

However, cyclosporine does seem to be effective when combined with steroids. In our own study, the combination of lower dose prednisone with cyclosporine improved the eye signs of 59% of the patients who had not responded sufficiently upon monotreatment with prednisone. Kahaly *et al.* performed a randomized clinical trial comparing this combination directly with prednisone alone, and found that cyclosporine with prednisone was even slightly more effective (26).

Cyclosporine therapy is not without risks, despite the fact that the studies mentioned above found that it was better tolerated than prednisone. Hypertrichosis, gingival hyperplasia and hypertension being the most frequent side-effects. There is, however, a serious risk for nephrotoxicity and monitoring of blood pressure, trough levels, serum creatinine and uric acid levels and urinary protein levels is mandatory. In general, lower doses of $\leq$5 mg/kg/d are now advocated in autoimmune diseases

Plasmapheresis

This method consists of the removal of large amounts (e.g. 2000 ml/day) of plasma in exchange for plasma, or sodium chloride. Thus, plasma exchange removes immunoglobulins, immune complexes, and any other humoral factor that might be involved in the pathogenesis of ophthalmopathy. It has been suggested to be effective in other autoimmune diseases, such as Goodpasture's Syndrome. The procedure is usually performed a number of times, and followed by immunosuppressive regimens.

Uncontrolled studies have reported benefit from this procedure (27), but properly controlled studies are not available to evaluate its effeicacy. One study showed improvement in NO SPECS class II signs and proptosis immediately after 4 plasma exchanges. The patients were then treated with high doses of steroids and azathioprine. The authors claimed that a more satisfactory response was observed in 24 patients treated with plasma exchanges, than in a "control" group treated with the above mentioned immunosuppressive regimen alone (28). Others found that plasma exchange given without subsequent corticosteroid therapy was ineffective.

Though the treatment is generally well tolerated, it is not without risk. It is also expensive and needs the collaboration of the dialysis department, precluding its routine use. It may be tried in desperate cases (5).

Other Immunosuppressive Therapies

Table 3 lists the response rates to the various frequently used modes of immunosuppression. In view of these figures, it is remarkable that only few of the currently available immunosuppressive drugs have actually been tested in ophthalmopathy patients. The reason for this might be that alternative therapies have proven to be ineffective. Randomized clinical trials have shown that both *ciamexon*, and *azathioprine* when applied as monotherapy have no beneficial effect (29,30). Although *cyclophosphamide* is sometimes used according to a recent European survey (31), there are no clinical studies supporting its value in thyroid-associated eye disease. Lastly, a randomized clinical trial demonstrated that *acupuncture* is of no benefit (32).

Summary Current Immunosuppressive Therapies

Both radiotherapy and corticosteroids have a good effect on visual acuity in patients suffering from optic nerve involvement. However, the other effects of current immunosuppression are more modest. None of the regimens have much effect on proptosis. Although studies invariably show a significant decrease in Hertel measurements, the mean gain is only 0.5-1.0 mm, which is clinically insignificant. Most treatments do have a beneficial effect on eye muscle motility and on soft tissue involvement, although complete regression is obtained only in a minority of patients. These results should be weighted against the side-effects associated with most therapies, leaving the treating physician with the difficult task to fare between Scylla and Charybdis.

Table 3. Response rates to frequently used therapeutic regimens (adapted from Marcocci *et al.*, and Bartalena *et al.*)

Treatment	No. of studies	No. of patients	No. of responders	response rate (%)
Oral prednisone	14	212	133	63
Iv steroids	11	157	121	77
Radiotherapy	23	603	357	59
Prednisone + Radiotherapy	2	49	35	71
Somatostatin analogues	7	51	38	75
IVIG	4	72	44	61

Despite the efforts to search for an alternative, corticosteroids and/or orbital radiotherapy remain the mainstay in immunosuppressive treatment of Graves' ophthalmopathy, and the only real alternative with a better efficacy seems to be the combination of both therapies. In very severe cases with optic nerve compression, a good alternative for an acute surgical decompression are the i.v. methylprednisolone pulses, or the combination of corticosteroids with radiotherapy (Table 3). In moderately severe patients (e.g. with constant diplopia) orbital radiotherapy and oral prednisone are the most widely used treatments. In view of the better tolerability of irradiation and the similar succes rate, we prefer radiotherapy in these patients.

When the disease is milder (e.g. inconstant diplopia), it is less certain that immunosuppressive treatment is actually of benefit to the patients. First, there is a rather strong tendency towards spontaneous improvement, as has been shown unequivocally in the two recent prospective trials which included a placebo treatment (sham-irradiation). Improvements were seen in 28 and 31% of these untreated patients (24,25). Secondly, even when immunosuppression did result in an improvement, 75% of the patients still need rehabilitative surgery. Thus, in the majority of patients medical treatment does not cure the disease and full rehabilitation is usually only achieved by surgery. This is not to say that immunosuppression is not useful, because another important reason for its use is the inactivation of the autoimmune attack (33). Rehabilititative surgery should not be done if the disease is still active (34), and immunosuppression will probably shorten the period of active disease, thus facilitating earlier surgery in comparison to observation.

Table 4. Recommendations for the use of the various immunosuppressive therapies based on the severity of the ophthalmopathy.

Severity	1st choice	2nd choice	alternatives in case of contraindications
Severe (optic nerve involvement)	i.v. Methylprednisolone pulses	steroids + radiotherapy	-steroids + CyA -plasmapheresis
Moderately severe	Radiotherapy	Oral steroids	Octreotide
Mild	Wait-and-see	Radiotherapy ?	Octreotide ?

CyA, cyclosporine

FUTURE DEVELOPMENTS

From the above it is evident that there is a clear need for an immunosuppressive therapy which is more potent and still well tolerated. There seem to be two approaches to achieve these goals in the future. First, the combination of steroids with radiotherapy is more effective than either one alone, and it might very well be that a combination of more therapies is even more effective. Secondly, the last decade has brought completely new tools for immunosuppression, interfering with immunomodulatory molecules such as cytokines or adhesion molecules.

Lessons From Rheumatoid Arthritis: Combined Immunosuppressive Therapies

Classically autoimmune diseases are divided into systemic and organ-specific immune disorders. Autoimmune thyroid diseases are considered to be organ-specific, but this may be questioned in the case of

Graves' disease, which involves several sites apart from the thyroid gland. Crohn's disease is classified as systemic, though intestinal disease is the prevailing phenotype. It appears that autoimmune disorders form a spectrum from completely local (type 1 diabetes mellitus) to entirely sysyemic (systemic lupus erythematosus). Using this view, Graves' disease and rheumatoid arthitis may not be so different from each other in pathogenesis as is commonly thought, implying that we could learn from recent innovations in this field.

Rheumatoid arthritis used to be treated according to a "pyramid" or "sequential" strategy, starting with non-steroidal anti-inflammatory drugs and followed by monotherapy with various immunosuppressive agents (35). This resembles the current practice in Graves' ophthalmopathy, where many centers use the various available treatments in a consecutive order (31). In rheumatoid arthtritis, this strategy has been replaced by an aggressive approach using combinations of multiple "disease-modifying" drugs in an early stage of the disease. Several large randomized clinical trials have shown the superiority of combinations of methotrexate (low-dose, given once weekly) plus cyclosporine, or plus steroids, or plus hydroxychloroquine (36).

Such combinations might also be envisioned in the treatment of thyroid-associated eye disease, since the mechanisms of action of the various treatments which have been found effective as monotherapy, is different. A rational combination would exist of a few cycles of high-dose i.v. Methylprednisolone pulses together with low-dose cyclosporine and and in combination with orbital irradiation. One group has reported benefit from such a combined approach (radiotherapy followed by azathioprine and steroids), though their study was not controlled (37).

New Immunomodulatory Drugs: Interfering In The Cytokine Network

Cytokines seem to play a key role in the pathogenesis of Graves' ophthalmopathy, and it has been suggested before that the patients may benefit from cytokine antagonist therapies (3,38,39). The cytokine network is complex and it is currently not clear which cytokines really play a pivotal role in the orbital immune attack. IL-2, IFN-γ, TNF-α, IL-4, IL-5, and IL-10 have been found of possible importance in *in vitro* studies (40). However, many other cytokines, growth factors (e.g. TGF-β, PDGF), and immunomodulatory molecules (CTLA-4) (41) may play a role as well, but have not been studied. Nevertheless, it is fascinating to speculate on the possibilities to block certain cytokine pathways. Especially now that a number of cytokine antagonists have been developed and applied succesfully in several conditions, most notably transplantation medicine, rheumatoid arthritis and inflammatory bowel diseases. Some of these cytokine antagonists and other agents interfering with the cytokine network are listed in Table 5.

Monoclonal Antibodies

One approach to interfere with the cytokine network is the use of monoclonal antibodies directed against cell-surface cytokine receptors (IL-2 Receptor or CD25), or against the cytokine itself (e.g. TNFα). The initial results with monoclonal antibodies were disappointing, mainly because of a high frequency of side-effects due to their xenogenetic nature (mostly murine). This problem has now been largely overcome by "humanizing" the immunoglobulins (42). With this approach, the variable region of the murine immunoglobulin is combined with the constant regions of human antibodies. This renders the antibody much less immunogenic, but also enhances the effector functions of the now human Fc region.

Table 5. New immunomodulatory drugs which interfere with the cytokine network.

Class	Name	Properties	Applications
Monoclonal antibodies	infliximab daclizumab	anti TNFα anti IL-2 Receptor	RA, Crohn transplantation
Recombinant cytokines	IL-10 IL-1 RA	Th1 suppression blocks IL-1	RA, Crohn RA
Immunoadhesions	CTLA-4-Ig	blocks B7 on APC's	animal models
Cytokine receptors	sIL-1R TNF-R I	blocks IL-1 blocks TNFα	RA RA, Crohn
Metalloproteinase inhibitors	Pentoxifylline Lisofylline GI 5402	anti TNF-α effects	GO MS, EAE animal models

RA, rheumatoid arthritis; Crohn, Crohn's disease, MS, multiple sclerosis; GO Graves' ophthalmopathy; EAE, experimental allergic encephalomyelitis

Several such monoclonal antibodies are now available and others will soon be. There is considerable experience with antibodies against TNFα in rheumatoid arthritis and in Crohn's disease. The anti-TNFα antibody Infliximab (Remicade, Centocor, USA) has a good clinical effect in rheumatoid arthritis patients, with a response in 77% with a duration of response of 3-8 weeks (43,44). Adding methotrexate (which has never been evaluated properly in Graves' ophthalmopathy!) appears to ehance the effect (45). In Crohn's disease a rapid clinical effect is seen in about two-thirds of the patients, again with a duration of response of 4-12 weeks (46,47). In both disorders, the monoclonal antibody therapy is remarkably well tolerated.

A last successful example is the use of a monoclonal antibody against the IL-2 receptor (daclizumab), which was used in combination with other new immunosuppressive drugs (tacrolimus and sirolimus) to prevent rejection of pancreatic islet transplantation (48,49).

Recombinant Human Cytokine Therapy

Another way to modulate the immune system consists of the administration of human cytokines which can inhibit the immune response. IL-10 is a good candidate. It is a so-called Th2 derived cytokine with a broad array of functions (50), and was initially described as "cytokine synthesis inhibitory factor" (44). It is currently tested in rheumatoid arthritis and the first resulst from phase II trials are promising, and the agent is well tolerated (44,50). The same holds true for the first preliminary results in patients with Crohn's disease (47).

Another molecule with potential merit in autoimmunity is the IL-1 receptor antagonist. In Graves' ophthalmopathy, IL-1Ra has been shown to inhibit IL-1 stimulated GAG synthesis by retro-orbital fibroblasts in culture (51). IL-1Ra has also been tried in clinical studies in rheumatoid arthritis. When given as daily subcutaneous injection for 24 weeks, it was found to be effective clinically after 4 weeks, with a rather good tolerability (52).

Immunoadhesion Molecules

Another fascinating approach is the fusion of the heavy chain IgG variable region to specific immunoligands, such as CTLA-4. The advantage of these design agents is their long circulating half-life due to the presence of the Fc region (53). A fusion of IgG with the ectodomain of CTLA-4 provides a high affinity ligand for the so-called B7 proteins. This CTLA-4-Ig then masks the B7 proteins on antigen presenting cells, which are the paramount co-stimulatory molecules necessary to induce a T-cell response. If these co-stimulatory molecules are blocked, T-cell anergy (and thus tolerance) will be induced (54). These fusion molecules are currently tested in animal models, and phase I clinical studies. Similar fusion molecules have been designed to target important homing molecules such as ICAM-1.

Cytokine Receptors

Naturally occurring cytokine receptors are also currently used to block certain pathways in the cytokine network. Soluble IL-1 receptors, just like IL-1Ra's can block IL-1function and have been used in rheumatoid arthritis (44). TNFα exerts its effect after binding to, and dimerization of two TNFα receptors on the cell surface: TNF-R I (also called p55) and TNF-R II (also called p75). These receptors also circulate in a soluble form after proteolytic cleavage, which function as natural inhibitors of TNFα. Human recombinant soluble TNF-R I has been found beneficial in animal models for rheumatoid arthritis and Crohn's disease, and clinical studies are now under way using a hybrid of TNF-R I and a high molecular weight polyethylene glycol (PEG) molecule (55).

Drugs With Effects on Cytokine Levels

Agents other than monoclonal antibodies, or immunoadhesins have been developed to interact with the immune system. Pentoxifylline is an example of this class of drugs. It has an inhibitory effect on TNFα (56), and on Natural Killer cells (57). This TNFα inhibiting effect may explain the beneficial effects observed in a recent, uncontrolled study in Graves' ophthalmopathy (58). However, there are much stronger TNFα inhibiting drugs currently available.

Metalloproteinase inhibitors are involved in the cleavage of cell-associated TNFα, and also in the shedding of the receptors type I and II for TNFα (59,60). A recent study found that the metalloproteinase inhibitor GI5402 (Glaxo Wellcome, Greenford, UK) strongly reduced LPS-induced

TNFα release, suggesting that this compound may be useful as a treatment of Crohn's disease or rheumatoid arthritis (61).

Lisofylline is a pentoxifylline derivative, which was found to inhibit the induction of experimental allergic encephalomyelitis (EAE) in mice via blocking of IL-12 receptor signaling subsequently inhibiting Th1 differentiation (62). A subsequent study from the same group, showed that lysofylline was stronger than pentoxifylline in reducing the number of TNFα secreting T cells, by inhibiting the transition of Th0 to Th1 via blocking of IL-12 (63). IL-12 is probably essential in the pathogenesis of some autoimmune disorders, for IL-12 knock-out mice are completely resistant to the development of EAE (a model for multiple sclerosis). IL-12 has been proposed to be a key inducer of Th1-mediated autoimmune diseases, also because many treatments shown to be effective in multiple sclerosis (corticosteroids, IVIG, pentoxifylline) all share the ability to suprress IL-12 production (64).

CONCLUDING REMARKS

New, alternative immunomodulating agents are being developed and tried at a pace fitting the new millenium. They are used in patients with autoimmune disorders like rheumatoid arthritis, Crohn's disease, and multiple sclerosis, which are more prevalent than Graves' ophthalmopathy and thought to more invalidating. This can be questioned seriously, because the quality of life of Graves' ophthalmopathy patients is more severely impaired than in patients with inflammatory bowel disease (65). It is probably time that thyroidologists open their eyes for the advances made in related autoimmune disorders.

REFERENCES

1. Marcocci C, Pinchera A, Prummel MF, Wiersinga WM. Immunosuppressive management of Graves' ophthalmopathy. In: Prummel MF (Ed.) Recent developments in Graves' ophthalmopathy. Kluwer Academic Publishers. Boston: 2000; 101-113.
2. Bahn RS, Heufelder AE. Pathogenesis of Graves' ophthalmopathy. N Engl J Med 1993; 329:1468-1475.
3. Bartalena L, Pinchera A, Marcocci C. Management of Graves' ophthalmopathy: Reality and perspectives. Endocr Rev 2000; 21:168-199.

4. Marcocci C, Tanda ML, Manetti L, et al. Intravenous and oral glucocorticoid therapy in patients with severe Graves' ophthalmopathy: Results of a randomized, single-blind, prospective study [abstract]. J Endocrinol Invest 1999; 22(Suppl. 6):104.
5. Wiersinga WM, Prummel MF. An evidence-based approach to the treatment of Graves' opthalmopathy. Endocrinol Metab Clin NA 2000; 29:297-319.
6. Prummel MF, Mourits MP, Blank L, Berghout A, Koorneef L, Wiersinga WM. Randomised double-blind trial of prednisone versus radiotherapy in Graves' ophthalmopathy. Lancet 1993; 342: 949-54.
7. Prummel MF, Mourits MPh, Berghout A, *et al.* Prednisone and Cyclosporine in the treatment of severe Graves' ophthalmopathy. N Engl J Med 1989; 321:1353-1359.
8. Dwyer JM. Manipulating the immune system with immune globulin. N Engl J Med 1992; 326:107-116.
9. Kekow J, Reinhold D, Pap T, Ansorge S. Intravenous immunoglobulins and transforming growth factor β. Lancet 1998; 351:184-185.
10. Kahaly G, Pitz S, Muller-Forell W, Hommel G. Randomized trial of intravenous immunoglobulins versus prednisolone in Graves' ophthalmopathy. Clin Exp Immunol 1996; 106:197-202.
11. Baschieri L, Antonelli A, Nardi S, Alberti B, Lepri A, Canapicchi R, Fallah P. Intravenous immunoglobulin versus corticosteroid in treatment of Graves' ophthalmopathy. Thyroid 1997; 7:579-585.
12. Picton P, Chisholm M. Aseptic meningitis associated with high dose immunoglobulin: case report. Br Med J 1997; 315:1203-1204.
13. Yu MW, Mason BL, Guo ZP, Tankersley DL, Nedjar S, Mitchell FD, Biswas RM. Hepatitits C transmission associated with intravenous immunoglobulins. Lancet 1997; 345:1173-1174.
14. Bartalena L, Marcocci C, Chiovato L, *et al.* Orbital cobalt irradiation combined with systemic corticosteroids for Graves' ophthalmopathy: comparison with systemic corticosteroids alone. J Clin Endocrinol Metab 1983; 56:1139.
15. Marcocci C, Bartalena L, Panicucci M, *et al.* Orbital cobalt irradiation combined with retrobulbar or systemic corticosteroids for Graves' ophthalmopathy: a comparative study. Clin Endocrinol 1987; 27:33.
16. Gerding MN, Van der Zant FM, Van Royen EA, *et al.* Octreotide-scintigraphy is a disease activity parameter in Graves' ophthalmopathy. Clin Endocrinol 1999; 50:373-379.
17. Wiersinga WM, Gerding MN, Prummel MF, Krenning EP. Octreotide scintigraphy in thyroidal and orbital Graves' disease. Thyroid 1998; 8: 433-436.
18. Chang TC, Kao SCS, Huang KM. Octreotide and Graves' ophthalmopathy and pretibial myxoedema. Br Med J 1992; 304:158.
19. Kung AWC, Michon J, Tai KS, Chan FL. The effect of somatostatin versus corticosteroid in the treatment of Graves' ophthalmopathy. Thyroid 1996; 6:381.
20. Krassas GE, Dumas A, Pontikides N, Kaltsas T. Somatostatin receptor scintigraphy and octreotide treatment in patients with thyroid eye disease. Clin Endocrinol 1995; 42:571.
21. Krassas GE, Kaltsas T, Dumas A, Pontikides N, Tolis G. Lanreotide in the treatment of patients with thyroid eye disease. Eur J Endocrinol 1997; 136:416.
22. Borel JF, Hiestand PC. Immunomodulation: particular pesrpectives. Transpl Proc 1999; 31:1464-1471.

23. Mihatchi MJ, Kyo M, Morozumi K, Yamaguchi Y, Nickeleit V, Ryffel B. The side-effects of ciclosporine-A and tacrolimus. Clin Nephrol 1998; 49:356-363.
24. Prummel MF, Terwee CB, Gerding MN, Blank L, Mourits MPh, Dekker FW, Wiersinga WM. A randomized placebo-controlled study on radiotherapy for mild Graves' ophthalmopathy: effects on clinical severity and quality of life. [abstract] 12th International Thyroid Congress. Oct 22-27, 2000; Kyoto, Japan.
25. Mourits Mph, Kempen-Hartveld M van, Garcia Garcia B, Koppeschaar HPF, Tick L, Terwee CB. Radiotherapy for Graves' orbitopathy: randomised placebo-controlled study. Lancet 2000; 355:1505-1509.
26. Kahaly G, Schrezenmeir J, Krause U, Schweikert B, Meuer S, Muller W. Ciclosporin and prednisone v. prednisone in treatment of Graves' ophthalmopathy: a controlled, randomized and prospective study. Eur J Clin Invest 1986; 16:415.
27. Glinoer D, Etienne-Decerf J, Schrooven M, *et al.* 1986 Beneficial effects of intensive plasma exchange followed by immunosuppressive therapy in severe Graves' ophthalmopathy. Acta Endocrinol (Copenh) 1986; 111:30.
28. De Rosa G, Menichella G, Della S, *et al.* Plasma exchange in Graves' ophthalmopathy. Prog Clin Biol Res 1990; 337:321.
29. Kahaly G, Lieb W, Muller-Forell W, *et al.* Ciamexone in endocrine orbitopathy: a randomized, double-blind, placebo-controlled study. Acta Endocrinol (Copenh) 1990; 122:13.
30. Perros P, Weightman DR, Crombie AL, Kendall-Taylor P. Azathioprine in the treatment of thyroid-associated ophthalmopathy. Acta Endocrinol (Copenh) 1990; 122:8
31. Weetman AP, Wiersinga WM. Current management of thyroid-associated ophthalmopathy in Europe. Results of an international survey. Clin Endocrinol 1998; 49:21-28.
32. Rogvi-Hansen B, Perrild H, Christensen T, Detmar S, Siersbaek-Nielsen K, Hansen J. Acupuncture in the treatment of Graves' ophthalmopathy. A blinded randomized study. Acta Endocrinol (Copenh) 191; 124:143.
33. Prummel MF, Wiersinga WM, Mourits Mph. Assessment of disease activity of Graves' ophthalmopathy. In: Prummel MF (ed), Recent developments in Graves' ophthalmopathy. Boston: Kluwer Academic Publishers 2000: 59-80
34. Mourits MPh, Rose GE, Garrity JA, Nardi M, Matton G, Koornneef L. Surgical management of Graves' ophthalmopathy. In: Prummel MF (Ed) Recent developments in Graves' ophthalmopathy. Boston: Kluwer Academic Publishers 2000:133-169.
35. Schiff M. Emerging treatments for Rheumatoid Arthritis. Am J Med 1997; 102 (Suppl. 1A):11S-15S.
36. Pincus T, O'Dell JR, Kremer JM. Combination therapy with multiple disease-modifying antirheumatic drugs in rheumatoid arthritis: a preventive strategy. Ann Int Med 1999; 131:768-774.
37. Claridge KG, Ghabrial R, Davis G, Tomlinson M, Goodman S, Harrad RA, Potts MJ. Combined radiotherapy and medical immunosuppression in the management of thyroid eye disease. Eye 1997; 11:717-722.
38. Bartalena L, Marcocci C, Pinchera A. Editrial: Cytokine antagonists: New ideas for the management of Graves' ophthalmopathy. J Clin Endocrinol Metab 1996; 81:446-448.

39. Prummel MF, Wiersinga WM. Immunomodulatory treatment of Graves' ophthalmopathy. Thyroid 1998; 8:545-548.
40. Heufelder AE, Weetman AP, Ludgate M, Bahn RS. Pathogenesis of Graves' ophthalmopathy. In: Prummel MF (Ed) Recent developments in Graves' ophthalmopathy. Boston: Kluwer Academic Publishers 2000:15-37.
41. Schwartz RS. The new immunology - The end of immunosuppressivee drug therapy? N Engl J Med 1999; 340:1754-1756.
42. Breedveld FC. Therapeutic monoclonal antibodies. Lancet 2000; 355:735-740.
43. Maini RN, Taylor PC. Anti-cytokine therapy for rheumatoid arthritis. Annu Rev Med 2000; 51:207-229.
44. Jorgensen C, Apparailly F, Sany J. Immunological evaluation of cytokine and anticytokine immunotherapy in vivo: what have we learnt? Ann Rheum Dis 1999; 58:136-141.
45. Maini R, St Clair EW, Breedveld F, Furst D, Kalden J, Weisman M, Smolen J, Emery P, Harriman G, Feldman M, Lipsky P. Infliximab (chimeric anti-tumour necrosis factor α monoclonal antibody) versus placebo in rheumatoid arthritis patients receiving concomitant methotrexate: a randomised phase III trial. Lancet 1999; 354:1932-1939.
46. Bell S, Kamm MA. Antibodies to tumour necrosis factor α as treatment for Crohn's disease. Lancet 2000; 355:858-857.
47. Van Deventer SJH. Immunomodulation of Crohn's disease. In: Tathman CG (Ed.): Biologic and gene therapy for autoimmune disease. Curr Dir Autoimmun Basel, Karger: 2000 (2):150-166.
48. Shapiro AMJ, Lakey JRT, Ryan EA, *et al.* Islet transplantation in seven patients with type 1 diabetes mellitus using a glucocorticoid-free immunosuppressive regimen. N Engl J Med 2000; 343:230-238.
49. Robertson RP. Successful islet transplantation for patients with diabetes - fact or fantasy? N Engl J Med 2000; 343:289-290.
50. St Clair EW. Interleukin-10: Therapeutic prospects in rheumatoid arthritis. In: Tathman CG (Ed.): Biologic and gene therapy for autoimmune disease. Curr Dir Autoimmun Basel, Karger: 2000 (2):129-149.
51. Tan GH, Dutton CM, Bahn RS. Interleukin-1 receptor antagonist and soluble interleukin-1 receptor inhibit interleukin-1induced glycosaminoglycan production in cultured human orbital fibroblasts from patients with Graves' ophthalmopathy. J Clin Endocrinol Metab. 1996; 81:449-452.
52. Bresnihan B. Treatment of rheumatoid arthritis with interleukin 1 receptor antagonist. Ann Rhem Dis 1999; 58 (Suppl. I):196-198.
53. Kim YS, Maslinski W, Zheng XX, Schachter AD, Strom TB. Immunoglobulin-cytokine fusion molecules: The new generation of immunomodulating agents. Transpl Proc 1998; 30:4031-4036.
54. Dick AD, Isaacs JD. Immunomodulation of autoimmune responses with monoclonal antibodies and immunoadhesins: treatment of ocular inflammatory disease in the next millennium. Br J Ophthalmol 1999; 83:1230-1234.
55. Edwards CK. PEGylated recombinant human soluble tumour necrosis factor receptor type I (r-Hu-sTNF-RI): novel high affinity TNF receptor designed for chronic inflammatory disease. Ann Rheum Dis 1999; 58 (Suppl. I):173-181.

56. Levi M, ten Cate H, Bauer KA, *et al.* Inhibition of endotoxin-induced activation of coagulation and fibrinolysis by pentoxifylline or by a monoclonal anti-tissue factor antibody in chimpanzees. J Clin Invest 1994; 93:114-120.
57. Nagy Z, Sipka R, Ocsovszki I, Balogh A, Mandi Y. Suppressive effect of pentoifylline on natural killer cell activity; experimental and clinical studies. Arch Pharmacol 1999; 359:228-234.
58. Balazs C, Kiss E, Vamos A, Molnar I, Farid NR. Beneficial effect of pentoxifylline on thyroid associated ophthalmopathy (TAO): a pilot study. J Clin Endocrinol Metab 1997; 82:1999-2002.
59. Woessner JF. Matrix metalloproteinase inhibition. From the Jurassic to the third millennium. Ann NY Acad Sci 1999; 878:388-403.
60. De B, Natchus MG, Cheng M, *et al.* The next generation of MMP inihibitors. Ann NY Acad Sci 1999; 878:40-60.
61. Dekkers PEP, Lauw FN, Ten Hove T, Te Velde AA, Lumley P, Bechere D, Van Deventer SJH, Van der Poll T. The effect of metalloproteinase inihibitor (GI5402) on Tumor Necrosis Factor-α (TNF-α) and TNF-α Receptors during human endotoxemia. Blood 1999; 94:2252-2258.
62. Bright JJ, Du C, Coon M, Sriram S, Klaus SJ. Prevention of experimental allergic encephalomyelitis via inhibition of IL-12 signaling and IL-12 mediated Th1 differnetiation: An effect of the novel anti-inflammatory drug Lysofylline. J Immunol 1998; 161:7015-7022.
63. Coon ME, Diegel M, Leshinsky N, Klaus SJ. Selective pharmacologic inhibition of murine and human IL-12-dependent Th1 differentiation and IL-12 signalling. J Immunol 1999; 163:6567-6574.
64. Karp CL, Biron CA, Irani DN. Interferon β in multiple sclerosis: is IL-12 suppression the key? Immunol Today 2000; 21:24-28.
65. Gerding MN, Terwee CB, Dekker FW, Koornneef L, Prummel MF, Wiersinga WM. Quality of life in patients with Graves' ophthalmopathy is markedly decreased: measurement by the medical outcomes study instrument. Thyroid 1997; 7: 885-889.

13

SURGICAL MANAGEMENT OF GRAVES' OPHTHALMOPATHY

Elizabeth A. Bradley, George B. Bartley and James A. Garrity
Mayo Clinic Department of Ophthalmology, 200 First Street, S.W., Rochester, MN 55905

Supported by an unrestricted grant from Research to Prevent Blindness, Inc., New York, New York.

INTRODUCTION

Most patients with Graves ophthalmopathy can be managed with observation or supportive measures alone. In a recent study of the treatment of Graves ophthalmopathy in an incident cohort, only 20% of patients required surgical intervention (1). The cumulative probability of undergoing ophthalmic surgery of any type increased from 5.0% within one year after the diagnosis of ophthalmopathy to 21.8% within ten years of diagnosis. Patients older than 50 years were significantly more likely to require surgery than were younger patients. Fortunately, many surgical procedures, including orbital decompression, strabismus surgery, and eyelid surgery, are available to restore ocular function and improve cosmesis in these patients. We review the rationale, indications, and basic technique for the most common surgical procedures used to treat Graves ophthalmopathy.

ORBITAL DECOMPRESSION

Many of the symptoms and signs of Graves ophthalmopathy result from expansion of the retrobulbar tissue within the rigid confines of the orbital cavity. Whereas non-surgical treatments such as steroids and orbital radiation attempt to resolve the volume-to-space discrepancy by shrinking the swollen tissues, surgical decompression expands the orbital volume to create more space for the orbital tissues. Surgical decompression is indicated when the retrobulbar tissue expansion results in severe proptosis with corneal ulceration, globe subluxation, or cosmetic disfigurement, or when the swollen tissues cause compressive optic neuropathy.

Because corneal ulceration resulting from proptosis can progress rapidly to corneal perforation with potential loss of the eye, this condition calls for emergent orbital decompression. Corneal ulceration is suggested by symptoms of intense ocular pain and signs of marked conjunctival injection, indistinct corneal light reflex, and a white plaque on the cornea (Figure 1). Corneal ulceration can result from either severe proptosis or eyelid retraction and lagophthalmos (inability to completely close the eyes), and therefore the relative contributions of these manifestations of Graves ophthalmopathy to the corneal disease must be determined. Patients with eyelid retraction alone can be treated with eyelid surgery, while those with proptosis require orbital decompression.

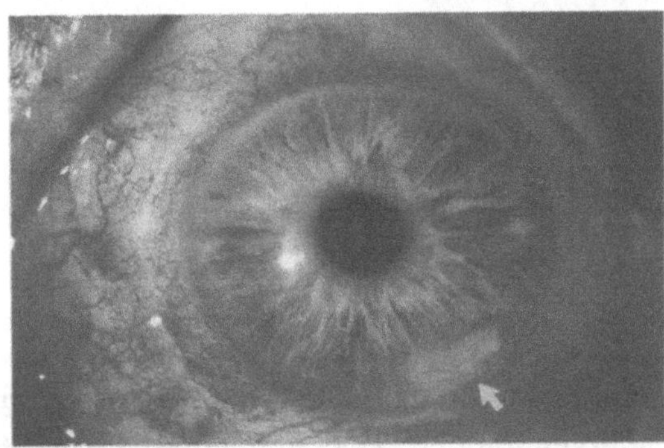

Figure 1. Corneal ulcer (arrow), near corneoscleral limbus, in a patient with Graves ophthalmopathy

Optic neuropathy is the most common indication for urgent orbital decompression. Optic neuropathy manifests as decreased visual acuity at both distance and near, and loss of peripheral visual field and color vision. The presence of an afferent pupillary defect is nearly diagnostic of a unilateral or asymmetric optic neuropathy. Examination of the optic nerve head may reveal a congested, swollen, or normal appearance in acute cases, and optic nerve pallor in the setting of a long-standing optic neuropathy. While corticosteroids are frequently employed for compressive optic neuropathy, their usefulness can be limited by recurrence of the optic neuropathy with corticosteroid taper. Orbital radiation can also effectively treat optic neuropathy. Among the available treatment modalities for optic neuropathy, orbital decompression offers the most prompt therapy.

Globe subluxation also indicates the need for surgical intervention for Graves ophthalmopathy. Subluxation occurs when the proptotic globe prolapses anterior to the eyelids. A frightening and painful experience for the patient, this condition is treatable through orbital decompression and eyelid surgery (Figure 2). Other indications for orbital decompression include severe orbital congestion, disfiguring proptosis or excessive proptosis prior to extraocular muscle surgery, steroid intolerance, and intractable pain. Because orbital decompression can affect ocular alignment and eyelid position, decompression surgery is performed in advance of either strabismus surgery or eyelid retraction repair.

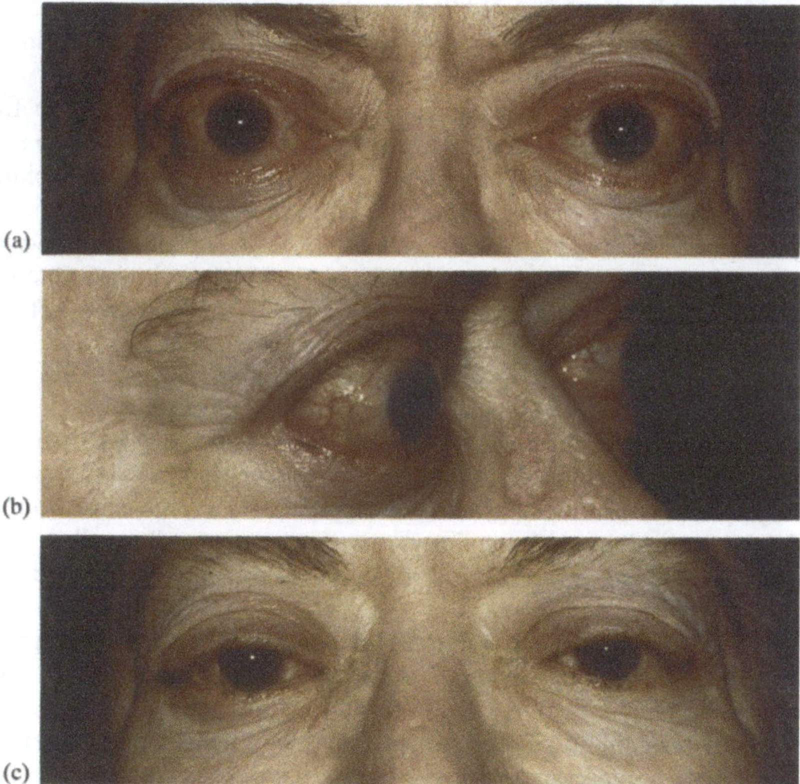

Figure 2. Graves ophthalmopathy with recurrent globe subluxation a, b. Severe proptosis and eyelid retraction resulting in recurrent episodes of globe subluxation. The patient was also forced to wear her eyeglasses low on her nose (note impression from nosepiece) to prevent contact between her proptotic globes and her eyeglasses. c. Three months after bilateral transantral decompression and one month after strabismus surgery and bilateral lateral tarsorrhaphies. (From Bradley EA, Garrity JA. The surgical management of Graves' ophthalmopathy. 1999. The Endocrinologist. 9(5):371-8, with permission.)

The orbit can be decompressed along any of its four walls, although the most effective decompression results from expansion into an adjacent sinus. This can be achieved either with decompression medially into the ethmoid sinuses, or inferiorly into the maxillary sinus. To maximize the amount of decompression, the medial wall and orbital floor can be decompressed simultaneously. Two-wall orbital decompression has been demonstrated in experimental and clinical studies to yield 3 to 6 mm of proptosis decompression (2), and is the most widely used means of orbital decompression. A variety of surgical approaches can be used to achieve a two-wall decompression. In the transantral approach, a hidden gingival incision allows access to the maxillary antrum. Both the medial wall and orbital floor can be decompressed through this single surgical incision. Other benefits of the transantral approach include the short operating room time and excellent posterior orbital access to treat optic neuropathy. The transcaruncular approach, in which an incision is made through the fleshy caruncle at the medial aspect of the eye, provides limited access to the medial wall. While posterior decompression is often difficult with this technique, additional inferior decompression can be gained by extending the incision along the posterior conjunctival surface of the lower eyelid. A two-walled decompression technique that has gained popularity since its introduction in 1990 is the transnasal endoscopic decompression (3). In addition to offering a hidden incision, endoscopic techniques provide excellent access to the orbital apex, and small case series have documented their efficacy in treating optic neuropathy. The ability to decompress the orbital floor, however, is more limited with the endoscopic approach than with the transantral or transconjunctival techniques. Surgical trials comparing the different two-walled techniques are lacking, and the approach taken at an institution is largely determined by surgeon interest and expertise. Regardless of the procedure employed, most orbital decompressions are performed under general anesthesia.

Other orbital decompression techniques include lateral decompression and fatty decompression. Because a lateral approach decompresses the orbital tissue into the temporal fossa instead of into a sinus, this approach typically offers smaller amounts of decompression than either medial or inferior decompression. Aggressive removal of the thick bone in the deep orbital wall, however, may achieve good decompression in some cases (4). Finally, removal of orbital fat has been shown to reduce proptosis by approximately 2 mm (5). This technique has also been reported to effectively treat optic neuropathy in a small case series, although prior treatment of these patients with corticosteroids and radiation may have contributed to their clinical improvement (6).

Of 428 consecutive patients with severe Graves ophthalmopathy who underwent transantral decompression at the Mayo Clinic, the most common indication for orbital decompression was optic neuropathy, seen in 217 (50.7%) of patients (7). Other indications for decompression included severe orbital inflammation/congestion (27.1%), excessive proptosis prior to extraocular muscle surgery (8.4%), disfiguring proptosis (7.9%), exposure keratitis (4.7%), and corticosteroid side effects (1.2%). Proptosis was reduced by a mean 4.7 mm. Nearly 90% of eyes with pre-operative visual acuity worse than 20/20 improved or remained the same, and 91% of visual field scotomas improved or resolved. Exposure keratitis improved or resolved in 92% of patients. 64% of patients who did not have pre-operative diplopia did develop diplopia post-operatively. However, at late follow-up, 92% of all patients had single vision, some after strabismus surgery or with the assistance of prism glasses.

Complications of orbital decompression observed in this series included lower eyelid entropion (8.9%), sinusitis (6%), persistent lip numbness (7.6%), cerebrospinal fluid leak (3.5%), and frontal lobe hematoma (0.2%). Other reported complications include blindness, orbital infection, nasolacrimal duct obstruction, and diminished olfaction (8,9).

EXTRAOCULAR MUSCLE SURGERY

Diplopia can be one of the most troubling aspects of Graves ophthalmopathy for both the patient and the physician. Fortunately, not all patients with Graves ophthalmopathy will experience diplopia during the course of their disease. In a population based study, diplopia was present at the time of diagnosis in 20 of 120 (17%) incident cases of Graves ophthalmopathy in Olmsted county, Minnesota from 1976 to 1990 (10). Of the 20 patients with diplopia, 4 were symptomatic when fatigued, 9 had diplopia at the extremes of gaze, 3 had continuous diplopia correctable with prisms and 4 had continuous diplopia unable to be corrected with prisms. During the follow-up period of this study, 51 (43%) of the incident cases had some evidence of extraocular muscle dysfunction. The cumulative probability of having strabismus surgery was approximately 6.2% at 5 years and 10.6% at 10 years for this study population. A report from the University of Iowa noted symptomatic diplopia in 25 of 175 (14%) patients with Graves ophthalmopathy seen over an 8 year period (11).

Patients with diplopia may report intermittent or continuous symptoms. Intermittent diplopia may become manifest with fatigue or in certain directions of gaze. While many patients are able to discern seeing two distinct images when symptomatic, others simply describe blurred vision or a sensation of visual distortion, or even dizziness. Thus, any type of visual symptom that clears when one eye is closed may represent ocular misalignment. Diplopia is most disabling when present in primary gaze (straight ahead) or in the reading position, because these are the two most useful fields of gaze. A simple set of questions can determine a patient's functional interference from diplopia (Table 1).

Table 1: Diplopia classification

- none
- intermittent, only when tired
- intermittent, only at extremes of gaze
- continuous, but can be corrected with prism in glasses
- continuous, cannot be corrected with prism in glasses

Nearly all diplopia in Graves ophthalmopathy is due to restriction of the extraocular muscles. Rarely, however, diplopia in Graves disease can result from paresis of an extraocular muscle due to associated myasthenia gravis. In these cases, the presence of ptosis and diplopia, as opposed to the typical eyelid retraction and diplopia of Graves ophthalmopathy, will usually raise the clinical suspicion for myasthenia gravis. Testing forced ductions, where forceps are used to grasp the topically anesthetized globe and the eye is moved in the field of motion for the affected muscle, can determine whether the muscle is restricted or paretic. Esotropia (eyes turned in) is related to restriction of the medial rectus muscle(s). Exotropia (eyes turned outward) is distinctly uncommon in Graves ophthalmopathy and should also raise the clinical suspicion for myasthenia gravis (12). Vertical diplopia and torsional diplopia are often a feature of Graves ophthalmopathy, and implicate either vertical rectus muscle or oblique muscle involvement. The relative contribution of each eye muscle can be assessed by measuring the ocular deviation in various positions of gaze. These measurements can be used to monitor the patients for disease progression or remission and, when indicated, to devise a surgical plan (13).

Surgical treatment is generally reserved for patients who have continuous diplopia that cannot be corrected with prisms or for patients who are treated with prism correction and wish to eliminate or decrease the requirement for prism. The goal of strabismus surgery is to restore single vision in primary gaze and in the reading position, recognizing that diplopia at the extremes of gaze will likely persist post-operatively. The timing of surgery is controversial. If the patient does not require orbital decompression, or has undergone orbital radiation therapy, then an interval of six months of clinical stability is suggested before considering extraocular muscle surgery.

In the setting of previous orbital decompression, however, we typically evaluate patients for strabismus surgery as early as 6 weeks after orbital decompression. Although we will defer surgery in the presence of continued orbital congestion or inflammation, in our experience this is only necessary in a small percentage of patients.

Strabismus surgery is typically an outpatient procedure. General anesthesia is our preference but local anesthesia can be used if one or two muscles on only one eye are being planned. Because of the extraocular muscle restriction, the most frequently performed surgical procedure is a recession, or weakening procedure (Figure 3), of the inferior rectus or medial rectus muscles.

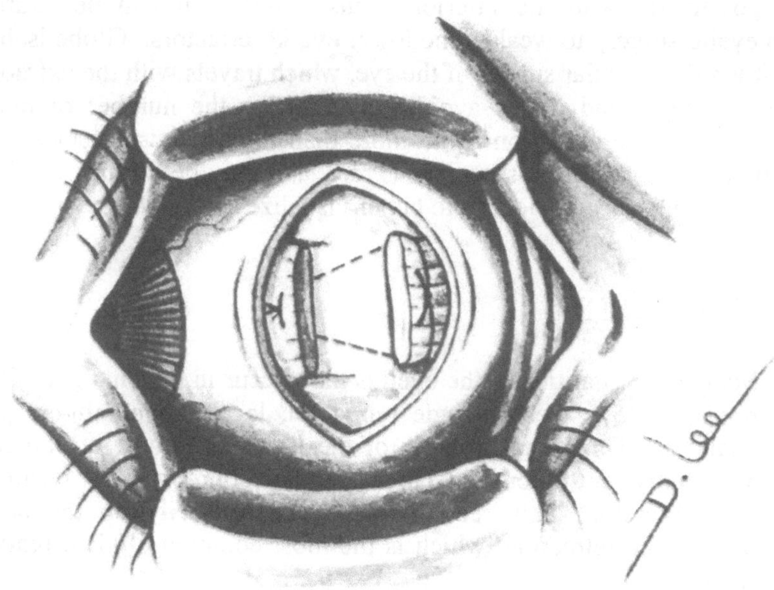

Figure 3. Recession of the left medial rectus muscle. The muscle has been detached from the globe, moved posteriorly (recessed), and reattached to the globe. This procedure physiologically weakens the muscle to reduce the effect of the restriction associated with the Grave's ophthalmopathy. (From Atlas of Extraocular Muscle Surgery. 1984. J.A. Dyer and D.A. Lee, editors. Praeger Scientific Publishers. By permission of Mayo Foundation)

If necessary, surgery can be repeated on the same muscle either to further recess or to advance the muscle (lessens some of the previous recession), in an effort to achieve single vision in primary gaze and in the reading position (14). A post-operative evaluation is performed in 6 weeks. If the goal of single vision in primary gaze and the reading position has been achieved, or if the residual deviation is small enough to be satisfactorily corrected with prisms, the patient can be considered for eyelid surgery, if indicated. In our review of 428 orbital decompressions performed at Mayo Clinic, 300 patients (70%) required at least one strabismus procedure following decompression. 92% of these 300 patients ultimately achieved single vision, although some patients required multiple surgeries or the use of prism glasses post-operatively (7).

Potential complications of strabismus surgery include residual diplopia, changes in eyelid position, ocular ischemia, and globe perforation. Additional surgery may be necessary if diplopia persists more than six weeks after surgery. Lower eyelid retraction is the most common post-operative alteration in eyelid position. It results from recession of the inferior rectus muscle, when the capsulopalpebral head of the lower eyelid retractors is moved posteriorly with the inferior rectus muscle. It can be addressed through eyelid surgery to weaken the lower eyelid retractors. Globe ischemia results when the vascular supply of the eye, which travels with the extraocular muscles, is interrupted. It is avoided by limiting the number of muscles involved in any one operation to no more than three rectus muscles. Globe perforation during strabismus surgery is rare, and may be minimized by the use of magnifying surgical loupes to better visualize suture placement.

EYELID SURGERY

Many abnormalities of the eyelids may occur in patients with Graves ophthalmopathy (15). These include retraction, lag, lagophthalmos, ptosis, dermatochalasis, edema, and prolapse of the lacrimal glands, orbital fat, or both. Additionally, entropion and lateral canthal obliquity may result from orbital decompression. This section will focus primarily on the surgical treatment of eyelid retraction, which is the most common clinical feature of Graves ophthalmopathy (16).

What is a normal eyelid position? The height of the eyelid fissure varies considerably in most patients from minute-to-minute depending on the level of alertness, emotional state, and volition. Normally, though, the upper eyelid rests approximately 1.5 mm below the superior corneoscleral limbus whereas the lower eyelid rests at about the level of the inferior limbus. (The limbus corresponds to the junction between the white sclera and the colored iris.) Retraction is present when the upper eyelid rests at or above the limbus or the lower eyelid sags below its corresponding ocular landmark; in other words, if there is "scleral show" at either the superior or inferior pole of the cornea (Figures 4 and 5). Upper eyelid retraction often is graded as mild (less than 2 mm), moderate (2 to 5 mm), or severe (greater than 5 mm). The comparable grades for the lower eyelid are mild (1 to 2 mm), moderate (3 mm), and severe (more than 3 mm) retraction. Mild and severe upper eyelid retraction tend to be more constant than moderate retraction, which may vary considerably even during the course of an examination. Lower eyelid retraction usually does not fluctuate from minute-to-minute.

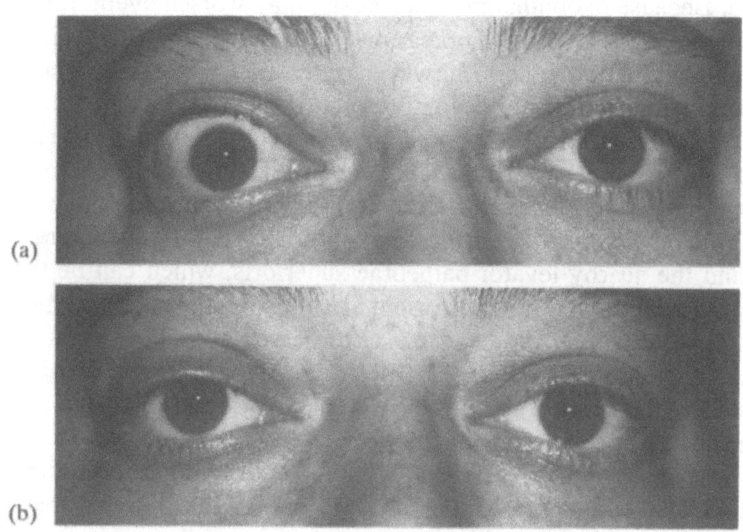

Figure 4. Moderate right upper eyelid retraction. a: Pre-operative appearance; b: After recession of right upper eyelid retractors (Muller muscle and the levator palpebrae superioris)

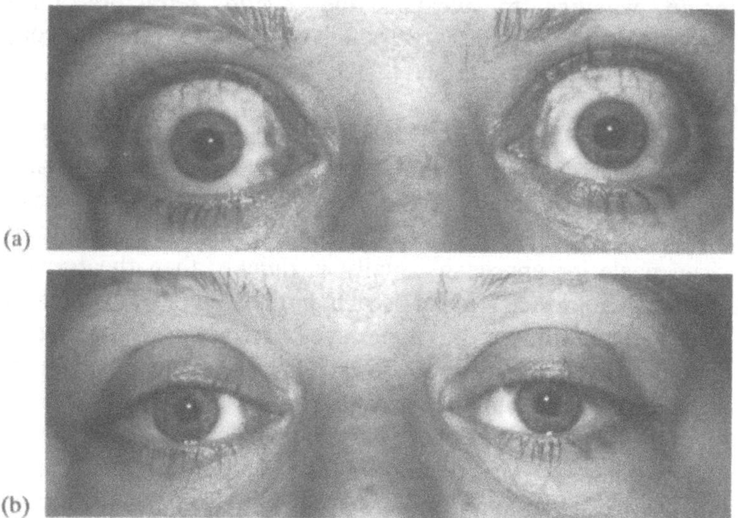

Figure 5: Severe bilateral upper eyelid retraction. a: Pre-operative appearance; b: After surgical repair

Occasionally, eyelid retraction and lagophthalmos are sufficiently severe to cause exposure and even ulceration of the cornea, mandating eyelid surgery on an emergent basis. Generally, though, eyelid retraction repair is elective and can be deferred until orbital decompression or strabismus operations, if needed, have been completed and thyroid dysfunction has been corrected. Because exophthalmos (proptosis) may worsen eyelid retraction, in some patients an orbital decompression will improve or even eliminate the eyelid malposition. In others, however, retraction persists or may become more prominent after orbital decompression if the globes "sink" down in the sockets (a condition termed hypoophthalmos or hypoglobus). As regards the relationship between strabismus and eyelid retraction, it is important to recognize that a "tight" inferior rectus muscle can cause the upper eyelid to retract. This results from compensatory stimulation of the ipsilateral superior rectus (and the nearby levator palpebrae superioris, which can be thought of as an extraocular muscle) as the patient attempts to elevate the globe. A chin-up head posture (tilting the head back) to decrease double vision may be a clue that the inferior rectus or recti are tight or overacting. In this circumstance, it often is appropriate to weaken the inferior rectus muscle (by recessing it) before considering surgery to decrease the eyelid retraction. Finally, because hyperthyroidism is associated with stimulation of the sympathetically innervated Muller muscle, one of the muscles that elevates the eyelid, a stable euthyroid state for several months is preferred before eyelid retraction repair is performed.

Once the timing for eyelid retraction repair is appropriate, the surgeon must decide whether to weaken the eyelid retractors through an anterior/external skin incision or through a posterior/internal conjunctival approach. Both methods are performed using local anesthesia, and each technique has pros and cons.

The external approach provides a familiar display of anatomic structures, allows recession of the levator palpebral superioris and Muller muscle under direct visualization, and permits the surgeon to excise excess fat and skin or to suspend a prolapsed lacrimal gland at the same sitting, if desired. The posterior approach usually is quicker than the transcutaneous method, avoids a skin incision (and scar), and has the advantage of recessing the conjunctiva in addition to the upper eyelid retractors. In some instances, a retracted upper eyelid may not "drop" intraoperatively even after the retractors have been completely released through an anterior approach, until the conjunctiva also is weakened by partial or complete division. Potential disadvantages of the posterior route include a greater risk of damaging the lacrimal gland ductules, the formation of pyogenic granulomas, more bleeding than the external approach, and the possibility that tissue planes may be confused if the surgeon is inexperienced in dissecting the eyelid when it is everted.

Waller's classic study of eyelid retraction provided valuable information that helps to determine an appropriate surgical plan (17). Myotomy, recession, or extirpation of Muller muscle usually lowers an eyelid approximately 1.5 mm. Transection of the attachments of the levator aponeurosis to the anterior tarsal surface provides, on average, an additional 0.5 mm of lid lowering. Mild upper eyelid retraction thus can be treated easily in most instances with a posterior (transconjunctival) approach. Relief of more than 2 mm of retraction usually requires transection of the primary insertions of the levator aponeurosis to the subcutaneous tissues. The surgeon should release the insertions judiciously and incrementally and must monitor the eyelid position frequently because considerable eyelid lowering may result from what seems to be minimal dissection.

Many surgeons prefer an external approach for severe retraction, in patients who have had previous surgery, or if lacrimal gland suspension or debulking of fat is desired. One should be aware of the advice of Harvey and coauthors, however, that the excision of redundant skin at the same time as the correction of eyelid retraction should be avoided in most cases (18). Although preoperatively it may seem that a considerable amount of redundant tissue can be removed safely, the eyelid skin is thin and may contract postoperatively, resulting in lagophthalmos and corneal exposure. Additionally, some patients who initially request correction of both eyelid retraction and eyelid fullness are satisfied with their appearance after eyelid retraction repair alone, precluding the need for subsequent blepharoplasty.

Mild degrees of lower eyelid retraction usually may be corrected simply by making a conjunctival incision at the inferior tarsal border and maximally recessing the lower eyelid retractors and the overlying conjunctiva. If possible, the eyelid should be placed on stretch for several days to counteract the gravitational tendency for the eyelid wound to heal back together. Although a spacer (a graft between the recessed eyelid retractors and their original insertion to keep the two tissue planes separated) is needed infrequently in the repair of upper eyelid retraction, such usually is necessary to correct lower eyelid retraction of greater than 2 mm. During the past decade, hard palate mucosa probably has been the most popular spacer. Hard palate mucosal grafts are autologous, easily harvested, and shrink only minimally. Additionally, unlike grafts of cartilage or donor sclera, hard palate spacers do not need to be epithelialized by the surrounding conjunctiva and do not result in a thickened lid (19,20). Recently, acellular dermal allografts have been used successfully as eyelid spacers and have the advantage of avoiding a second surgical site (21).

A lateral tarsorrhaphy may be used to treat upper or lower eyelid retraction, or both. Because a broad adhesion between the eyelids is aesthetically displeasing and obscures peripheral vision, most surgeons now use a tarsorrhaphy only as a minor adjunct to recession of the eyelid retractors and not as the primary procedure. The technique of lateral tarsorrhaphy described by Stamler and Tse is simple and effective and has the advantage of reversibility even though it is designed to be permanent (22).

The most common problem associated with the surgical treatment of eyelid retraction in Graves ophthalmopathy is an imperfect postoperative eyelid level. Patients usually are more forgiving of residual retraction than of postoperative blepharoptosis; a "bright-eyed" appearance is preferable to "sleepy eyes." Additionally, it is easier and more predictable to recess the levator aponeurosis secondarily to address residual retraction than it is to advance the levator if eyelid ptosis has occurred. Therefore, the intraoperative eyelid position usually is set at the desired final level or perhaps just slightly higher. If the eyelid is ptotic in the operating room, it almost always will remain so postoperatively.

In addition to residual retraction or iatrogenic blepharoptosis, abnormalities of the eyelid contour or crease may detract from an otherwise satisfactory result. Examples include nasal ptosis, temporal flare, asymmetric eyelid folds, or a flat eyelid contour. Droopiness of the nasal portion of the eyelid is relatively uncommon and may be minimized by being conservative when recessing the eyelid retractors in this area. In contrast, residual temporal flare is likely unless the lateral horn of the levator aponeurosis is partially or completely disinserted. Asymmetry of the eyelid creases or folds may cause eyelids that are equal in height to appear too high or too low. Weakening the retractors through a skin incision may allow for re-formation of the eyelid crease in the desired position. One must be aware that manipulation of the levator aponeurosis, either transcutaneously or transconjunctivally, may "westernize" an Asian eyelid, which may not be pleasing to the patient. A flat eyelid contour may result from excessive recession of the eyelid retractors in the central portion of the eyelid or from inadequate recession of the retractors nasally, especially in patients who have undergone orbital decompression (23).

CONCLUSION

The majority of patients with Graves ophthalmopathy do not require surgical treatment. For those who do, orbital decompression, strabismus surgery and eyelid surgery can improve visual function and the patient's appearance. (Figure 6)

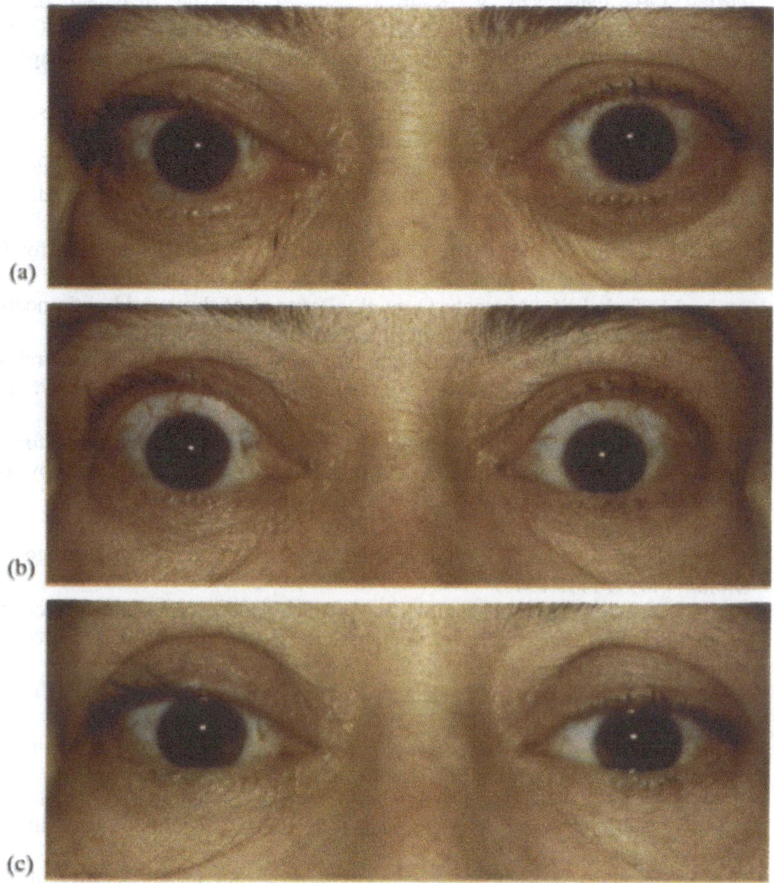

Figure 6: Graves ophthalmopathy with disfiguring proptosis and eyelid retraction. a. Preoperative appearance with bilateral proptosis, upper and lower eyelid retraction, and eyelid fullness; b. Postoperative appearance following transantral orbital decompression. The proptosis and lower eyelid retraction are less, but the upper eyelid retraction appears worse due to the inferior movement of the globes with decompression; c. Post-operative appearance following upper eyelid retraction repair. (From Bradley EA, Garrity JA. The surgical management of Graves' ophthalmopathy. 1999. The Endocrinologist. 9(5):371-8, with permission.)

REFERENCES

1. Bartley GB, Fatourechi V, Kadrmas EF, et al. The treatment of Graves ophthalmopathy in an incidence cohort. Am J Ophthalmology 1996; 121:200-6.
2. Kennerdell JS, Maroon JC, and Buerger GF. Comprehensive surgical management of proptosis in dysthyroid orbitopathy. Orbit 1987;. 6:153-8.
3. Kennedy DW, Goodstein ML, Miller NR, et al. Endoscopic transnasal orbital decompression. Arch Otolaryngol Head Neck Surg 1990; 116:275-82.
4. Goldberg RA, Kim AJ, and Kerivan KM. The lacrimal keyhole, orbital door jamb, and basin of the inferior orbital fissure. Three areas of deep bone in the lateral orbit. Arch Ophthalmol 1998; 116(12):1618-24.
5. Trokel S, Kazim M, and Moore S. Orbital fat removal: decompression for Graves orbitopathy. Ophthalmology 1993; 100:674-82.
6. Kazim M, Trokel SL, Acaroglu G, et al. Reversal of dysthyroid optic neuropathy following orbital fat decompression. Br. J. Ophthalmol. 2000; 84:600-5
7. Garrity JA, Fatourechi V, Bergstralh EJ, et al. Results of transantral orbital decompression in 428 patients with severe Graves ophthalmopathy. Am. J. Ophthalmology 1993; 116:533-47.
8. Mourits M, Koornneef L, Wiersinga WM, et al. Orbital decompression for Graves ophthalmopathy by inferomedial, by inferomedial plus lateral, and by coronal approach. Ophthalmology 1990; 97:636-41.
9. Lund VJ, Larkin G, Gells P, et al. Orbital decompression for thyroid disease: a comparison of external and endoscopic techniques. The Journal of Laryngology and Otology 1997; 111:1051-5.
10. Bartley GB. The epidemiologic characteristics and clinical course of ophthalmopathy associated with autoimmune thyroid disease in Olmsted county, Minnesota. Trans Am Ophthalmol Soc 1994; 92:477-588.
11. Scott WE, Thalacker JA. Diagnosis and treatment of thyroid myopathy. Ophthalmology 1981; 88:493-8.
12. Vargas ME, Warren FA, Kupersmith MJ. Exotropia as a sign of myasthenia gravis in dysthyroid ophthalmopathy. Br J Ophthalmol 1993; 77:822-3.
13. Younge BR. Eye examination techniques in Graves ophthalmopathy. In The Eye and Orbit in Thyroid Disease. C.A.Gorman, R.R. Waller, and J.A. Dyer, editors. New York: Raven Press. 143-153, 1984.
14. Dyer JA. Ocular Muscle Surgery. In The Eye and Orbit in Thyroid Disease. C.A.Gorman, R.R. Waller, and J.A. Dyer, editors. New York: Raven Press. 253-261, 1984.
15. Bartley GB. The eyelids in Graves ophthalmopathy. In Principles and Practice of Ophthalmic Plastic and Reconstructive Surgery. S. Bosniak, editor. Philadelphia: W.B. Saunders. 514-524, 1996.
16. Bartley GB, Fatourechi V, Kadrmas EF, et al. Clinical features of Graves ophthalmopathy in an incidence cohort. Am J Ophthalmol 1996; 121:284-90.
17. Waller RR. Eyelid malpositions in Graves ophthalmopathy. Trans Am Ophthalmol Soc 1982; 80:855-930.
18. Harvey JT, Corin S, Nixon D, Veloudios A.. Modified levator aponeurosis recession for upper eyelid retraction in Graves disease. Ophthalmic Surg 1991; 22:313-7.
19. Bartley GB, Kay PP. Posterior lamellar eyelid reconstruction with a hard palate mucosal graft. Am J Ophthalmol 1989; 107:609-12.
20. Kersten RC, Kulwin DR, Levartovsky S, et al. Management of lower-lid retraction with hard-palate mucosa grafting. Arch Ophthalmol 1990; 108:1339-43.
21. Rubin PAD, Fay AM, Remulla HD, Maus M. Ophthalmic plastic applications of acellular dermal allografts. Ophthalmology. 1999; 106:2091-7.

22. Stamler JF, Tse DT. A simple and reliable technique for permanent lateral tarsorrhaphy. Arch Ophthalmol 1990; 108:125-7.
23. van den Bosch, WA, Tjon-Fo-Sang MJ, Lemij HG. Eyeball position in Graves orbitopathy and its significance for eyelid surgery. Ophthalmic Plast Reconstr Surg 1998; 14:328-35.

14

ORBITAL RADIOTHERAPY: AN UPDATE

Henry B. Burch
Chief, Thyroid Clinic, Walter Reed Army Medical Center, Associate Professor of Medicine, Uniformed Services University of the Health Sciences, Bethesda, Maryland

INTRODUCTION

Targeted orbital supervoltage radiation for Graves' ophthalmopathy was begun in an attempt to deliver local therapy to sensitized lymphocytes believed responsible for the retroorbital autoimmune response (1). The lack of a satisfactory alternative therapy was the motivation for the use of radiotherapy at the time, a situation that has unfortunately improved only marginally over the past 25 years (2). A recent survey of members of the European Thyroid Association found that 23% of respondents would use orbital irradiation either alone or in combination with corticosteroids in severe ophthalmopathy, and nearly 50% of respondents would do so when considering rapidly progressing ophthalmopathy (3).

PROPOSED MECHANISMS OF ACTION

The application of orbital radiotherapy to the treatment of Graves' ophthalmopathy is based upon the radiosensitivity of lymphocytes to the destructive effects of radiation (4). In addition, in vitro studies have demonstrated an inhibition of cutaneous fibroblast proliferation after exposure to ionizing radiation (5). No studies have examined the in vitro effect of ionizing radiation on either orbital lymphocytes or fibroblasts obtained from Graves' ophthalmopathy patients. Interestingly, cultured human synovial fibroblasts obtained from patients with rheumatoid arthritis show a decreased proliferation rate but an enhanced production of hyaluronic acid after exposure to ionizing radiation (6).

TECHNIQUE

The use of megavoltage linear accelerators has allowed the delivery of well-collimated, high-energy therapy to the involved retroorbital structures, minimizing irradiation of adjacent structures such as the skin and lens (7). Most centers using this technique have delivered 20 Gy (2000 rads) to each eye given in 10 fractions over 2 weeks. The patient's head is fixed using a head shell to prevent movement. The dose is calculated at the midline and delivered by lateral ports angled 3-10° posteriorly, in order to prevent inclusion of the anterior chamber and retina of the contralateral eye (Figure 1). The irradiation field is approximately 4 x 4 cm, with an anterior border just behind the fleshy lateral canthus, and a posterior border just in front of the sella turcica, with exact treatment fields individualized according to pretreatment computed tomography scanning. Although marked bilateral differences in proptosis are uncommon, patients with significant asymmetry require additional angling to adjust the extent of the treatment field.

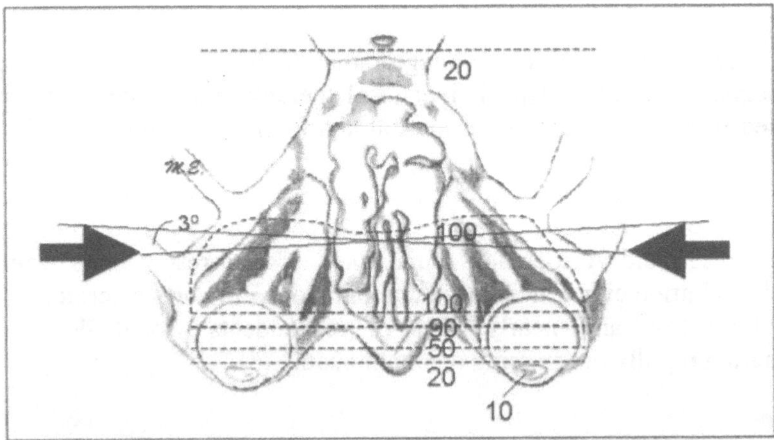

Figure 1. Orbital radiotherapy technique. Shown are the radiation ports and approximate percentage of total dose delivered to individual zones, with ten percent or less delivered to the lens and less than twenty percent delivered to the sella turcica. Fields are angled posteriorly to minimize contralateral lens exposure.

Alternative approaches have also been examined. Beam splitting rather than posterior angulation has been utilized to decrease lens exposure still further (8). Variation in the amount (or fractionation of radiation delivered) has not provided additional benefit. For example, an attempt to increase the total dose delivered to 30 Gy was not beneficial in one study (9). Recently, three different dosing regimens were compared in a randomized trial (10). A standard regimen of 20 Gy over 10 days at 2 Gy/ day was compared to 10 Gy over 10 days at 1 Gy/day, or to 20 Gy at 1 Gy/ week over 20 weeks. The latter, more protracted course appeared to produce a greater reduction in soft tissue changes and associated symptoms at 24 weeks. However, the apparent superiority of this regimen may relate more to the proximity of the end of treatment at 20 weeks to the measurements made at 24 weeks rather than to the provision of any long-term advantage. Patients in the prolonged therapy group had a lower incidence of radiation-induced conjunctivitis than patients treated with the other two regimens (10).

SIDE EFFECTS AND CONTRAINDICATIONS

Table 1 lists potential and theoretical adverse effects from orbital radiation for Graves' ophthalmopathy and their relative frequency. These include cataract formation, radiation retinopathy, skin irritation, loss of temporal hair at the entry ports, a transient aggravation of soft-tissue inflammation, and a theoretical risk for secondary oncogenesis. Radiation-induced cataracts occur with radiation doses to the lens of approximately 15 Gy, a dose far in excess of that occurring with shielding techniques, fractionation, and beam collimation currently in use for the treatment of Graves' ophthalmopathy (8). For higher exposures, the average latent period for cataract formation is 2 years, with a range of 0.5 to 2.5 years (11). Retinopathy and optic neuropathy are also unlikely to occur with properly delivered radiation therapy, since doses of 30-40 Gy are generally required to produce this degree of damage. Three patients with retinopathy resulting in blindness after radiation therapy for Graves' ophthalmopathy were found on reassessment to have received approximately 40 Gy in 4 Gy fractions (8). Conditions that may predispose to retinopathy, such as diabetes mellitus or chemotherapy are generally considered contraindications to orbital radiotherapy (12).

Retinopathy following radiation therapy has several unique features that are demonstrable with fluorescein angiography (13). Transient worsening of soft-tissue inflammation during the course of orbital radiotherapy occurs at a rate of 10-20% of treated patients, and can be prevented with the use of concurrent corticosteroids (11). Temporal hair loss and skin irritation after radiotherapy for Graves' ophthalmopathy occurs in approximately 5-15% of treated patients (14). The theoretical risk of oncogenesis following radiation therapy has been calculated at 0.3% to 1.2% (15). Tumor formation as a result of radiation exposure is a serious concern, but has not been reported to date within the duration of follow-up available in Graves' ophthalmopathy patients.

Table 1. Potential and Theoretical Adverse Effects From Orbital Radiotherapy for Graves' ophthalmopathy

Adverse effect	Frequency	Comment
Worsened soft tissue inflammation	Common	Transient, blocked with concurrent corticosteroids
Skin irritation	Common	Minor
Temporal hair loss	Common	Minor
Lens opacification	Rare	Dose-related
Retinopathy	Rare	Dose-related
Secondary tumors	Not reported	Prolonged follow-up studies needed

LITERATURE SUMMARY

Observational Studies

Over a dozen non-randomized trials have been published dealing with orbital irradiation therapy for Graves' ophthalmopathy (Table 1). The first series using megavoltage irradiation was published by researchers at the Stanford University Medical Center in the 1970s (1). These authors have since published data on over 300 patients treated with megavoltage irradiation for Graves' ophthalmopathy (9,16,17). Approximately one third of patients were treated concurrently with corticosteroids. Soft tissue improvement occurred in 80% of patients affected, proptosis regression in 51%, eye muscle function improvement in 56%, and vision improved in 67% of affected patients following orbital irradiation. Despite this improvement, 29% of patients required one or more eye surgeries following orbital irradiation, most performed to correct extraocular muscle dysfunction. Seventy-six percent of patients taking concurrent corticosteroids were able to discontinue these drugs within several months of completing orbital irradiation. Prognostic factors indicating a less favorable response included male gender, older age, the need for concurrent antithyroid therapy, and no history of prior hyperthyroidism (9).

Another study reported the effects of orbital irradiation in 62 patients with Graves' ophthalmopathy of 1 to 17 month duration (mean 7.5 months) (18). These authors noted onset of improvement at a mean of 14 days after initiation of radiation therapy, with maximal effect of therapy observed at a mean of 5.6 months. Among 14 patients with objective evidence of optic neuropathy, 10 patients improved or stabilized, allowing discontinuation of corticosteroids, the remaining 4 patients required decompression surgery. Following radiotherapy, 21 patients (34%) required one or more eye surgeries including 4 patients requiring orbital decompression, 12 undergoing eye muscle surgery, and ten receiving eyelid surgery. A favorable response was obtained in 65% of patients with ocular symptoms for less than 6 months, compared to 50% of patients with symptoms for greater than 6 months, but this difference did not achieve statistical significance.

Another non-randomized trial provided therapeutic outcome in 39 patients undergoing orbital irradiation for Graves' ophthalmopathy (19). Disease duration varied widely, with a mean duration of 20.4 months. The outcome of therapy was assessed at 6 months following orbital irradiation and rated as "excellent", "good", "fair", and "no response," with careful recording of change in class within the NO SPECS classification system. Two-thirds of patients were classified as responders, among whom 23% had a "good" response and 16 (41%) had a "fair" response. Improvement was noted in all classes of the NO SPECS system although minimal improvement in proptosis was noted. Responders had eye manifestations for a mean duration of 17 months compared to a mean of 26.5 months in non-responders, although the difference was not significant. No correlation was found between outcome and such factors as age, gender, or pre-treatment ophthalmopathy index. Another study examined outcome following radiotherapy in 20 patients with moderately severe Graves' ophthalmopathy (20). Five patients were treated concurrently with prednisone. Among patients with a mean duration of disease of 4.8 years, only 35% of patients showed a significant improvement in an ophthalmopathy index score. The peak effect of treatment was observed within 2-3 weeks in this study. Following irradiation, prednisone dosage was reduced from a mean of 14 mg daily to 4 mg daily without exacerbation.

Recent observational reports have provided a focused assessment of the effects of orbital radiotherapy on unique aspects of Graves' ophthalmopathy, including optic neuropathy and extraocular muscle function. One report involving 12 consecutive patients with optic neuropathy due to Graves' ophthalmopathy showed improvement in optic nerve function in 8 of 10 patients with complete data available after a period of follow-up ranging from 5 to 50 months (21). Improvement was noted either during or within 2 weeks of completing radiation therapy, with color vision better in 10 of 13 affected eyes and normalization of an afferent pupillary defect in 7 of 10 affected patients. However, one patient with an early improvement later experienced worsening optic nerve function at approximately 2 months. Another report provided data on 36 patients with restricted eye muscle range of motion due to Graves' ophthalmopathy and found that 46% of affected eyes showed no improvement in upward gaze while 54% experienced an average improvement of 6° of upward gaze at 6 months after therapy (22).

Differences between populations studied in the various non-randomized trials of radiotherapy in Graves' ophthalmopathy hamper direct comparison and summation of data. Such variations include the activity, duration, and severity of disease, the concurrent use and dose of corticosteroid therapy, and the degree of heterogeneity of patients within individual studies (2). An even larger impediment to interpretation of non-randomized trials is an inability to accurately distinguish treatment effect from spontaneous disease regression, as is characteristic of Graves' ophthalmopathy. Table 2 summarizes the results from 15 selected observational studies on orbital radiotherapy for Graves' ophthalmopathy.

Comparison studies

A 1983 non-randomized study compared combination orbital cobalt irradiation and corticosteroids to corticosteroids alone in 36 and 12 patients, respectively (24). Methylprednisolone was administered with an initial dose of 70-80 mg daily for three weeks and then tapered over a 5-6 month period. Orbital irradiation was delivered using the standard two-week regimen, DS, decompression surgery; CS, corticosteroids; XRT, orbital irradiation; NS, not stated; pts, patients; N/A, not applicable; VF, visual fields [a]Percent of patients showing improvement among those affected and followed; [b]Percent of patients followed; includes 6 cataract procedures without ill effects. Eye changes six months after therapy were compared to baseline using an ophthalmopathy index. Resolution or partial improvement in soft tissue changes was noted in 35 of 36 (97%) patients with combination therapy and in 100% of 12 patients treated with methylprednisolone alone. Proptosis decreased by greater than 2 mm in 19 of 34 (56%) patients treated with combination therapy and in 45% of 11 patients using corticosteroids alone. Extraocular muscle dysfunction improved in 93% of 28 patients receiving radiation plus methylprednisolone, compared to 56% of patients taking this drug alone. A total of 72% of patients in the combination therapy group experienced an "excellent" or "good" response, whereas no "excellent" responses and 25% "good" responses were found in the corticosteroid alone group. The decrease in the ophthalmopathy index was greater in the combined therapy group than the medical therapy alone group ($p < .005$). Patients with a duration of eye involvement of less than 2 years were more likely to respond than patients with disease of longer duration.

Table 2. **Results from Non-Randomized Trials**

Study Author (Year)	Ref. No	n	Soft Tissue	Proptosis (%)[a]	Eye Muscle (%)[a]	Vision (%)[a]	Overall Response (% of n)	Concurrent Therapy	Further Therapy Required (% of n)
Ravin (1975)	23	37	improved in "many pts"	32	11%	89	NS	CS 18%	DS 3% corneal transplant 3%
Teng (1980)	20	20	9 pts (?%)	25	1 pt (?%)	N/A	35	CS 25%	25% CS; dose was reduced in 4 of 5
Bartalena (1983)	24	36	97	56	93	100	97; 72 good or excellent	CS 100%	8% CS 3% DS
Hurbli (1985)	18	62	NS	23	74	57	56	CS 23%	34% eye surgery
Olivotto (1985)	25	28	93	26	43	100	68 excellent or good	CS tapered during XRT	50% eye surgery 14% CS
Van Ouwerkerk (1985)	26	24	100	mean 5.0 mm in 1st 11 pts	78	NS	NS	CS 75%	NS
Konishi (1986)	27	17	6 pts (?%)	5 pts (?%)	8 pts (?%)	4 pts (?%)	59 good or moderate	NS	18% CS
Palmer (1987)	28	29	78	52	24	67	48	CS 34%	45% eye surgery; 10% CS
Pigeon (1987)	29	21	76	47	32	N/A	57 excellent or good	CS 67%	24% had aggravation avg 5 mo after XRT
Wiersinga (1988)	19	39	NS	NS	NS	NS	64	CS 5%	NS
Peterson (1990)	9 17	31 1	80	51	56	65	NS	CS 32%	29% eye surgery[b]
Kriss (1989)									8% CS
Sandler (1989)	30	35	NS	NS	NS	78	71 did not require DS or CS	CS 80%	40% eye surgery (17% DS) 29% CS
Lloyd (1992)	31	36	22 pts (?%)	14 pts (?%)	15 pts (?%)	NS	92 disease "arrested"	None	NS
Wilson (1995)	22	33	85%	NS	54%	NS	NS	No CS for 6 mo. prior	67% strabismus surgery
Claridge (1997)	32	40				100		77.5% CS and/or azathioprine	47.5% eye surgery

DS, decompression surgery; CS, corticosteroids; XRT, orbital irradiation; NS, not stated; pts, patients; NA, not applicable; VF, visual fields
[a]Percent of patients showing improvement among those affected and followed; [b]Percent of patients followed; includes 6 cataract procedures

A 1993 randomized trial compared the efficacy of orbital radiation to corticosteroids alone in 56 patients with moderately severe Graves' ophthalmopathy (34). Patients had not received prior therapy for ophthalmopathy and were euthyroid for at least two months before study entry. Patients with optic neuropathy or corneal abrasions were excluded. The corticosteroid group received prednisone at 60 mg/d for two weeks, then 40 mg/d for two weeks, 20 mg/d for 2 weeks followed by a gradual taper by weekly decrements of 2.5 mg/d. Radiotherapy was given using a standard dose of 2 Gy in ten fractions. Objective measurements included lid aperture measurement, serial exophthalmometer readings, visual acuity assessment, and extraocular eye movements measured using a Maddox cross, and eye muscle thickness as assessed with computed tomography. Patients were assigned a total eye score based on the NOSPECS classification system. In addition, patients provided a subjective eye score, rating their condition on a scale of 1 to 10. Patients were assessed at baseline and then at 4, 12, and 24 weeks after initiation of therapy. Overall response was similar in the two groups, with 50% of prednisone-treated patients showing improvement in NOSPECS category compared to 46% or irradiated patients. Significant improvement of the subjective eye score occurred in both groups. Soft-tissue inflammation improved in slightly more patients treated with prednisone than with radiotherapy (Figure 2). The overall rate of improvement was slightly faster in the prednisone group. Mean eye elevation improved by at least 5° in 7 prednisone-treated and 8 irradiated patients. Proptosis did not change in either group, and ultimately rehabilitative surgery was required in 79% of prednisone-treated and 71% of irradiated patients, respectively. Baseline patient characteristics were not predictive of ultimate response to either therapy. Adverse side effects occurred in 25 of 28 prednisone-treated patients compared to 15 of 28 irradiated patients.

On the basis of these two comparison trials, radiation therapy compares favorably to corticosteroid therapy and appears better tolerated. Neither radiation therapy nor corticosteroid therapy results in sufficient reduction of proptosis or improvement in extraocular muscle dysfunction to obviate the need for corrective surgery.

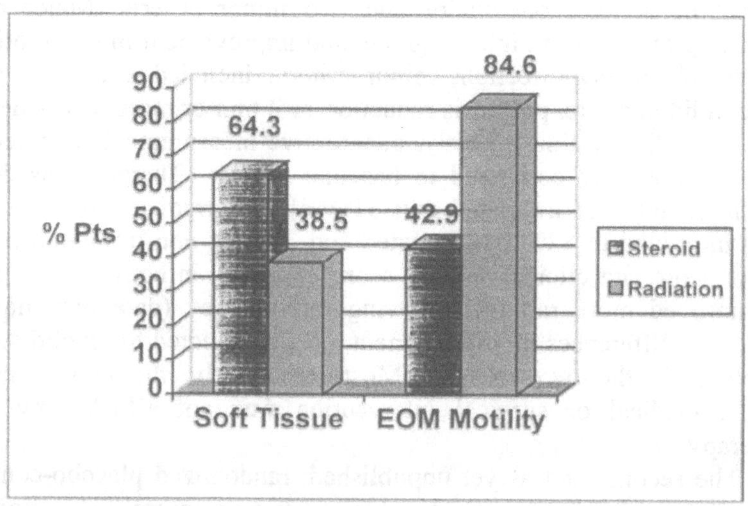

Figure 2. Type of improvement seen in patients with response to therapy. Overall improvement rates were 50% for steroid-treated patients and 46% for radiotherapy patients. *Derived from* Prummel MF, Mourits MP, Blank L, et al. Randomized double-blind trial of prednisone versus radiotherapy in Graves' ophthalmopathy. Lancet 1993; 342:949.

Randomized placebo-controlled trials

Two prospective randomized placebo (sham irradiation)-controlled trials assessing the efficacy of radiotherapy in patients with Graves' ophthalmopathy have been completed to date (35,36), although one has been published in abstract form only at the time of this writing.

The first study was a double-blind randomized trial comparing orbital radiotherapy to sham-irradiation, with 30 patients in each arm (35). Patients were excluded if they had mild eye disease or optic neuropathy. No patient had received prior therapy for ophthalmopathy or radioiodine for hyperthyroidism, and patients were maintained in the euthyroid state throughout the study period. Irradiated patients received 20 Gy divided into 10 fractions. The effect of therapy was assessed with a comparison of baseline features to those at 4, 12, and 24 weeks. Specific measurements included eyelid aperture, an eyelid swelling scale, patient photographs, exophthalmometer readings, extraocular motility as assessed by perimetry, visual field testing using a Maddox Cross and headlamp, corneal staining with bimicroscopy, and visual acuity using a Snellen chart. A patient self assessment using a subjective eye score, and a physician's subjective assessment of disease using an activity score were also recorded. Treatment outcome was determined at week 24. A successful response required the fulfillment of at least one major and two minor criteria. Major criteria included improvement in diplopia grade, and improvement in eye motility of more than 8° in any direction; minor criteria included 2 mm or greater decrease in lid aperture, proptosis reduction of 2 mm or more, and a decrease in class of eyelid swelling. Lastly, quantitative measurements and scores at each time point were compared to baseline values. Therapy was deemed successful in 60% of irradiated and 31% of non-irradiated patients. Eye motility improved in 82% of irradiated and 27% of non-irradiated patients. Symptom score and clinical activity score improved in both groups, but the latter improved more rapidly following radiotherapy (data not shown by authors). No differences in improvement rates were noted for eyelid swelling or proptosis in the two groups. Most importantly, the requirement for additional medical or surgical intervention was not affected by orbital radiotherapy.

The second, and as yet unpublished, randomized placebo-controlled trial was designed to use a patient as his or her own control (36). Forty-two euthyroid patients with bilateral Graves' ophthalmopathy who had not received corticosteroids for a minimum of two weeks received irradiation to a single orbit, followed by an observation period of 6 months before receiving irradiation to the remaining orbit. Patients with optic neuropathy or prior surgical or radiotherapy to the orbits were excluded. In addition to allowing a comparison of a patient's treated and untreated eyes, the study design permitted an assessment of response to delayed therapy, performed at a later stage in the course of disease. Careful quantitative assessment was performed at 3-month intervals, including thyroid function testing, measurements of lid fissures and proptosis, extraocular muscle motility measurement, visual acuity measurement, funduscopic and slit lamp examination, and a calculation of orbital fat and extraocular muscle volume using computed tomography. At 6 months, the authors noted no difference in orbital fat volume, extraocular muscle volume, eye motility, lid fissure width, or proptosis in the treated and untreated eyes. While a complete summary of this second randomized trial awaits its publication, it is apparent that this study does not demonstrate substantial improvement in orbital volume or eye muscle function following radiotherapy (36).

On the basis of these two randomized placebo-controlled trials, improvement in the measured parameters of Graves' ophthalmopathy after orbital radiotherapy appears to be modest at best. The improvement in ocular motility found in the first trial, although *statistically* significant, may not have been *functionally* significant, given the need for subsequent intervention. This finding is not incongruous with the assertion that rather than obviating the need for surgery, orbital radiotherapy hastens attainment of a plateau stage, at which time surgical intervention may proceed (12,37). It is worth noting that while maximizing the use of quantifiable measurement and preventing harm in these two placebo-controlled trials, soft tissue inflammation and optic neuropathy--two elements of Graves' ophthalmopathy generally cited to respond well to radiotherapy--were largely ignored or excluded from analysis. Specifically, among soft tissue changes with Graves' ophthalmopathy, only lid edema was included in the criteria used to define a positive response in the first study, and no data on soft tissue changes was provided in the second study. Both studies excluded patients with optic neuropathy rather than risk randomizing such patients to a no treatment arm.

CONCLUSIONS AND RECOMMENDATIONS

How does one account for the disparity between the broad benefit attributed to radiotherapy for Graves' ophthalmopathy in well over a dozen non-randomized trials and the more modest or non-existent benefit described in the two recent placebo-controlled randomized trials? Do the latest findings compel clinicians to abandon radiotherapy for Graves' ophthalmopathy? In this author's opinion, radiotherapy should not be removed from the already limited arsenal against Graves' ophthalmopathy. This is based on three arguments, including: 1) published expert opinion and repeated clinical observation of observed benefit; 2) randomized trial findings of similar effectiveness of radiotherapy and corticosteroids; and 3) the marginal benefits noted in the published placebo-controlled randomized trial, despite the de-emphasis upon or exclusion of soft tissue changes and optic neuropathy, respectively. On the other hand, an expectation of more than mild-to-moderate improvement or an ability to obviate surgical intervention after orbital radiotherapy for Graves' ophthalmopathy would seem unrealistic and not supported by the current literature in this area.

Is further study needed in this area? A quantitative technique for measuring change in orbital inflammation may enhance our ability to discern potential benefit not measured using traditional techniques. In this regard, further randomized trials using either T2-weighted MR images (38) or octreotide scanning (39,40) before and after orbital radiotherapy to supplement traditional measurement may provide further evidence for or against the continued use of this modality in patients with Graves' ophthalmopathy.

REFERENCES

1. Donaldson SS, Bagshaw MA, Kriss JP. Supervoltage orbital radiotherapy for Graves' ophthalmopathy. J Clin Endocrinol Metab 1973; 37: 276-285.
2. Burch HB, Wartofsky L. Graves' ophthalmopathy: Current concepts regarding pathogenesis and management. Endo Rev 1993; 14: 747-793.
3. Weetman AP; Wiersinga WM. Current management of thyroid-associated ophthalmopathy in Europe. results of an international survey. Clin Endocrinol (Oxf) 1998 Jul;49(1):21-8.
4. Harris G, Cramp WA, Edwards JC, George AM, Sabovljev SA, Hart L, Hughes GR, Denman AM, Yatvin MB. Radiosensitivity of peripheral blood lymphocytes in autoimmune disease. Int J Radiat Biol Relat Stud Phys Chem Med. 1985 Jun;47(6):689-99.
5. Cole J, Arlett CF, Green MH, Harcourt SA, Priestley A, Henderson L, Cole H, James SE, Richmond F. Comparative human cellular radiosensitivity: II. The survival following gamma-irradiation of unstimulated (G0) T-lymphocytes, T-lymphocyte lines, lymphoblastoid cell lines and fibroblasts from normal donors, from ataxia-telangiectasia patients and from ataxia-telangiectasia heterozygotes. Int J Radiat Biol 1988 Dec;54(6):929-43.
6. Yaron M, Yaron I, Levita M, Herzberg M. Hyaluronic acid production by irradiated human synovial fibroblasts. Arthritis Rheum 1977 Mar;20(2):702-8.
7. Char DH. Thyroid eye disease: Natural history and response to hyperthyroidism treatment. In: Thyroid Eye Disease, Char DH (Ed), Churchill Livingstone Inc., New York, 1990; pp 111-122.
8. Smitt MC, Donaldson SS. Radiation therapy for benign disease of the orbit. Semin Radiat Oncol 1999 Apr;9(2):179-89.
9. Peterson IA, Kriss JP, McDougall IR, Donaldson SS. Prognostic factors in the radiotherapy of Graves' ophthalmopathy. Int J Radiat Oncol, Biol, Phys 1990; 19: 259-264.
10. Kahaly GJ, Rosler HP, Pitz S, Hommel G. Low- versus high-dose radiotherapy for Graves' ophthalmopathy: a randomized, single blind trial. J Clin Endocrinol Metab 2000 Jan;85(1):102-8.
11. Bartalena L, Marcocci C, Manetti L, Tanda ML, Dell'Unto E, , Rocchi R, Cartei F, Pinchera A. Orbital radiotherapy for Graves' ophthalmopathy. Thyroid 1998; 8:439-441.
12. DeGroot LJ, Gorman CA, Pinchera A, Bartalena L Marcocci C, Wiersinga WM, Prummel MF, Wartofsky L Marocci C. Therapeutic controversies. Retro-orbital radiation and radioactive iodide ablation of the thyroid may be good for Graves' ophthalmopathy. J Clin Endocrinol Metab 1995 Feb;80(2):339-40.
13. Kahaly GJ, Roesler HP, Kutzner J, Pitz S, Muller-Forell W, Beyer J, Mann W. Radiotherapy for thyroid-associated orbitopathy. Exp Clin Endocrinol Diabetes 1999;107 Suppl 5:S201-7.
14. Mourits MP, van Kempen-Harteveld ML, Garcia MB, Koppeschaar HP, Tick L, Terwee CB. Radiotherapy for Graves' orbitopathy: randomized placebo-controlled study. Lancet 2000 Apr 29;355(9214):1505-9.
15. Snijders-Keilholz A, De Keizer RJ, Goslings BM, Van Dam EW, Jansen JT, Broerse JJ. Probable risk of tumour induction after retro-orbital irradiation for Graves' ophthalmopathy. Radiother Oncol 1996 Jan;38(1):69-71.
16. Donaldson SS, Bagshaw MA, Kriss JP. Orbital radiotherapy for ophthalmopathy of Graves' disease. N Engl J Med 1974; 290: 805-806(letter).

17. Kriss JP, Peterson IA, Donaldson SS, McDougall IR. Supervoltage orbital radiotherapy for progressive Graves' ophthalmopathy: Results of a twenty year experience. Acta Endocrinol (Copenh) 1989; 121(Suppl 2): 154-159.
18. Hurbli T, Char DH, Harris J, Weaver K, Greenspan F, Sheline G. Radiation therapy for thyroid eye disease. Am J Ophthalmol 1985; 99: 633-637.
19. Wiersinga WM, Smit T, Schuster-Uttenhoeve ALJ, van der Gaag R, Koornneef L. Therapeutic outcome of prednisone medication and of orbital irradiation in patients with Graves' ophthalmopathy. Ophthalmologica 1988; 197: 75-84.
20. Teng CS, Crombie AL, Hall R, Ross WM. An evaluation of supervoltage orbital irradiation for Graves' ophthalmopathy. Clin Endocrinol 1980; 13: 545-551.
21. Rush S, Winterkorn JM, Zak R. Objective evaluation of improvement in optic neuropathy following radiation therapy for thyroid eye disease. Int J Radiat Oncol Biol Phys 2000 Apr 1;47(1):191-4
22. Wilson WB, Prochoda M. Radiotherapy for thyroid orbitopathy. Effects on extraocular muscle balance. Arch Ophthalmol 1995 Nov;113(11):1420-5.
23. Ravin JG, Sisson JC, Knapp WT. Orbital radiation for the ocular changes of Graves' disease. Am J Ophthalmol 1975; 79: 285-288.
24. Bartalena L, Marcocci C, Chiovato L, Lepri A, Andreani D, Cavallacci G, Baschieri L, Pinchera A. Orbital cobalt irradiation combined with systemic corticosteroids for Graves' ophthalmopathy: comparison with systemic corticosteroids alone. J Clin Endocrinol Metab 1983; 56: 1139-1144.
25. Olivotto IA, Ludgate CM, Allen LH, Rootman J. Supervoltage radiotherapy for Graves' ophthalmopathy: CCABC technique and results. Int Radiation Oncol Biol Phys 1985; 11: 2085-2090.
26. van Ouwerkerk BM, Wijngaarde R, Hennemann G, van Andel JG, Krenning EP. Radiotherapy of severe ophthalmic Graves' disease. J Endocrinol Invest 1985; 8: 241-247.
27. Konishi J, IIda Y, Kasagi K, Misaki T, Arai K, Endo K, Amemiya T, Abe M, Torizuka K. Clinical evaluation of radiotherapy for Graves' ophthalmopathy. Endocrinol Jpn 1986; 33: 637-644.
28. Palmer D, Greenberg P, Cornwell P, Parker RG. Radiation therapy for Graves' ophthalmopathy: a retrospective analysis. Int J Radiat Oncol, Biol, Phys 1987; 13: 1815-1820.
29. Pigeon P, Orgiazzi J, Berthezene F, Gerard JP, Haguenauer JP, Mornex R. High voltage orbital radiotherapy and surgical orbital decompression in the management of Graves' ophthalmopathy. Horm Res 1987; 26: 172-176.
30. Sandler HM, Rubenstein JH, Fowble BL, Sergott RC, Savino PJ, Bosley TM. Results of radiotherapy for thyroid ophthalmopathy. Int J Radiation Oncol Biol Phys 1989; 17: 823-827.
31. Lloyd WC, Leone CR. Supervoltage orbital radiotherapy in 36 cases of Graves' disease. Am J Ophthalmol 1992; 113: 374-380.
32. Claridge KG, Ghabrial R, Davis G, Tomlinson M, Goodman S, Harrad RA, Potts MJ. Combined radiotherapy and medical immunosuppression in the management of thyroid eye disease. Eye 1997;11 (Pt 5):717-22.
34. Prummel MF, Mourits MP, Blank L, Berghout A, Koornneef L, Wiersinga WM. Randomized double-blind trial of prednisone versus radiotherapy in Graves' ophthalmopathy. Lancet 1993 Oct 16;342(8877):949-54.
35. Mourits MP, van Kempen-Harteveld ML, Garcia MB, Koppeschaar HP, Tick L, Terwee CB. Radiotherapy for Graves' orbitopathy: randomized placebo-controlled study. Lancet. 2000 Apr 29;355(9214):1505-9.

36. Gorman C, Jarrity J, Fatourechi V, Bahn RS, Peterson I, Stafford S, Earle J, Forbes G, Kline R, Bergstralh E, Offord K, Rademacher D, Stanley N, Bartley G. A prospective randomized, double-blind controlled study of orbital radiotherapy for Graves' ophthalmopathy. Presented at the 72nd Annual Meeting of The American Thyroid Association, Palm Beach, Florida, 1999.
37. Wiersinga WM. Immunosuppressive treatment of Graves' ophthalmopathy. Trends in Endocrinol Metab 1990; 1: 377-381.
38. Bailey CC, Kabala J, Laitt R, Goddard P, Hoh HB, Potts MJ, Harrad RA. Magnetic resonance imaging in thyroid eye disease. Eye. 1996;10 (Pt 5):617-9.
39. Gerding MN, van der Zant FM, van Royen EA, Koornneef L, Krenning EP, Wiersinga WM, Prummel MF. Octreotide-scintigraphy is a disease-activity parameter in Graves' ophthalmopathy. Clin Endocrinol (Oxf). 1999 Mar;50(3):373-9.
40. Somatostatin receptor scintigraphy to predict the clinical evolution and therapeutic response of thyroid-associated ophthalmopathy. Eur J Nucl Med. 1999 May;26(5):511-7.

INDEX

Note: Page numbers in *italics* refer to illustrations; page numbers followed by *t* refer to tables.

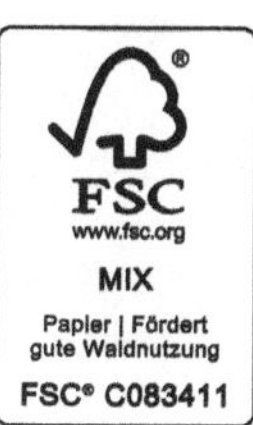

Zeitfracht Medien GmbH
Ferdinand-Jühlke-Straße 7
99095 Erfurt, Deutschland
produktsicherheit@kolibri360.de